DEDICATION

*In memory of our dear friend and
colleague Dr. Robert Susil*

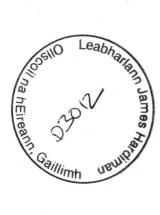

PREFACE

It is our pleasure to introduce the first edition of *Radiation Oncology: A Question-Based Review*. This handbook is the product of a collaborative effort between senior residents and attending physicians at the Department of Radiation Oncology and Molecular Radiation Sciences at the Johns Hopkins Hospital and many other institutions across the country. The book's question-based format, rather than serving as a comprehensive reference, is meant to provide the reader with a quick and user-friendly means for self-assessment on the most salient topics in modern radiation oncology practice. The primary focus of this text is to aid advanced and motivated medical students, residents, and practicing radiation oncologists in building upon existing knowledge and further mastering the complex and heterogeneous body of knowledge that clinical radiation oncology represents.

This publication covers in detail all the major sites and cancer types currently treated with radiotherapy with an emphasis on treatment recommendations and the evidence behind them. Because this book is also meant to serve as a study guide for residents and junior radiation oncologists preparing for their written and oral board examinations, we have also included detailed questions on the natural history, epidemiology, diagnosis, staging, and treatment-related side effects for each cancer type. Additionally, interspersed within each chapter are numerous mnemonics as well as many useful facts from other disciplines such as radiology, anatomy, and medical oncology. Finally, every chapter has undergone a comprehensive revision by experienced faculty physicians.

We believe this text will play an important role in the instruction of future radiation oncologists. Whether they need a rapid way to begin learning the fundamentals of radiation oncology, or require a more in-depth review of the evidence-based treatment approaches for each cancer type, we hope that *Radiation Oncology: A Question-Based Review* will prove to be an invaluable and high-yield learning tool.

The Editors

CONTRIBUTORS

Michelle Alonso-Basanta, MD, PhD
Helene Blum Assistant Professor
Department of Radiation Oncology
Hospital of the University of Pennsylvania
Philadelphia, Pennsylvania

Fariba Asrari, MD
Clinical Associate in Radiation Oncology
Senior Radiation Oncologist
Department of Radiation Oncology and
    Molecular Radiation Sciences
Johns Hopkins University
    School of Medicine
Baltimore, Maryland

Gopal K. Bajaj, MD
Director of Head and Neck Radiation
Department of Radiation Oncology
Inova Fairfax Hospital
Falls Church, Virginia

Justin E. Bekelman, MD
Assistant Professor
Department of Radiation Oncology
Hospital of the University of Pennsylvania
Philadelphia, Pennsylvania

M. Kara Bucci, MD
Assistant Professor
Department of Radiation Oncology
The University of Texas MD Anderson
    Cancer Center
Houston, Texas

Kevin Camphausen, MD
Chief
Department of Radiation Oncology
National Cancer Institute
Bethesda, Maryland

Timothy A. Chan, MD, PhD
Assistant Professor
Department of Radiation Oncology
Memorial Sloan-Kettering Cancer Center
New York, New York

Joe Y. Chang, MD, PhD
Associate Professor
Department of Radiation Oncology
The University of Texas MD Anderson
    Cancer Center
Houston, Texas

John P. Christodouleas, MD, MPH
Assistant Professor
Department of Radiation Oncology
Hospital of the University of Pennsylvania
Philadelphia, Pennsylvania

Deborah E. Citrin, MD
Investigator
Department of Radiation Oncology
    Branch
Attending Physician
Department of Radiation Oncology
National Cancer Institute
Bethesda, Maryland

Theodore L. DeWeese, MD
Professor
Department of Radiation Oncology and
　Molecular Radiation Sciences
Johns Hopkins University
Chief
Department of Radiation Oncology and
　Molecular Sciences
Johns Hopkins Hospital
Baltimore, Maryland

Roland Engel, MD
Radiation Oncology Element Chief
Department of Radiation Oncology
David Grant Medical Center
Travis Air Force Base, California

Deborah A. Frassica, MD
Associate Professor
Department of Radiation Oncology and
　Molecular Radiation Sciences
Johns Hopkins University
Baltimore, Maryland

Eli Glatstein, MD
Vice Chairman
Department of Radiation Oncology
Hospital of the University of Pennsylvania
Philadelphia, Pennsylvania

Thomas J. Guzzo, MD
Assistant Professor of Urology and
　Surgery
Department of Surgery, Division of
　Urology
Hospital of the University of Pennsylvania
Philadelphia, Pennsylvania

Naomi B. Haas, MD
Associate Professor
Leader, Prostate Program
Division of Hematology and Oncology
Abramson Cancer Center
Hospital of the University of Pennsylvania
Philadelphia, Pennsylvania

Russell K. Hales, MD
Department of Radiation Oncology and
　Molecular Radiation Sciences
Johns Hopkins University
Baltimore, Maryland

Joseph M. Herman, MD, MSC
Assistant Professor
Department of Radiation Oncology and
　Molecular Radiation Sciences
Johns Hopkins University School of
　Medicine
Baltimore, Maryland

Boris Hristov, MD
Staff Radiation Oncologist
Radiation Therapy
David Grant Medical Center
Travis Air Force Base, California

Salma Jabbour, MD
Assistant Professor
Department of Radiation Oncology
Cancer Institute of New Jersey-
University of Medicine and Dentistry
　of New Jersey
New Brunswick, New Jersey

Melenda D. Jeter, MD, MPH
Associate Professor
Department of Radiation Oncology
The University of Texas MD Anderson
　Cancer Center
Houston, Texas

Atif Khan, MD
Assistant Professor
Department of Radiation Oncology
University of Medicine and Dentistry
　of New Jersey
Robert Wood Johnson Medical School
Member
Department of Radiation Oncology
Cancer Institute of New Jersey
New Brunswick, New Jersey

Ritsuko Komaki, MD
Professor
Department of Radiation Oncology
The University of Texas MD Anderson
 Cancer Center
Houston, Texas

Vincent J. Lee, MD
Associate Staff Physician
Department of Radiation Oncology
Taussig Cancer Institute
Cleveland Clinic Foundation
Cleveland, Ohio

Zhongxing Liao, MD
Professor
Department of Radiation Oncology
University of Texas
Center Medical Director
The University of Texas MD Anderson
 Cancer Center
Houston, Texas

Alexander Lin, MD
Assistant Professor
Department of Radiation Oncology
Hospital of the University of Pennsylvania
Philadelphia, Pennsylvania

Lilie Lin, MD
Assistant Professor
Department of Radiation Oncology
Hospital of the University of Pennsylvania
Philadelphia, Pennsylvania

Steven H. Lin, MD, PhD
Assistant Professor
Department of Radiation Oncology
The University of Texas MD Anderson
 Cancer Center
Houston, Texas

Robert A. Lustig, MD, FACR
Professor of Clinical Radiation Oncology
Director of Clinical Operations
Department of Radiation Oncology
Hospital of the University of Pennsylvania
Philadelphia, Pennsylvania

Anita Mahajan, MD
Associate Professor
Division of Radiation Oncology
The University of Texas MD Anderson
 Cancer Center
Houston, Texas

Charles H. Matthews, MD, MBA
Fourth Year Resident
Department of Radiation Oncology &
 Molecular Radiation Science
Johns Hopkins University
Baltimore, Maryland

William P. O'Meara, MD
Attending Physician
Department of Radiation Oncology
National Naval Medical Center
Bethesda, Maryland

Daniel G. Petereit, MD
Associate Professor
Department of Human Oncology
University of Wisconsin
Madison, Wisconsin
Radiation Oncologist
Regional Cancer Care Institute
Rapid City Regional Hospital
Rapid City, South Dakota

John P. Plastaras, MD, PhD
Assistant Professor
Department of Radiation Oncology
Hospital of the University of Pennsylvania
Philadelphia, Pennsylvania

Robert Prosnitz, MD
Radiation Oncologist
Department of Radiation Oncology
Hospital of the University of Pennsylvania
Philadelphia, Pennsylvania

Kristin Janson Redmond, MD, MPH
Instructor
Department of Radiation Oncology &
    Molecular Radiation Sciences
Johns Hopkins University
Baltimore, Maryland

Ramesh Rengan, MD, PhD
Assistant Professor
Department of Radiation Oncology
Hospital of the University of Pennsylvania
Philadelphia, Pennsylvania

Daniele Rigamonti, MD, FACS
Professor and Director of Stereotactic
    Radiosurgery
Department of Neurosurgery
Department of Radiation Oncology and
    Molecular Radiation Sciences
John Hopkins University
Baltimore, Maryland

Howard M. Sandler, MD, MS
Ronald H. Bloom Family Chair in
    Cancer Therapeutics and Chairman
Department of Radiation Oncology
Cedars-Sinai Medical Center
Los Angeles, California

Giuseppe Sanguineti, MD
Associate Professor
Department of Radiation Oncology and
    Molecular Radiation Sciences
Johns Hopkins University
Radiation Oncologist
The Johns Hopkins Hospital
Baltimore, Maryland

Ori Shokek, MD
Staff Radiation Oncologist
Department of Radiation Oncology
York Cancer Center
York, Pennsylvania

Benjamin D. Smith, MD
Assistant Professor
Department of Radiation Oncology
The University of Texas MD Anderson
    Cancer Center
Houston, Texas

Danny Y. Song, MD
Assistant Professor
Department of Radiation Oncology and
    Molecular Radiation Sciences
Johns Hopkins University
Baltimore, Maryland

Bronwyn R. Stall, MD
Assistant Professor of Radiology/
    Radiological Services
Department of Radiology/Radiological
    Services
Uniformed Services University of the
    Health Sciences
F. Edward Hebert School of Medicine
Bethesda, Maryland
Staff Physician
Department of Radiation Oncology
Walter Reed Army Medical Center
Washington, DC

Robert C. Susil, MD, PhD*
Resident
Department of Radiation Oncology and
    Molecular Radiation Sciences
Johns Hopkins University School of
    Medicine
Baltimore, Maryland

Michael J. Swartz, MD
Attending Radiation Oncologist
Department of Radiation Oncology
John T. Vucurevich Cancer Care Institute
Rapid City, South Dakota

Owen C. Thomas, MD, PhD
Resident
Department of Radiation Oncology and
    Molecular Radiation Sciences
Johns Hopkins University
Baltimore, Maryland

Brent A. Tinnel, MD
Teaching Faculty
National Capital Consortium Radiation
    Oncology Residency Program
Uniformed Services University of the
    Health Sciences
Bethesda, Maryland
Chief
Department of Radiation Oncology
    Service
Walter Reed Army Medical Center
Washington, DC

Richard Tuli, MD, PhD
Resident
Department of Radiation Oncology and
    Molecular Radiation Sciences
Johns Hopkins University
Baltimore, Maryland

Neha Vapiwala, MD
Assistant Professor
Department of Radiation Oncology
Hospital of the University of Pennsylvania
Philadelphia, Pennsylvania

James Welsh, MD
Assistant Professor
Department of Radiation Oncology
The University of Texas MD Anderson
    Cancer Center
Houston, Texas

Moody D. Wharam, Jr., MD
Professor
Department of Radiation Oncology and
    Molecular Radiation Sciences
Johns Hopkins University
Baltimore, Maryland

Shiao Y. Woo, MD, FACR
Professor and Chairman
Department of Radiation Oncology
University of Louisville
Louisville, Kentucky

Tse-Kuan Yu, MD, PhD
Assistant Professor
Department of Radiation Oncology
The University of Texas MD Anderson
    Cancer Center
Houston, Texas

Richard C. Zellars, MD
Assistant Professor
Department of Radiation Oncology and
    Molecular Radiation Sciences
Johns Hopkins University School of
    Medicine
Baltimore, Maryland

Jing Zeng, MD
Resident
Department of Radiation Oncology and
    Molecular Radiation Sciences
Johns Hopkins Medical Institutions
Baltimore, Maryland

Abbrev	Full Spell-Out
2D	two-dimensional
3D	three-dimensional
3D-CRT	three-dimensional conformal radiation therapy
5-FU	5-fluoro uracil
ABMT	autologous bone marrow transplant
abnl	abnormal
ACTH	adrenocorticotropic hormone
ADH	antidiuretic hormone
adj	adjuvant
Adr	Adriamycin
AFP	alpha-feto protein
AIDS	acquired immune deficiency syndrome
AJCC	American Joint Committee on Cancer
aka	also known as
alk phos	alkaline phosphatase
am	morning (ante meridian)
ANC	absolute neutrophil count (lab)
ant	anterior
anterolat	anterolateral
AP	anterior-posterior
APC	adenomatous polyposis coli (gene mutation)
ARUBA	A Randomized Trial of Unruptured Brain Arteriovenous Malformations
ASCUS	atypical squamous cells of unknown significance
ASTRO	American Society for Therapeutic Radiation and Oncology
AUC	area under the curve
avg	average
BAT	B-mode acquisition and targeting
b/c	because
β-HCG	beta-human chorionic gonadotropin
bid	twice daily

(continued)

Abbrev	Full Spell-Out
bilat	bilateral
BM	bone marrow
BMI	body mass index
BMP	basic metabolic panel
BMT	bone marrow transplant
BTSG	Brain Tumor Study Group
Bx	biopsy/biopsies
C	cervical (spine level)
CA 19-9	cancer antigen 19-9
CA 125	cancer antigen 125
CALGB	Cancer and Leukemia Group B
C/A/P	chest/abdomen/pelvis
CBC	complete blood count (lab)
CCCG	Colorectal Cancer Collaborative Group
cCR	clinical complete response
CD	cone-down
CD4	cluster of differentiation 4 (for immune cells)
CEA	carcinoembryonic antigen
CESS	Cooperative Ewing Sarcoma Study
CHART	Continuous Hyperfractionated Accelerated Radiotherapy Trial
chemo	chemotherapy
CHF	congestive heart failure
CIN	cervical intraepithelial neoplasia
CIS	carcinoma in situ
cm	centimeter/centimeters
CMP	complete metabolic panel (lab)
c-myc	(gene)
cN0	clinically node-negative
CN	cranial nerve
CNS	central nervous system
Co-60	cobalt-60
COG	Children's Oncology Group
contralat	contralateral
Cr	creatinine
CR	complete response
CRT	chemoradiation
CSF	cerebrospinal fluid
CSI	craniospinal irradiation
CSM	cancer-specific mortality
CSS	cause-specific survival
CT	computed tomography
CTV	clinical target volume
CXR	chest x-ray
D/C	discontinue/discontinued
D&C	dilation and curettage
DCC	deleted in colorectal cancer (gene)

Abbrev	Full Spell-Out
DDx	differential diagnosis
DFS	diseasefree survival
DLCO	lung diffusion capacity testing
DM	distant metastasis
DMFS	distant metastasisfree survival
DOI	depth of invasion
DRE	digital rectal examination
DSS	disease-specific survival
DVH	dose volume histogram
DVT	deep venous thrombosis
Dx	diagnosis/diagnoses
Dz	disease/diseases
EB	external beam
EBRT	external beam radiation therapy
EBV	Epstein-Barr virus
ECE	extracapsular extension
ECOG	Eastern Cooperative Oncology Group
EFS	eventfree survival
e.g.	for example
EGFR	epidermal growth factor receptor
ENI	elective nodal irradiation
EORTC	European Organisation for Research and Treatment of Cancer
ESR	erythrocyte sedimentation rate (lab)
et al.	and others
EUA	exam under anesthesia
EUS	endoscopic ultrasound
exam	examination
FDA	Food and Drug Administration
FDG	fluorine-18 2-fluoro-2-deoxy-D-glucose
FEV	forced expiratory volume
FFS	failurefree survival
FIGO	International Federation of Gynecology and Obstetrics
FISH	fluorescence in situ hybridization
FKHR	Forkhead (drosophilia) homolog 1 (rhabdomyosarcoma) (gene)
FLAIR	fluid attenuation inversion recovery
F:M	female to male ratio
FN rate	false-negative rate
FNA	fine needle aspiration
FOLFOX	5-FU/leukovorin/oxaliplatin
FPR	false-positive rate
FSH	follicle-stimulating hormone
FSR	fractionated stereotactic radiotherapy
fx	fraction/fractions

(continued)

Abbrev	Full Spell-Out
MRC	Medical Research Council
MRI	magnetic resonance imaging
MS	median survival
MTD	maximum tolerated/tolerable dose
MVA	multivariate analysis
N/C	nuclear to cytoplasm ratio
NCCN	National Comprehensive Cancer Network
NCCTG	North Central Cancer Treatment Group
NCI	National Cancer Institute
NCIC	National Cancer Institute of Canada
NED	no evidence of disease
NEJM	*New England Journal of Medicine*
neoadj	neoadjuvant
NF	neurofibromatosis
NPV	negative predictive value
NR	no response
NSABP	National Surgical Adjuvant Breast and Bowel Project
NSAID	nonsteroidal anti-inflammatory drug
NSS	not statistically significant
NTR	near-total resection
n/v	nausea/vomiting
NZ	New Zealand
OR	odds ratio
ORR	overall response rate
OS	overall survival
PA	posterior-anterior
PAP	Papanicolau
PCI	prophylactic cranial irradiation
PCP	pneumocystic pneumonia
PCR	polymerase chain reaction
pCR	pathologic complete response
PDGFR	platelet-derived growth factor receptor
PEG (tube)	percutanous endoscopic gastrostomy tube
periop	perioperative
PET	positron emission tomography
PFS	progressionfree survival
PFT	pulmonary function test
Plt	platelets
pm	afternoon (post meridian)
pN0	pathologically node negative
PNET	primitive neuroectodermal tumor
PNI	perineural invasion
PORT	postoperative radiation therapy
post	posterior
posterolat	posterolateral
postop	postoperative

Abbrev	Full Spell-Out
PPV	positive predictive value
PR	partial response
preop	preoperative
PSA	prostate-specific antigen
pt/pts	patient/patients
PTHrP	parathyroid hormone-related peptide
PT	prothrombin time
PTV	planning target volume
PUVA	psoralen and long-wave ultraviolet radiation
q	every
qd	daily
QOL	quality of life
RAO	right anterior oblique
RBE	relative biologic effectiveness
RCT	randomized controlled trial
rcv	receive/received
RFS	relapsefree survival
RLL	right lower lobe
RML	right middle lobe
r/o	rule out
RPO	right posterior oblique
RR	relative risk
RT	radiation or radiation therapy
RTOG	Radiation Therapy Oncology Group
RUL	right upper lobe
RUQ	right upper quadrant
Rx	prescription/prescriptions
S	sacral (spine level)
SBO	small bowel obstruction
SEER	Surveillance Epidemiology and End Results (data)
SFOP	French Society of Pediatric Oncology
SIADH	syndrome of inappropriate secretion of antidiuretic hormone
SIL	squamous intraepithelial lesion
SQ	subcutaneous
s/p	status post
SPECT	single photon emission computed tomography
SRS	stereotactic radiosurgery
SS	statistically significant
SSD	source to skin distance
STD	sexually transmitted disease
STR	subtotal resection
sup	superior
SVC	superior vena cava

(continued)

PART I Pediatrics

1

Rhabdomyosarcoma

Steven H. Lin and Moody D. Wharam, Jr.

▌Background

What are the 3 most commonly tested rhabdomyosarcoma (RMS) cases on the radiation oncology oral boards?

Bladder (trigone), parameningeal (PM), and orbit

What are the 2 incidence age peaks of RMS and their associated histologies?

2–6 yo (embryonal) and **15–19 yo (alveolar)**

What is the estimated overall annual incidence of RMS in the U.S.?

350 cases/yr of RMS in the U.S., 3% of all childhood cancers (#1 soft tissue sarcoma)

What are the most common sites of RMS? List them in order of approximate frequency in %.

Most common sites of RMS:
  1. H&N 40% (PM 25%, orbit 9%, non-PM 6%)
  2. GU 30%
  3. Extremity 15%
  4. Trunk 15%

What are the most common sites of mets?

Bone, BM, and lung

What % of pts present with mets? What types are prone to have hematogenous mets?

15% of pts present with mets. The prostate, trunk, and extremities are prone to hematogenous mets.

What is the most common origin of RMS?

Mesenchymal stem cells. Sporadic RMS is the most common.

What genetic syndromes and environmental risk factors are associated with RMS?

Genetic syndromes: Beckwith-Wiedemann syndrome (BWS), Li Fraumeni, and NF-1
Environmental risk factors: parental marijuana/cocaine use and prior RT

What are the 4 major histologies of RMS and their associated subtypes (if any)?

Major histologies of RMS and subtypes:
1. Embryonal (classic, spindle cell, and botryoid)
2. Alveolar
3. Pleomorphic
4. Undifferentiated

What genetic change is associated with embryonal RMS?

LOH 11p15.5 (embryonal) is associated with **IGF2 gene deletion,** seen in BWS; also abnormalities in chromosomes 2, 8, 12, and 13 are associated with MYCN, MDM2, CDK4, CDKN2A (p16), CDKN2B, and TP53 genes.

What translocations are associated with alveolar RMS? What are the genes involved in the fusion?

Alveolar RMS is associated with **t(2:13)** (70%) and **t(1,13)** (20%). Genes involved are **PAX3 or PAX7 with FKHR.**

Which is the most common histology of RMS in infants? Young children? Adolescents? Adults?

Most common RMS histology **(by age group):**
Infants: botryoid
Young children: embryonal
Adolescents: alveolar
Adults: pleomorphic

Which histologies are most commonly associated with each organ site (H&N, GU, extremities/trunk)?

Most common RMS histologies **(by site):**
Head & Neck: embryonal
Genitourinary: botryoid
Extremities/Trunk: alveolar

What is the most important cytogenetic tumor marker for RMS?

MyoD (and other myogenic proteins: actin, myosin, desmin, myoglobin)

List the histologies of RMS in terms of prognosis from best to worst.

RMS histologies **(by prognosis**—best to worst):
1. Spindle cell and botryoid
2. Classic embryonal
3. Alveolar
4. Undifferentiated

What are the ~5-yr OS rates for each of the histologic subtypes?

~5-yr OS **(by histology):**
Botryoid: 95%
Spindle cell: 88%
Embryonal: 66%
Alveolar: 54%
Undifferentiated: 40%

Which sites require LND b/c of a high propensity for LN mets? What is the risk of LN mets for these sites?

The following sites are associated with >**20%** LN mets rate and thus require LND:
Paratesticular (PT): (only if >10 yo)
Bladder: pelvic
Head & Neck: nasopharynx (NPX), LND typically not done for NPX
Extremities: upper extremity (UE) (axillary) and lower extremity (LE) (inguinal/femoral)

Which International Rhabdomyosarcoma Study (IRS) called for routine LN sampling in RMS of the extremity?

IRS-IV (*Neville HL et al., J Ped Surg 2000*): 139 extremity pts, 10% cN+, 50% pN+; **of those cN0, 17% were pN+.**

What are considered nonregional mets/LNs for various sites (upper extremity [UE], lower extremity [LE], pelvic organs [PT, vagina, uterus])?

Nonregional LN stations by primary site:
UE: scalene node
Pelvic (PT/vagina/uterus): inguinal
Retroperitoneal (RP): para-aortic (P-A) (except if immediately adjacent)
LE: iliacs/P-A

What are the 4 favorable organ sites and their ~3-yr OS rate?

Favorable organ sites:
1. Orbit
2. Non-PM H&N
3. Non-prostate/bladder GU
4. Biliary

The ~3-yr OS is **94%.**

What is the estimated 3-yr OS for RMS arising from unfavorable sites (PM H&N, prostate, bladder, extremities/ trunk)?

For unfavorable sites, overall ~3-yr OS is **70%.**

What are the PM H&N sites?

PM H&N sites:
Middle ear
Mastoid
Nasal cavity
Nasopharynx
Infratemporal f**O**ssa
Pterygopalatine f**O**ssa
Paranasal sinuses
Parapharyngeal space

(Mnemonic: MMNNOOPP)

What are the non-PM H&N sites?

Scalp, cheek, parotid, oral cavity, oropharynx, and larynx

According to IRS I–II analysis, which RMS site was shown to carry the highest risk for LN mets?

The **prostate** (~40% with LN+ Dz) was shown to have the highest risk for LN mets.

IRS-III: What did it answer?

Group I–II UH: better with vincristine/Adriamycin/cyclophosphamide (VAdrC) alternating with VAC + RT, than RT + VA or VAC.

Group II–III favorable site: VA + RT adequate

Group II–III unfavorable site and group IV FH/UH: VAC + RT; no benefit adding Adr

WBRT prophylaxis did not reduce CNS relapse.

There was an improved bladder preservation rate and OS in the multimodality Tx of special pelvic sites.

Who did not get RT in IRS-III?

Group I FH and group III special pelvic sites (if CR after chemo) did not get RT.

In IRS-III, the OS was mainly driven by what groups of pts?

Group I–II UH getting VAdrC alternating with VAC and group III FH special pelvic sites

What did IRS-III demonstrate about the Tx of special pelvic sites?

Pelvic site I (bladder dome, vagina, uterus): VAdrC alternating with VAC × 2 yrs → second-look surgery (SLS) at 20 wks → if PR, then RT at wk 20 + Adriamycin/etoposide × 2 cycles; if CR, no RT and continue chemo.

Pelvic site II (bladder neck/trigone, prostate): VAdrC alternating with VAC × 2 yrs → RT (wk 6) → SLS at 20 wks.

Bladder preservation rate 60% vs. 25% (IRS-I–II) and better OS rate (83% vs. 72%).

IRS-IV: What did it answer?

IRS-IV focused on improving outcome for group III: utility of adding IE to VAC, and bid RT (1.1 Gy bid to 59.4 Gy) vs. conventional RT (1.8–50.4 Gy).

Qd RT remains standard.

VAC remains standard, even for the alveolar type.

However, **for group IV, VAC + IE is standard** (IE vs. vincristine/melphalan).

What trial utilized WBRT prophylaxis for high-risk PM RMS, and how did it differ from other IRS trials?

IRS-II–III, with whole brain to 30 Gy with intrathecal chemo, all started day 0. IRS-IV started day 0 but did not treat the whole brain—just to the involved field on day 0.

Now **IRS-VI,** no day 0 RT for high-risk PM (base of skull invasion, CN palsy); RT starts wk 4 (except intracranial extension in intermediate-risk and metastatic PM).

What did *Wolden et al.* data show about the importance of RT in clinical group (CG)-I UH RMS?

Wolden et al. (*JCO 1999*) analyzed **IRS-I–III,** RT vs. no RT in **CG-I** pts: showed only a trend to improved FFS and no OS with RT in FH; however, **in CG-I UH, RT improved FFS and OS.**

What are the 2 subsets of low-risk pts on IRS-VI?

Subsets of low-risk pts on IRS-VI:
  Subset I (treated with VA + RT on **IRS-III–IV**): stage 1, CG-I–II, orbit CG-III, stage 2, CG-I–II. Now treated with VAC × 4 cycles **(reduced chemo) → 4 cycles VA + RT.***
  Subset II (treated with VAC + RT on IRS-III–IV): stage 1, CG-III (nonorbit), stage 3 CG-I–II. Now treated with VAC × 4 cycles **(reduced chemo) → 12 cycles VA + RT.***

What are the major study questions for intermediate-risk pts in IRS-VI?

VAC vs. VAC alternating with vincristine/irinotecan (VI); timing of RT (wk 4 vs. wk 10, **IRS-IV**)

What are the major study questions for high-risk pts in IRS-VI?

VAC alternating with IE using interval dose compression; ability to improve LC in metastatic RMS by using VI with RT.

What is the timing of RT in IRS-V?

Low risk: **wk 3**
Intermediate risk: **wk 12**
High risk: **wk 15**

What is the timing of RT in IRS-VI?

Low risk: **wk 13**
Intermediate risk: **wk 4**
High risk: **wk 20**

What are secondary objective questions for RT in IRS-VI?

Whether 36 Gy is adequate for N0, R1 and if 45 Gy is adequate for orbital RMS

What is the dose for CG-I with FH?

0 Gy. No RT is required for CG-I with FH.

What study provided the rationale for reduced RT doses of 36 Gy in IRS-V–VI?

MSKCC retrospective review (*Mandell L et al., JCO 1990*): in only 32 CG-II pts, no difference in LC between <40 Gy vs. >40 Gy.

All pts with initial nodal involvement, regardless of response to induction therapy or SLS, must get what?

RT to **41.4 Gy if R0-R1** resected; all gross or suspected **gross Dz** treated to **50.4 Gy.**

RT is NEVER omitted for node+ Dz.

---

*However, bear in mind that CG-I, FH, stage 1–3 rcv no RT, just chemo.

What is the max allowed dose to the whole heart? Whole abdomen/pelvis?

The max dose to the whole heart is **30.6 Gy.** The max dose to the whole abdomen/pelvis is **24 Gy** (at 1.5 Gy/fx).

What is the dose limit to the lungs, if less than one half of the combined lung volume is in the PTV?

In this situation, the dose limit to the lung is **15 Gy** (in 1.5 Gy/fx).

What is a major side effect of VAC besides myelosuppression?

Veno-occlusive Dz of the liver

TABLE 1.1 Radiation Doses for Favorable Histology Tumors (per IRS-VI ARST0331, Ongoing)	
Stage 1, clinical group I	No radiotherapy
Stage 1, clinical group II, N0	Conventional RT: 36 Gy
Stage 1, clinical group II, N1	Conventional RT: 41.4 Gy
Stage 1, clinical group III	Conventional RT: 45 Gy (orbit only)
Stage 1, clinical group III	Conventional RT: 50.4 Gy (nonorbit)
Stage 2, clinical group I	No radiotherapy
Stage 2, clinical group II, N0	Conventional RT: 36 Gy
Stage 3, clinical group I	No radiotherapy
Stage 3, clinical group II, N0	Conventional RT: 36 Gy
Stage 3, clinical group II, N1	Conventional RT: 41.4 Gy

RT, radiation therapy.
For certain clinical group III pts, the radiotherapy dose may be modified by the use of 2nd-look surgery.
Source: http://members.childrensoncologygroup.org (ARST0331).

TABLE 1.2 Radiation Doses for Unfavorable Histology Tumors (per IRS-VI ARST0531, Ongoing)	
Clinical Group	*Dose*
Group I, alveolar only	36 Gy
Group II, node negative	36 Gy
Group II, node positive	41.4 Gy
Group III, alveolar, orbit only	45 Gy
Group III, all others	50.4 Gy

TABLE 1.3 Principles of Radiation Therapy (per IRS-VI, Ongoing)

<u>Low risk</u>: Surgery 1st, then chemo. If group I → chemo only, no RT. All pts with initial +node must get RT regardless of response to induction chemo or SLS (at least 41.4 Gy, 50.4 Gy to gross Dz). Vincristine is given with RT and dactinomycin is given at wk 13 prior to RT, but they are not given concurrently.

Target volume: GTV—pre-Tx volume + involved LN; CTV = GTV + 1 cm; PTV = CTV + 0.5 cm. For CG-III to 50.4 Gy, CD at 36 Gy to pre-Tx GTV + 0.5 cm (CTV), with PTV = CTV + 0.5 cm. The planning organ-at-risk volume is based on organs at risk; GTV can be defined by exam, CT, MRI, or PET.

Timing: RT begins wk 13 after postop chemo. The exceptions are those who get SLS and those with vaginal primaries. For those who get SLS, RT starts after surgery at wk 13 (to allow time for healing).

All pts with initial CG-III in a favorable site (stage I, except orbit and paratesticular sites) should be considered for SLS at wk 13.

<u>Intermediate risk</u>: RT given at wk 4 (compare with data from wk 10 on IRS-IV). IMRT/proton/brachytherapy/electron and PET imaging are all allowed. CRT = VC or VI concurrently. Simulation occurs before wk 4 to begin on time.

Margins: CD after 36 Gy for tumors with "pushing" rather than invasive (lung, intestine, bladder). Boost to 50.4 Gy with new GTV representing response + 1 cm (CTV) and 0.5 cm (PTV). If 36 or 41.4 Gy, there is no volume reduction. GTV is pre-Tx volume + margin, except intrathoracic or intra-abdominal tumors (GTV as pre-Tx volume excluding intrathoracic or intra-abdominal/pelvic tumor from which it was debulked, since these are "pushing" borders).

Timing: All at wk 4. Emergency RT for *symptomatic cord compression* and high-risk PM (intracranial extension) can be given on wk 1 (day 1). Management of BOS erosion and CN palsy was not specified in the protocol, so it can be managed according to the discretion of the radiation oncologist.

<u>High risk</u>: RT given on wk 20 to primary and metastatic sites (except high-risk PM sites with IC extension and emergency RT).

High-risk PM sites with only BOS and/or CN palsy will get RT at wk 20. PM sites with intracranial extension will rcv RT at wk 1 (day 0) (but within 2 wks of the 1st cycle of chemo to start RT) and Tx to the metastatic site at wk 20 (unless the metastatic site is within the same Tx port as the primary). Emergency RT for cord compression is on day 0.

CRT: VI is given concurrently with RT, starting on wk 19 (day 0 if an emergency or PM with IC). *Alternative:* VC, if VI is not tolerable.

Margins: CD after 36 Gy for tumors with "pushing" rather than invasive (lung, intestine, bladder). Boost to 50.4 Gy with new GTV representing response + 1 cm (CTV) and 0.5 cm (PTV). If 36 or 41.4 Gy, GTV is pre-Tx volume + margin.

(continued)

| TABLE 1.3 | Principles of Radiation Therapy (per IRS-VI, Ongoing) *(Continued)* |

Bilat whole lung 15 Gy (10 fx) for pulmonary mets or pleural effusion (can boost to gross Dz) to 50.4 Gy.

IRS, International Rhabdomyosarcoma Study; chemo, chemotherapy; RT, radiation therapy; pt, patient; +node, positive node; SLS, second-look surgery; Gy, Gray; Dz, disease; wk, week; GTV, gross target volume; Tx, treatment; LN, lymph node; CTV, clinical target volume; cm, centimeter; PTV, planning target volume; CG, clinical group; CD, cone down; exam, examination; CT, computed tomography; MRI, magnetic resonance imaging; PET, positron emission tomography; postop, postoperative; IMRT, intensity modulated radiation therapy; CRT, chemoradiation; VC, vincristine/Cytoxan; VI, vincristine/irinotecan; PM, parameningeal; BOS, base of skull; CN, cranial nerve; IC, internal carotid; rcv, receive; bilat, bilateral; fx, fraction; met, metastasis.

| TABLE 1.4 | Principles of Surgery (per IRS-VI, Ongoing) |

1. WLE with margin preferred, no amputation for group IV setting. The rest get incisional or core Bx (orbit, PM H&N).
2. Sentinal LN Bx should be done for extremity sites.
3. Needle Bx or open Bx can be done; an aggressive LN sample is most appropriate.
4. Definitive surgery can be carried out after initial Bx or noncancer surgery. This subsequent PRE is followed by local adj therapy based on pathology from the definitive PRE.
5. A subsequent delayed resection can be done after chemo and RT (for initial Bx only) if the tumor has diminished enough to make resection feasible. SLS takes place on wk 13 (except orbit, PT).
6. If residual tumor persists after SLS, subsequent-look procedures can be done after further therapy, if the tumor appears resectable. SLS should be done to max extent if it is cosmetically and functionally feasible.
7. H&N sites: no neck dissection unless there is clinical involvement.
8. PT: Only ipsi RP LN dissection should be done. Do not do radical bilat regional node dissection. Regional LNs are ipsi iliac and RP nodes up to the hilum of the ipsi kidney. Orchiectomy and resection of the entire spermatic cord is via inguinal excision. Bx can take place prior to excision (but must ensure there is no spillage).
9. GU (bladder/prostate): if laparotomy is preformed, then iliac/para-aortic node sample should be done, and any other clinically involved site(s) should be biopsied. Bladder preservation rate is 50%–60%. Partial cystectomy should be done for bladder dome tumors.
10. Elective LND is not indicated except for extremities and PT lesions. Open Bx or LN sampling should be done for any gross enlarged nodes.

WLE, wide local excision; Bx, biopsy; PM, parameningeal; H&N, head and neck; LN, lymph node; PRE, pretreatment re-excision; adj, adjuvant; chemo, chemotherapy; RT, radiation therapy; SLS, second-look surgery; wk, week; PT, paratesticular; max, maximum; ipsi, ipsilateral; RP, retroperitoneal; bilat, bilateral; GU, genitourinary; LND, lymph node dissection.

2

Ewing Sarcoma

John P. Christodouleas and
Moody D. Wharam, Jr.

Background

What is the annual incidence of Ewing sarcoma (EWS) in the U.S.? How common is it relative to other bone tumors?	**200 cases/yr** of EWS in the U.S.; **2nd most common bone tumor** (osteosarcoma #1)
What is the median age of presentation of EWS?	The median age of EWS is **14–15 yrs.**
Is EWS associated with congenital Dz?	**No.** However, it can occur as a 2nd malignant neoplasm.
What is the racial and gender predilction?	EWS is more common in **whites** (>90% of cases) and among **males** (1.5:1).
What is the embryologic tissue of origin in EWS?	**Neuroectodermal tissue** is the embryonic tissue of origin for EWS.
What is the most common genetic change seen in EWS?	**t(11:22)** in 90%, FLI1(11): EWS(22). Other minor translocations include t(21,22) and t(7,22).
What other neoplasms are associated with the EWS translocation?	PNET, malignant melanoma of soft parts, and desmoplastic small round cell tumor (DSRCT)
Which exon fusion in t(11,22) is most common, and why is this important?	The most common fusion is **exon 7** of EWS and **exon 6** of FLI1 in 60% of cases. It is **associated with a lower proliferative rate and better prognosis.**
What type of cell morphology is expected to be seen in EWS?	**Small round blue cells** should be seen in EWS.
What constitutes the Ewing family of tumors?	**EWS** (osseous and extraosseous), **PNET, DSRCT,** and **Askin tumor**

What other tumors also have small round blue cells?	**L**ymphoma **E**wing **A**cute lymphoblastic leukemia **R**habdomyosarcoma **N**euroblastoma (NB) **N**euroepithelioma **M**edulloblastoma **R**etinoblastoma (Mnemonic: **LEARN NMR**)
What markers help differentiate EWS from other small round blue tumors?	Markers that differentiate EWS: 1. Vimentin 2. HBA-71 3. β2-microglobulin 4. ↑c-myc (vs. n-myc in NB)
How is PNET similar to and different from EWS histologically?	PNET and EWS have similar translocations and are both CD99 (MIC2)+ and vimentin+. However, **PNET is NSE+**, S100+, more differentiated, and has more neuroendocrine features. **EWS is NSE–** and S100 variable.
What major factors have been classically associated with a poor prognosis in EWS?	**M**ale gender **A**ge >15 yrs (>17 yrs in some) Pelvic/axial **S**ite or rib origin **S**ize (>8 cm per St. Jude or >100 cc per **CESS-81**) **S**tage (metastatic) ↑**LDH** Poor **response** to chemo (>10% viable tumor) (Mnemonic: **MASSSive LDH response**)
What is Askin tumor?	Askin tumor is **nonosseous PNET of the chest wall** (worse prognosis than other sites).
What % of EWS pts present with mets?	**20%–25%** of EWS pts present with mets. Mets typically occur in the **lung** (40%–50%) > **bone**
Where do mets typically occur?	(25%–40%) ≥ **BM** (~25%) and LNs (<10%).
What % of pts with localized Dz vs. lung mets have BM micromets?	25% (localized) vs. 40% (lung mets)

■ Workup/Staging

What is the typical clinical presentation with EWS?	Pain (96% of cases) and swelling (63% of cases) are most common → fever (21%) and fractures (16%).

What Sx at presentation portends a particularly poor prognosis in EWS?

Pts who present with **fever** (21% of cases) tend to have a poor prognosis.

What is the most commonly involved site in EWS at presentation?

Extremities (53%) > **axial skeleton** (47%). The **lower extremity** is the most common region, and the **femur** is most common site (~20% of cases).

If an EWS tumor presents centrally, what is the most common site?

The **pelvis** (20% of cases) is more common than the axial skeleton (12% of cases).

List the general workup for a pt who presents with an extremity mass.

Extremity mass workup: H&P, plain x-ray, MRI/CT primary, and core needle Bx or incisional Bx. Once a Dx of a sarcoma (EWS) is confirmed, complete the workup with CBC, BMP, LDH, ESR, LFTs, CXR, CT chest, bone scan or PET/CT, and BM Bx.

What are the characteristic findings on plain x-ray in EWS? How does this compare to osteosarcoma?

Classically, EWS shows an **"onion skin"** reaction on plain films, whereas osteosarcoma is associated with a "sunburst" appearance. The **Codman triangle,** an area of new subperiosteal bone as a result of periosteal lifting by underlying tumor, can be seen in both EWS and osteosarcoma.

How is EWS staged?

No standard staging system exists. Tumors are either localized or metastatic.

In EWS, what is meant by expendable bones? Name 3.

Expendable bones are ones that can be resected with minimal morbidity, such as:
1. Proximal fibula
2. Ribs
3. Distal four fifths of clavicle
4. Body of scapula
5. Iliac wings

■ Treatment/Prognosis

Summarize the current Tx paradigm for EWS.

EWS Tx paradigm: **induction—vincristine/Actinomycin D/Cytoxan (VAC) or vincristine/Actinomycin D/Cytoxan/Adriamycin (VACAdr) alternating with ifosfamide/etoposide (IE)** → **local therapy at wk 12** (surgery +/− RT or definitive RT) → **further adj chemo to wk 48.** Surgery when possible, give PORT when necessary, and whole lung irradiation (WLI) for lung mets.

Estimate the 5-yr OS for localized EWS.

5-yr OS for localized EWS is **60%–80%.**

What are the RT doses given for EWS in the definitive vs. the postop setting?

<u>Definitive</u>: **55.8 Gy**
<u>Postop</u>: **50.4 Gy for microscopic**/tumor spill and **55.8 Gy for gross** residual; **45 Gy for vertebral body** involvement

What is the LF rate for EWS after definitive RT?

Overall, **5%–25%;** worse with pelvic sites (LF 15%–70%); worse with large (>8 cm) lesions (LF 20%)

What are considered adequate surgical margins in EWS?

Per COG protocol **AEWS0031,** adequate margins are >1 cm for bone, >0.5 cm for soft tissue, and >0.20 cm for fascia.

What are 3 indications for adj RT after surgery in EWS?

+Margin, tumor spill, and >10% viable tumor after induction chemo (poor chemo response)

Is there a difference in LC between EWS pts who rcv preop RT vs. postop RT vs. definitive RT?

Yes. *Schuck et al.* performed a secondary analysis of 1,085 pts in **CESS-81 and -86** and **EICESS 92** and found no difference in LF between preop and postop RT (5.3% vs. 7.5%), but LF was significantly worse in the definitive RT arm (26%). However, there was a strong negative selection bias against the definitive RT cohort. There was no difference in LF between RT alone and surgery + post-RT if only partial resection was achieved. Preop RT may improve LC if STR is deemed likely. (*IJROBP 2003*)

When is surgery preferred to RT as a local therapy in EWS?

Surgery is preferred when expendable bones are involved, if there is a pathologic fracture, and when there is a lower extremity lesion in a child (<10 yo).

What Tx were compared in IESS-1? Summarize the study's major results (OS, RFS, and LR).

IESS-1 compared induction VAC alone to VACAdr and VAC + prophylactic WLI. 5-yr OS was significantly worse in the VAC alone arm (28%) compared to VACAdr (65%) or VAC + WLI (53%). 5-yr OS was not significantly different between VACAdr and VAC + WLI. However, the VACAdr arm had an improved 5-yr RFS (60%) compared to VAC + WLI (44%). 5-yr LR was not significantly different between arms (~15%). (*Nesbit ME et al., JCO 1990*)

In IESS-1, what site had the worst prognosis?

In **IESS-1,** pts with pelvic primaries had significantly worse 5-yr OS (pelvic 34% vs. nonpelvic 57%). (*Nesbit ME et al., JCO 1990*)

What Tx were compared in IESS-2? Summarize the study's major results (OS).

IESS-2 compared induction high-dose intermittent (HDI) VACAdr to moderate-dose continuous (MDC) VACAdr in nonpelvic tumors. HDI given q3wks vs. MDC given weekly. **5-yr OS favored the HDI arm** (77% vs. 63%). (*Burgert EO et al., JCO 1990*)

What Tx were compared in INT-0091 (IESS-3)? Summarize the study's major results (OS and LR).

INT-0091 compared induction **VACAdr to VACAdr alternating with IE.** The study enrolled pts with EWS, PNET of bone and primitive sarcoma of bone, and pts with both localized and metastatic Dz. In pts with nonmetastatic Dz, induction VACAdr alternating with IE improved 5-yr OS (72% vs. 61%) and 5-yr LR **(5% vs. 15%).** There was no 5-yr OS advantage in the VACAdr alternating with IE arm for pts with metastatic Dz at presentation (~34%). (*Grier HE et al., NEJM 2003*)

When was local therapy given in INT-0091?

In **INT-0091**, local therapy (surgery +/− PORT or RT alone) was given at **wk 12.**

How was RT given in INT-0091 compared to IESS-1–2?

> **INT-0091:** definitive RT was given with IE to **GTV + 3-cm** margin to 45 Gy → CD to postchemo volume to 55.8 Gy. For PORT, if R0, then no PORT; if R1, then 45 Gy (initial GTV + 1 cm); if R2, then 55.8 Gy.
> **IESS-1–2:** definitive RT to **whole bone** to 45–50 Gy → CD to 55–60 Gy

In INT-0091, what pt characteristics were associated with the largest benefit from the addition of alternating IE?

In **INT-0092,** benefit from the addition of alternating IE was associated with **pelvic tumors, large tumors, and age <17 yrs.**

In INT-0091, for pts with pelvic primaries, did LR differ between surgery alone, surgery + PORT, and definitive RT?

In **INT-0091,** for pts with pelvic primaries, **LR did not differ** by local therapy (~**15%**). (*Yock TI et al., JCO 2006*)

What RT Tx techniques were compared in POG 8346? Summarize the study's major results.

In **POG 8346,** osseous EWS pts who rcv definitive RT for local therapy after induction chemo were randomized to **whole bone RT (39.6 Gy → 55.8 Gy boost to GTV + 2 cm) vs. involved-field RT (GTV + 2 cm to 55.8 Gy).** All pts then rvc maintenance chemo. The RT Tx techniques had similar 5-yr EFS (~38%) and LC (~53%). (*Donaldson SS et al., IJROBP 1998*)

What are 2 Tx options in EWS pts with lung mets?

In addition to chemo, **consider WLI or surgical resection (if <5 mets)** in EWS pts with lung mets.

What 2 key retrospective studies support the use of WLI in pts with metastatic EWS?

<u>EICESS secondary analyses</u>: *Paulussen et al.* reviewed the outcomes of EWS pts with (a) isolated pulmonary mets or (b) combined lung + bone/BM mets who were treated +/− WLI as part of a series of protocols from the EICESS. WLI was associated with improved EFS in both subgroups. (*Ann Oncol 1998*)

<u>St. Jude retrospective study</u>: *Rodriguez-Galindo et al.* reviewed outcomes in EWS pts with isolated pulmonary recurrence. Pts who rcv WLI had improved 5-yr postrecurrence survival (30% vs. 17%). (*Cancer 2002*)

What doses and technique are used for WLI in EWS?

The WLI dose in EWS depends on age: if <14 yo, then **15 Gy (1.5 Gy/fx); if ≥14 yo, then 18 Gy.**

Describe the field borders used in WLI for EWS.

<u>Superior-Inferior</u>: 1 cm above 1st rib to L2
<u>Lateral</u>: 1 cm lat rib cage
Block PA kidney at 7.5 Gy.

Is there a difference in prognosis for metastatic EWS pts who present with isolated lung mets, bone-only mets, or both?

Yes. Metastatic EWS pts who present with either isolated pulmonary mets or skeletal mets have a similar EFS. However, EFS is significantly worse in pts with both.

5-yr OS for metastatic EWS:
    Lung mets: ~35%
    Bone/BM mets: ~25%
    Lung 1 bone/BM mets: ~15%

(Paulussen M et al., *Ann Oncol 2009*)

What evidence supports the use of hemithorax RT in chest wall EWS?

Schuck A et al. retrospectively reviewed 138 pts with localized chest wall EWS treated in **CESS-86** and **EICESS 92.** 42 pts rcv hemithorax RT. If <14 yo, then 15 Gy; otherwise, 20 Gy at 1.5 Gy/fx or 1.25 Gy bid. All RT pts rcv a boost to the primary site of 45–60 Gy. Despite worse baseline prognostic factors in the hemithorax RT cohort, 7-yr EFS trended in its favor (63% vs. 46%). Improvements in EFS appeared to be due to reductions in pulmonary mets. A major criticism of this study is that the RT group had superior chemo. (*IJROBP 2002*)

Does hyperfractionation improve outcomes in EWS?

No. CESS-86 randomized localized osseous EWS pts being treated with definitive RT to conventional fractionation (60 Gy in 1.8 Gy–2.0 Gy/fx) during a chemo break or split-course hyperfractionated RT concurrently with chemo. Hyperfractionated RT was 1.6 Gy bid to 60 Gy with a 12-day break after the initial 22.4 Gy and 44.8 Gy. LC was somewhat higher in the hyperfractionation arm (86% vs. 76%), but the difference was not SS. Benefits of this altered fractionation may have been lost due to the Tx breaks. (*Dunst J et al., IJROBP 1995*)

In EWS, how are the Tx volumes defined, and what are the margins used for the following scenarios?
1. **Bone-only lesion**
2. **Bone lesion with soft tissue extension**
3. **Postop setting**

In EWS, **RT volumes depend on the chemo response.**
1. **Bone only:** treat prechemo GTV + 2 cm to block margin (1-cm CTV, 0.5-cm PTV) to 55.8 Gy.
2. **Bone with soft tissue extension:** treat prechemo GTV + 2 cm to 45 Gy, then CD to initial/prechemo bone and postchemo soft tissue extent + 2 cm to 55.8 Gy.
3. **Postop setting:** treat preop, prechemo volume (except pushing borders in areas of lung or intestines) + 2 cm to 45 Gy, then CD to postop residual + 2 cm to 55.8 Gy.

In EWS pts with resected node+ Dz, what RT dose is used to treat the nodal bed?

In EWS pts with resected node+ Dz, treat the nodal bed to **50.4 Gy.**

Based on the SFOP (France) metastatic EWS protocol, what was the 5-yr EFS with the addition of high-dose busulfan and melphalan as consolidation?

High-dose oral busulfan and melphalan was used → stem cell rescue as consolidation after 5 cycles Cytoxan/Adr and 2 cycles IE → local therapy (surgery and/or RT). 5-yr EFS was 52% for lung-only mets and 36% for bone-only mets (no BM involvement). With BM involvement, survival was **4%.** (*Oberlin O et al., JCO 2006*)

Based on the SFOP (France) metastatic EWS protocol, how was local therapy delivered?

Local therapy was delivered either before or after consolidative high-dose chemo. RT was given alone or after incomplete resection (55–60 Gy). RT after R0 resection was given if >5% viable cells were seen (40 Gy). If <5% viable cells were seen, no RT was given. (*Oberlin O et al., JCO 2006*)

What study demonstrated the prognostic importance of LOH 1p + 16q for Wilms?

NWTS-5 analysis (*Grundy PE et al., JCO 2005*). For favorable histology (FH), LOH 1p or 16q is associated with ↑ RR of relapse. LOH of both ↑ RR of relapse + death.

What are the UH subtypes in Wilms?

Anaplastic (focal or diffuse), clear cell sarcoma, and rhabdoid (~10% of cases)

What is considered FH?

Typical features without anaplastic or sarcomatous features (~90% of cases)

How is focal anaplasia defined?

Focal anaplasia is sharply localized within the primary tumor, without atypia in the rest of the tumor.

What are the 4 sets of criteria used to define DA?

Criteria to define DA:
1. Nonlocalized
2. Localized with severe nuclear unrest elsewhere in the tumor
3. Anaplasia outside the tumor capsule or mets
4. Anaplasia revealed by random Bx

What is the stage-by-stage 4-yr OS for anaplastic/UH WT?

4-yr OS for anaplastic/UH Wilms:
Stage I: 83%
Stage II: 83%
Stage III: 65%
Stage IV: 33%

(*Dome JS et al., JCO 2006*)

How does the 4-yr OS compare between focal and diffuse anaplasia?

Overall: 97% vs. 50%
Stage I: 100%
Stage II: 93% vs. 55%
Stage III: 90% vs. 45%
Stage IV: 80% vs. 4%

Which histology has the worst prognosis?

Rhabdoid histology has the worst prognosis.

What are the typical presenting Sx in Wilms? How does this compare to NB?

Asymptomatic abdominal mass (83%) → abdominal pain (37%), HTN (25%, due to ↑ renin), hematuria (25%), fever, anemia (due to ↓ erythropoietin)
NB most commonly presents with systemic Sx.

(Mnemonic: **W**ilms are **W**ell, **N**euroblastomas are **N**ot well)

▨ Workup/Staging

What is the typical workup for an abdominal mass of unclear etiology in a child?

Abdominal mass workup: H&P (focusing on congenital defects), labs, UA (including urinary catecholamines), abdominal US, CXR, and CT C/A/P

What is the recommended 1st-line imaging modality for an abdominal mass?

US is the recommended 1st-line study for imaging the abdomen.

With a Dx of Wilms, what other imaging modalities are used for staging purposes?

CT or MRI head (for rhabdoid and clear cell histologies) and **bone scan** (for clear cell). Typical appearance on CT is a large mass with pseudocapsule.

With a Dx of Wilms, what 2 chest imaging modalities can be employed for staging purposes?

Both **CXR and CT** are used for chest imaging. Lesions seen on CT but not visible on CXR may be treated more conservatively than lung mets visible on CXR.

Pts with what histologic subtypes need BM Bx?

Pts with **clear cell and rhabdoid** subtypes require BM Bx.

> **Rhabdoid:** 10%–15% will have PNET in brain (atypical teratoid rhabdoid tumors)
> **Clear cell:** to r/o brain mets

Pts with what histologic subtypes require MRI of the head as part of their workup?

Under what circumstances should Bx be performed?

Do not Bx unless the tumor is unresectable or bilat Dz. If Bx is necessary, use a **post approach** to avoid contaminating the abdomen.

On what issues should the surgeon comment at the time of surgery?

Involvement of regional nodes, opposite kidney, peritoneum, liver, renal vein/IVC. Also, if there is tumor spillage and if it is confined to the ipsi flank.

What % of pts present with bilat Dz?

7% of pts present with bilat Dz.

What % of pts present with multifocal Dz?

12% of pts present with multifocal Dz.

What % of pts present with renal vein invasion?

10% of pts present with renal vein invasion.

What % of pts present with LN involvement?

20% of pts present with LN involvement.

What % of pts present with mets, and what are some common sites of mets?

10% of pts present with mets; lung (80%) → liver → bone, brain (clear cell), LN (outside abdomen and pelvis)

How commonly is calcification seen in Wilms?

Calcification is seen in 10%–15% of cases but is seen in 85% of NB cases.

How many stages are there in Wilms?

There are **5 stages** in Wilms.

Summarize the staging of WT.

Stage I (40% of pts): limited to kidney

Stage II (20%): extension to outside capsule, vessel involvement >2 mm

Stage III (20%): R1-R2 resection, +LN, local spillage or diffuse peritoneal spillage, Bx (including FNA), +implants, +margin, transected tumor thrombus, piecemeal resection, unresectable tumor

Stage IV (10%): hematogenous mets or LN+ outside the abdomen/pelvis

Stage V (4%–8%): bilat Dz; each side staged independently

Is adrenal involvement considered a met?

No. Adrenal involvement is considered local extension.

▌ Treatment/Prognosis

What is the Tx paradigm for WT in the U.S?

WT Tx paradigm: inital surgical resection → risk-adapted adj chemo +/− RT

What is the major difference between the International Society of Pediatric Oncology (SIOP) Tx paradigm (European cooperative group) and the National Wilms Tumor Study (NWTS) paradigm (American cooperative group)?

SIOP trials incorporate **preop therapy** (CRT), whereas the NWTS trials do not.

Under what circumstance is the SIOP paradigm favored in the U.S.?

In **unresectable or bilat Wilms,** preop chemo is used.

What are the indications for postop RT in the current COG protocols (AREN0532,533)?

Indications for postop RT depend on **histology and stage:**
  Favorable histology: stages III–IV
  Unfavorable histology: stages I–IV

What chemotherapeutic agents are typically used in Wilms?

Vincristine, Actinomycin D (Adr/VP-16/Cytoxan/ carboplatin added in UH)

What did the early NWTS-1 and NWTS-2 studies show?

1. Vincristine and Actinomycin D (VA) are better together than either alone.
2. RT is not needed for stage I FH pts, but when given it should start within 9 days of surgery.
3. There was no RT dose response from 10–40 Gy.

What study demonstrated that whole abdomen irradiation (WAI) is not needed for local spillage?

NWTS-1; flank fields suffice if spillage is local.

What study demonstrated that adding Adr to VA benefited group 2–4 pts?

NWTS-2; adding Adr benefited group 2–4 FH, especially group 2–4 UH pts (OS 38% vs. 78%).

Which study demonstrated that 10 wks was equal to 6 mos of chemo for stage I pts?

NWTS-3; 4-yr OS was 96%–97%.

Which study showed that stage II FH pts do not need RT as long as VA is given?

NWTS-3 (4 arm: vincristine/Actinomycin D/ Adriamycin [VAAdr] vs. VA vs. +/− RT → 4-yr OS ~90%–95%, no difference)

What study eliminated Adr from stage II FH?

NWTS-3. VA alone was sufficient.

What study demonstrated that 10 Gy was equal to 20 Gy if Adr was added to stage III pts?

NWTS-3 demonstrated the noninferiority of lower RT doses with Adr.

What study addressed the addition of Cytoxan to VAAdr for high-risk pts?

NWTS-3. Cytoxan improved outcome in UH stage II–IV but not FH stage IV.

What study addressed pulse-intense (PI) chemo?

NWTS-4. 6 mos of PI was equal to 15 mos of conventional chemo.

What are the main advantages of PI chemo?

With PI chemo, there is ↓ **hematologic toxicity** and ↓ **total cost** b/c fewer drugs are used.

What study found that local spillage (old stage II) without RT results in a ↑ LR?

NWTS-4; ↑ LR, but no difference in OS; so, moved to stage III for FH (need adj RT)

What question does NWTS-5 address? (*Dome JS et al., JCO 2006*)

Nonrandomized, assesses prognostic importance of LOH 1p + 16q

For which pts did NWTS-5 show ↑ (13.5%) rates of relapse with nephrectomy alone and without adj chemo?

Stage I FH, pts <2 yo, and tumors <550 g. Most (>70%) were salvaged successfully, however.

What is the outcome for relapsed Wilms treated with VA only for stage I or II Dz?

4-yr EFS/OS: 71% (stage I) vs. 82% (stage II). Pt salvaged with surgery, RT, and chemo with vincristine/Adr/Cytoxan/etoposide. Lung mets only, 4-yr EFS/OS: 68% (stage I) vs. 81% (stage II).

What about relapsed stage III–IV Dz?

Relapse after stage III–IV Tx is worse (4-yr EFS/OS: 42% vs. 48%, respectively), lung only mets: 4-yr EFS/OS: 49% vs. 53%, respectively. (*Green DM et al., Ped Blood Cancer 2007; Malogolowkin M et al., Ped Blood Cancer 2008*)

▪ Toxicity

What is the dose constraint for the kidney?

One third of contralat kidney <14.4 Gy

What is the dose constraint for the liver?

One half of uninvolved liver <19.8 Gy; with liver mets, 75% of liver ≤30.6 Gy

Pts are at risk for what late effects with flank RT? WLI?

Scoliosis of the spine, muscular hypoplasia, kyphosis, iliac wing hypoplasia, SBO, veno-occlusive Dz of the liver; breast hypoplasia (four fifths of females who get WLI will have underdeveloped breasts), pneumonitis, CHF, 2nd malignancy, and renal failure

What is the risk of SBO at 15 yrs after flank/abdominal RT?

The risk of SBO at 15 yrs is **15%.**

What is the risk of a 2nd malignancy at 15 yrs?

The risk of a 2nd malignancy at 15 yrs is **1.6%–2%.**

The re-irradiation tolerance of which organ decreases with time after initial RT?

Re-irradiation tolerance of the **kidney** decreases with time.

What is the TD 5/5 for an entire kidney?

The TD 5/5 is **23 Gy.**

What is the cumulative maximal total dose (including prior RT) for WT pts?

30.6 Gy (if <3 yrs) or 39.5 Gy (if >3 yrs)

TABLE 3.1 Current Children's Oncology Group Wilms Protocol (AREN0532/533)

Goals: Reduce Tx-related toxicity in low-risk tumors and improve outcome for high-risk tumors with chemo intensification.

Tumor Risk Classification	Multimodality Treatment
Very low risk FH WT >2 yrs, stage I FH, <550 g	Surgery, *no* therapy if central pathology review and LN sampling
Low-risk FH WT ≥2 yrs, stage I FH, ≥550 g	Surgery, no RT, regimen EE4A
Standard-risk FH WT	Surgery, regimen DD4A
Stage I-II FH with LOH	Surgery, RT, regimen DD4A
Stage III FH without LOH	
Stage III-IV FH with LOH	Surgery, RT, regimen M, WLI
Stage IV FH (slow/incomplete responders)	
Stage IV FH: CR of lung mets at wk 6/DD4A (rapid early responders)	Surgery, RT, regimen DD4A; no WLI
Stage I-III FA	Surgery, RT, regimen DD4A
Stages I DA	
Stage IV FA	Surgery, RT, regimen UH1
Stage II-IV DA	
Stage IV CCSK	
Stage IV RTK	
Stage I-III CCSK	Surgery, RT, regimen 1

FH, favorable histology; WT, Wilms tumor; LN, lymph node; RT, radiation therapy; LOH, loss of heterozygocity; WLI, whole lung irradiation; CR, complete response; FA, focal anaplasia; DA, diffuse anaplasia; CCSK, clear cell sarcoma of the kidney; RTK, rhabdoid tumor of the kidney.

TABLE 3.2 Chemotherapy Regimens on AREN0532/533 Protocols

Regimen	Agents
EE4A	VCR/AMD
DD4A	VCR/AMD/ADR
M	VCR/AMD/ADR; CY/ETOP
I	VCR/DOX/CY; CY/ETOP
UH1	CY/CARBO/ETOP; VCR/DOX/CY

VCR, vincristine; AMD, dactinomycin; ADR, Adriamycin; CY, Cytoxan; ETOP, etoposide; DOX, doxorubicin; CARBO, carboplatin.

TABLE 3.3 Radiation Planning and Doses on Protocols AREN0532/533

RT timing: Concurrent with VCR, surgery day 1, RT ≤day 10 (max day 14).
Exception: Medical contraindication or delay in central pathology review.

RT field design:

I. **Flank RT:** GTV = preop CT/MRI (tumor and involved kidney).

$$CTV + PTV = ≤1 \text{ cm}$$

Medial border across midline to include vertebral bodies + 1-cm margin but sparing contralat kidney. Other field borders placed at edge of PTV. Use AP/PA.

If + PA and removed, then treat entire PA chain to 10.8 Gy.

If + residual Dz, then boost with 10.8 Gy after initial 10.8 Gy (3D-CRT, GTV = postop volume).

Dose limits: Two thirds contralat kidney to 14.4 Gy, one half of undiseased liver to 19.8 Gy.

II. **WAI:** CTV = entire peritoneal cavity from diaphragm to pelvic diaphragm.
Superior border: 1 cm above dome of diaphragm.
Inferior border: Bottom of oburator foramen.
Laterally: 1 cm beyond lat abdominal wall; block femoral heads.
Dose 10.5 Gy (1.5 Gy/fx) except for diffuse anaplasia or rhabdoid tumors (dose is 19.8 Gy, shield kidney to keep <14.4 Gy).

III. **WLI:** CTV includes lungs, mediastinum, and pleural recesses. PTV = CTV + 1 cm.
Inf border at L1, sup border 1 cm above 1st rib, block humeral heads.
Can boost after 12 Gy (1.5 Gy/fx) (10.5 Gy for <12 mos) for persistent Dz after 2 wks → +7.5 Gy (19.5 Gy) to residual with conformal fields.

IV. **Liver mets:** Surgery for solitary mets, excised to -margins. Whole liver RT for diffuse liver mets to 19.8 Gy (with additional 5.4-10.8 Gy at discretion).

V. **Brain:** WBRT to 21.6 Gy (30.6 Gy if >16 yo). If 21.6 Gy → conformal RT boost with additional 10.8 Gy.

VI. **Bone:** GTV + 3-cm margin, AP/PA to 25.2 Gy (30.6 Gy if >16 yo).

VII. **Unresected nodes:** Cover entire LN chain to 19.8 Gy (30.6 Gy if >16 yo), with optional 5.4–10.8 Gy boost. If removed +PA LN, use 10.8 Gy to cover.

RT, radiation therapy; VCR, vincristine; max, maximum; GTV, gross target volume; preop, preoperative; CT/MRI, computed tomography/magnetic resonance imaging; CTV, clinical target volume; PTV, planning target volume; cm, centimeter; contralat, contralateral; AP/PA, anterior-posterior/posterior-anterior; +, positive; Gy, Gray; Dz, disease; 3D-CRT, three-dimensional conformal radiation therapy; postop, postoperative; WAI, whole abdomen irradiation; lat, lateral; fx, fractions; WLI, whole lung irradiation; inf, inferior; sup, superior; mos, months; wks, weeks; mets, metastasis; −, negative; WBRT, whole brain radiation therapy; yo, years old; LN, lymph node.

4

Neuroblastoma

John P. Christodouleas and Moody D. Wharam, Jr.

▉ Background

What are the 3 types of neuroblastic tumors?

3 types of neuroblastic tumors:
1. Neuroblastoma (NB)
2. Ganglioneuroblastoma
3. Ganglioneuroma

These tumors differ in the degree of cellular maturation.

What is the most common malignancy in infants?

NB is the most common malignancy in infants.

Estimate the annual incidence of NB in the U.S.

There are ~**650 cases/yr** of NB in the U.S.

What is the median age at Dx for NB?

The median age at Dx is **17 mos**.

Name 3 genetic syndromes associated with NB.

3 genetic syndromes associated with NB:
1. NF
2. Hirschsprung Dz
3. Fetal hydantoin syndrome

What tests have been used to screen infants for NB?

Historically, infants were screened for NB using **urinary catecholamines (vanillylmandelic acid/ homovanillic acid).**

Does screening improve survival in NB?

This is **controversial.** Screening infants for NB with urinary catecholamines has been evaluated in multiple studies; however, the value of catecholamine-based screening is limited by its false+ rate and b/c a significant % of infant NBs spontaneously regress.

What markers distinguish NB from other small round blue tumors?

NB-specific markers:
1. Neuron-specific enolase
2. Synaptophysin
3. Neurofilament

What is the cell of origin for NB?

NB arises from **neural crest cells of the sympathetic ganglion.**

What % of NB pts have detectable urinary catecholamines?

90% of pts have detectable urinary catecholamines.

What genetic changes are associated with n-myc amplification?

Double-minute chromatin bodies and homogeneously staining regions are associated with n-myc amplification.

What are the genetic/chromatin changes that portend a poor prognosis in NB?

Genetic/chromatin changes with a poor prognosis in NB:
1. **N-myc amplification**
2. LOH 1p + 11q
3. Diploid DNA
4. ↑ telomerase activity

In which pts does DNA content *not* have prognostic importance?

DNA content does not have prognostic importance in **metastatic pts.**

What % of NB pts present with n-myc amplification?

30%–40% of pts present with n-myc amplification.

What % of NB pts present with 1p deletions?

70% of pts present with 1p deletions.

What is the genetic variation on 6p22 that is associated with clinically aggressive NB?

Homozygosity for 3 single nucleotide polymorphisms on 6p22 is associated with stage IV Dz, n-myc amplification, and Dz relapse. (*Maris JM et al., NEJM 2008*)

What are the most common sites of presentation for NB?

Adrenal medulla > paraspinal > post mediastinum

In what age group is thoracic presentation of NB more common?

Thoracic NB is more common in **infants.**

How does NB presentation differ from Wilms?

There are **more systemic Sx in NB.** (Mnemonic: **W**ilms are **W**ell, **N**euroblastomas are **N**ot well)

What are some presenting Sx of NB?

Along with the presentation of a mass, NB may be associated with **constitutional Sx** (fever, malaise, pain, weight loss), periorbital ecchymosis **("raccoon eyes")**, **"blueberry muffin" sign** (nontender blue skin mets), scalp nodules, bone pain, irritable/ill appearance, diarrhea (↑ vasoactive intestinal peptide), Horner syndrome, opsomyoclonus truncal ataxia (rare paraneoplastic syndrome of ataxia, random eye movement, and myoclonic jerking associated with early stage but persists after cure), and Kerner-Morrison syndrome (diarrhea, low K).

What % of NB pts present with mets?	**75%** of all NB pts present with mets.
A 2 yo presents with an abdominal mass and lung mets. What is the most likely Dx?	Wilms. **NB rarely metastasizes to the lungs!**
What are the most common sites of mets for NB?	NB commonly metastasizes to **bone (~50%), LNs (35%)**, BM, liver, skin, and orbits. **Lung mets are rare.**
What are the most common bony sites of metastatic Dz in NB?	**Bones of the skull and orbit** (proptosis, ecchymosis, scalp mass)
Which is more likely to exhibit calcifications on x-ray: Wilms or NB?	**NB (85%)** is more likely to exhibit calcifications.
What are the classic histologic findings seen in NB?	**Homer-Wright pseudorosettes,** hemorrhage, and calcification

■ Workup/Staging

Outline the workup for pts with suspected NB.	Suspected NB workup: 1. H&P 2. Labs (CBC, LFTs, serum markers, UA, urine catechol) 3. Imaging (bone scan, CT C/A/P, abdominal US, MRI abdomen/liver/spine, I-131 metaiodobenzylguanidine [MIBG] scan 4. BM Bx 5. Pathology (DNA content, n-myc amplification, and cytogenetics)
Why is a BM Bx important in the workup of NB?	BM Bx may obviate the need for primary site surgery if the testing is positive and the clinical picture is clear.
What % of NB pts have uptake on an I-131 MIBG scan?	**~90%** of NB pts have uptake on an I-131 MIBG scan.
What are the currently used NB staging systems?	As of 2010, most cooperative group trials use the **International Neuroblastoma Staging System (INSS),** which involves the extent of surgical resection. However, a new staging system that uses only pre-Tx factors has been developed: the **International Neuroblastoma Risk Group (INRG).** These 2 staging systems will likely be used concurrently to allow for comparisons between trials. (*Monclair T et al., JCO 2009*)

Summarize the INSS staging system.

Stage 1: unilat localized tumor s/p GTR +/− microscopic residual Dz; ipsi LN−, though LNs attached and removed with the primary may be involved

Stage 2A: unilat localized tumor s/p STR only; ipsi LN−, though LNs attached and removed with the primary may be involved

Stage 2B: unilat localized tumor s/p GTR or STR with involved nonadherent ipsi LNs; enlarged contralat LN−.

Stage 3: unresectable localized tumor extending across the midline +/− regional LN involvement; unilat localized tumor with contralat regional LN involvement

Stage 4: distant Dz except as defined by stage 4S

Stage 4S: localized unilat primary as defined by stage 1, 2A, or 2B; distant Dz limited to the liver, skin, and/or <10% of BM in infants <1 yo

Summarize the INRG staging system.

In the **INRG system,** locoregional tumors are staged **L1** or **L2** based on the absence or presence of 1 or more of 20 image-defined radiographic findings (IDRFs). These IDRFs generally affect whether or not a tumor is surgically resectable and to what degree. The authors of the INRG system avoided the terms resectable and unresectable since that may depend more on the surgeon's style and subjective judgment. **Metastatic tumors** are defined as stage **M**, except for stage **MS**, in which mets are confined to the skin, liver, and/or BM in pts <18 mos old. (*Monclair T et al., JCO 2009*)

What is the INRG stage of an 8-mo-old pt with metastatic Dz to bone only?

An 8-mo-old pt with metastatic Dz to bone only is INRG **stage M** (only BM, liver, and skin mets qualify for stage MS).

What is the INSS stage of a 14-mo-old pt with metastatic Dz to BM only?

A 14-mo-old pt with metastatic Dz to bone marrow only is INSS **stage 4** (only pts <12 mos old qualify for stage 4S).

What 2 clinical factors are most predictive of cure in NB?

The 2 clinical factors most predictive of cure are **age** and **stage at Dx**.

In children with metastatic Dz, what is the most important prognostic factor?

In children with metastatic Dz, **age (<1 yo best)** is the strongest prognostic factor, even more so than n-myc.

The Shimada classification system divides NB into what 2 categories? What 5 features are used to classify pts in this system?

The Shimada classification system divides NB into **favorable histology** (FH) and **unfavorable histology** (UH). Favorable factors:

Stroma-rich (Schwann cell stroma)
Age (young)
Differentiation (well differentiated)
Mitotic/karyorrhectic index (low)
Nodularity (nonnodular)

(Mnemonic: Dr. Shimada has a **SAD MiNd**)

What 5 factors are used to classify NB pts into low-, intermediate-, and high-risk groups per the COG?

5 factors used to classify NB in COG low-, intermediate- and high-risk groups:

1. **S**tage, INSS
2. **A**ge
3. **N**-myc status
4. **D**NA ploidy
5. **S**himada classification

(Mnemonic: **SANDS** [Table 4.1])

What features make NB pts with stage 4S Dz intermediate risk?

NB stage 4S pts are intermediate risk if tumors are **not n-myc amplified** and are **either Shimada UH or have diploid DNA.**

What feature makes NB pts with stage 4S Dz high risk?

NB stage 4S pts are high risk if tumors are **n-myc amplified.**

What risk group is a NB pt with stage I Dz and n-myc amplification?

All stage I NB pts are **low risk.**

Can a pt with n-myc amplification be classified as intermediate risk?

No. All NB pts with n-myc are either low risk or high risk.

In which COG risk group do NB pts most commonly present?

NB pts are most commonly **high risk (55%)** → low risk (30%).

■ Treatment/Prognosis

Estimate the 3-yr OS for low-, intermediate-, and high-risk NB.

NB 3-yr OS by risk group:
Low risk: 95%–100%
Intermediate risk: 75%–98%
High risk: <30%

What is the Tx paradigm for low-risk NB?

Low-risk NB Tx paradigm: surgery alone with chemo reserved for persistent or recurrent Dz

What is the Tx paradigm for intermediate-risk NB?

Intermediate-risk NB Tx paradigm: surgery → short- or long-course chemo depending on biologic factors +/− 2nd surgery if needed

What is the role of RT in the Tx of intermediate-risk NB?

In intermediate-risk pts, RT is typically reserved for those who are symptomatic due to tumor bulk and are not responding to initial chemo, such as pts with respiratory distress due to hepatomegaly or with neurologic compromise due to cord compression. RT is not indicated as a consolidative therapy even with persistent Dz.

Indications for RT based on **A3961**: Symptomatic palliation, viable residual Dz in Tx-refractory pts, and recurrent Dz. Local Tx is to 24 Gy.

What is the Tx for unfavorable 4S (intermediate-risk) Dz?

The Tx is **chemo × 8 cycles**.

What is the Tx paradigm for high-risk NB?

High-risk NB Tx paradigm: induction chemo, then resection, then high-dose chemo and stem cell transplant → **consolidation RT**, then oral cis-retinoic acid

What is the Tx paradigm for low-risk stage 4S NB, and what study supports this approach?

Low-risk stage 4S NB Tx paradigm: Bx → supportive care. Chemo and/or RT are reserved for rapidly growing or symptomatic Dz. A subgroup analysis of **CCG 3881** showed that supportive care is sufficient for 57% of pts. The protocol resulted in a 5-yr EFS of 86% and an OS of 92%. (*Nickerson HJ et al., JCO 2000*)

What studies support the use of observation (without resection) in infants with localized NB without n-myc amplification?

The use of observation (without resection) in infants with localized NB without n-myc amplification was evaluated in the German GPOH trials **NB95-S and NB97.** Of 93 pts with gross Dz, 44 had spontaneous regression. OS and DM-free survival were no different from outcomes of pts treated with surgery or chemo in these trials (3-yr OS 99%, DM-free survival 94%). (*Hero B et al., JCO 2008*)

In high-risk NB, what tissues are targeted during RT and to what dose?

Per current **COG0532,** high-risk NB pts are treated with RT to their **postchemo, preop tumor bed** to a total dose of **21.6 Gy in 1.8 Gy/fx if GTR** and 36.0 Gy (21.6 Gy to preop GTV → 14.4 Gy boost) **if gross residual.**

In high-risk NB, should elective nodal RT be given?

No. In high-risk NB, only clinically+ or pathologically+ LN regions are covered in the RT volumes.

What study indirectly demonstrated an RT dose response in high-risk NB?

Haas-Kogan et al. performed a secondary analysis of **CCG 3891** and found that high-risk NB pts who rcv 10 Gy local EBRT + 10 Gy total body irradiation (TBI) as part of a transplant preparation regimen had better LC than pts who did not get TBI (or a transplant) (5-yr LRR was 22% vs. 52%) (*IJROBP 2003*).

These results support the current use of 21.6 Gy in high-risk protocols.

What study demonstrated the benefits of high-dose chemo → BMT as well as adj cis-retinoic acid in high-risk NB?

In **CCG 3891,** 379 high-risk NB pts were treated with induction chemo → surgery and 10 Gy to gross residual. Pts were then randomized to 3 cycles of nonmyeloablative chemo vs. myeloablative chemo, TBI, and BMT. Pts underwent secondary randomization to observation vs. cis-retinoic acid × 6 mos. Both the myeloablative chemo and cis-retinoic acid improved OS. 5-yr OS for pts who rcv both was 59%. (*Matthay KK et al., JCO 2009*)

What is the appropriate Tx for NB pts with cord compression?

Consider chemo initially for NB-related cord compression. Unresponsive Dz can be treated with surgery or RT.

What is the RT dose and dose/fx used for NB pts being treated for symptomatic cord compression?

For symptomatic cord compression:
1. If pt is <3 yo, treat to 9 Gy (1.8 Gy/fx).
2. If pt is ≥3 yo, treat to 21.6 Gy (1.8 Gy/fx).

What is the RT dose and dose/fx used for NB pts being treated for symptomatic hepatomegaly?

Symptomatic hepatomegaly is treated to 4.5 Gy **(1.5 Gy × 3).**

What chemo drugs are typically used in NB?

Chemo drugs typically used in NB:
1. Cytoxan
2. Doxorubicin
3. Etoposide
4. Carboplatin
5. Ifosfamide

What is the role of I-131 MIBG in NB?

I-131 MIBG can be used for refractory NB, based on a promising phase II study showing a 36% response rate. (*Matthay KK et al., JCO 2007*)

■ Toxicity

In NB, what dose constraint is used for the contralat kidney?

Limit the dose to the entire contralat kidney to **<15 Gy.**

In NB, what dose constraint is used for the liver?

Limit liver V15 to **<66 %.**

In NB, what dose contraint is used for the lung?

Limit lung V15 to **<66%.**

What are 2 tumor-related factors that correlate with an increased risk for mets?	**Thickness** (relates to invasion of optic nerve, uvea, orbit, choroid) and **size** of lesion
What is trilat RB? How common is it? What is the prognosis?	Trilat RB is **bilat RB + CNS midline PNET** (pineal or suprasellar), representing **3%–9% of hereditary RB** (rare). It is **uniformly fatal.**
How does RB present grossly?	Endophytic mass (projects into vitreous) and less frequently exophytic
What % of cases are bilat at presentation?	**10%–15%** of RB cases are bilat.
How do pts present with RB in the U.S. vs. in developing countries?	<u>In the U.S.</u>: **leukocoria** > strabismus > painful glaucoma, and irritability. Leukocoria refers to an abnl white reflection from the retina. <u>In developing countries</u>: proptosis, orbital mass, and mets (more advanced)
What are the major negative prognostic factors in RB?	Delay in Dx >6 mos of age, Hx of intraocular surgery leading to seeding, cataracts, thick tumors, and Hx of RT (because such pts are fairly advanced)

■ Workup/Staging

What is the DDx for pts who present with leukocoria?	Hyperlastic primary vitreous, retrolental fibrodysplasia, Coat Dz, congenital cataracts, toxocariasis, and toxoplasmosis
Is Bx done for RB?	**Generally not.** Because of the fear of seeding, the Dx is established clinically.
What is the typical workup for pts with an intraocular mass?	Intraocular mass workup: H&P (EUA, max dilated pupil, scleral indentation), labs, US/CT/MRI
When are bone scan, BM Bx, and LP indicated?	If the tumor is not confined to the globe (with deep invasion), BM Bx, LP, and bone scan are indicated.
What % of RBs are calcified?	**90%** of RBs are calcified.
What is the most commonly used staging system for RB? For what does this system predict?	**Reese-Ellsworth grouping system;** used to predict for **visual preservation after EBRT** (does *not* predict for survival)
What staging system is used in ongoing COG protocols?	The **International Classification for Intraocular Retinoblastoma** is used for staging in ongoing COG protocols.
Summarize the International Classification for Intraocular Retinoblastoma.	**Group A:** all tumors ≤3 mm, confined to retina, and ≥3 mm from foveola and ≥1.5 mm from optic disc

Group B: all tumors confined to retina, clear sub-retinal fluid <3 mm from tumor with no subretinal seeding

Group C: discrete tumors, subretinal fluid without seeding involving up to one fourth of retina, local fine vitreous seeding close to discrete tumor, local subretinal seeding <3 mm from tumor

Group D: massive or diffuse tumors; subretinal fluid or diffuse vitreous seeding; retinal detachment; diffuse or massive Dz including greasy seeds or avascular tumor masses; subretinal seeding may include subretinal plaques or tumor nodules

Group E: presence of any of the following features: tumor touching lens, tumor ant to ant vitreous surface involving ciliary body or ant segment, diffuse infiltrating RB, neovascular glaucoma, opaque media from hemorrhage, tumor necrosis with aseptic orbital cellulites, phthisis bulbi (shrunken, nonfunctional eye)

■ Treatment/Prognosis

What is the Tx paradigm for unilat intraocular RB?	Unilat intraocular RB Tx paradigm: preserve eye with chemoreduction × 6 cycles (vincristine/carboplatin/etoposide [VCE]) → focal therapy (if needed)
What are some focal therapies used for RB?	Enucleation, EBRT or brachytherapy (plaque), cryotherapy, photocoagulation (laser), thermochemo (thermal + carboplatin), sub-Tenon injection of carboplatin (preferred approach at the Johns Hopkins Hospital)
To what does "sub-Tenon" injection refer?	Injection of agents into eye through the **capsule of Tenon** (thin outer membrane enveloping the eye)
When can cryotherapy/laser be used in RB?	**Small lesions,** at least 4 disc diameters from the fovea/optic disc
What is the generally accepted Tx breakdown based on the international RB groupings?	UCSF (*Lin P et al., Am J Ophthalmol 2009*): **Group A:** focal therapy only (laser, cryotherapy, hyperthermia, brachytherapy) **Group B:** vincristine + carboplatin × 6 cycles; focal therapy after 2–6 cycles **Group C:** VCE × 6 cycles; focal therapy **Group D:** same as group C; EBRT **Group E:** enucleation; 3-agent chemo

What are the diagnostic histopathologic characteristics of LCH?

Birbeck granules on electron microscopy and **CD1a/ S100** positivity are typical for LCH.

What is the normal function of Langerhans cells? Where are they normally found?

Langerhans cells serve as **antigen presenting cells to lymphocytes** and are typically found in **skin, mucosa, spleen, and lymphatics.**

What organs are typically involved in LCH?

Bones (children) and lungs (adults), but LCH can present in any organ (e.g., liver, skin, etc.).

What defines good risk groups vs. poor risk groups?

Good risk: unifocal lesion in bone (local therapy)
Poor risk: <2 yo with organ dysfunction

What is Hand-Schuller-Christian Dz?

Hand-Schuller-Christian Dz refers to the proliferation of hystiocytes that results in **exophthalmos, skull lesions, diabetes insipidus** (DI), **and hemangiomas** (poor prognosis).

How does LCH relate to other histiocytosis entities like eosinophilic granuloma, Letterer-Siwe Dz, Hand-Schuller-Christian Dz, and histiocytosis X?

Eosinophilic granuloma is an older term for focal LCH, while the eponyms represent multifocal Dz. Histiocytosis X is the older term for LCH.

■ Workup/Staging

In what age group are widespread seborrheic rash in the scalp/groin, +LAD, and liver involvement seen with LCH?

These Sx are seen in LCH pts <**2 yo.**

For what age group is DI a common presentation of LCH?

>**2 yo** (20%–50%). In this group, bone (pain +/− soft tissue mass), lung, oral mucous membrane, and cerebral involvement by LCH can be seen.

Is bone scan useful for LCH? Why?

No. LCH bone lesions are usually purely lytic.

What type of workup is necessary?

LCH workup: H&P, labs, skeletal survey (lucency in the medullary cavity), and Bx

What is the appearance of LCH lesions on plain radiograph?

LCH lesions appear **lytic** or **"punched-out"** on plain radiograph.

What staging system is used for LCH?

The **Greenberger staging system** (I–V, based on age and extent of involvement) is used for LCH.

■ Staging/Prognosis

What are the indications for RT in LCH?

No signs of local healing, relapse after surgery, if other local therapy (i.e., curettage) is not appropriate, potential compromise of critical structures from expansile bone lesions, pain relief, and DI

What is the largest series supporting RT for DI from LCH?

Mayo data (*Kilpatrick SE et al., Cancer 1995*): 45 pts. There was a 36% rate of DI improvement with RT.

Within how many days after Dx should RT be given for DI?

RT should be administered within **14 days** of DI Dx. (*Kilpatrick SE et al., Cancer 1995*)

When is RT not indicated in LCH?

RT is not indicated for **sclerotic LCH lesions and collapsed vertebral lesions** (only indicated if such lesions are painful).

What data supports the use of RT for localized osseous LCH lesions?

German meta-analysis (*Olschwski T et al., Strahlenther Onkol 2006*): LC was 96% and CR was 93% for single-system Dz with RT.

What are commonly used doses and volumes for LCH?

DI: **15 Gy** to pituitary/hypothalamus
Bone (small margin): **5–10 Gy**
Adults: **15–24 Gy** (in 2 Gy/fx)

When is chemo used in LCH?

Multisystem Dz (e.g., if fever, pain, severe skin involvement, failure to thrive, and organ dysfunction)

What systemic agents are used for LCH?

Prednisone (1ˢᵗ line), then vinblastine or etoposide. Single-agent chemo is as good as multiagent chemo. Vincristine can also be used.

How are asymptomatic, organ-confined LCH lesions managed?

Asymptomatic LCH lesions are typically **observed.**

How is a symptomatic bony LCH lesion managed?

A symptomatic bony LCH lesion is typically managed by surgery **(or curettage, excision) and/or local injection of steroids.**

How are symptomatic LCH skin lesions managed?

Symptomatic LCH skin lesions are managed by **topical therapy with nitrogen mustard or systemic therapy (steroids).**

How is LCH of the eye, ear, spine, or weight-bearing bones managed?

LCH of these areas is managed by s**ystemic steroids or local RT.**

How is asymptomatic multifocal LCH Dz with organ dysfunction managed?

Such asymptomatic LCH Dz is typically **observed.**

What are common cytogenetic abnormalities in MB?	Common cytogenetic abnormalities in MB: 1. **Deletion of 17p** (40%–50%) 2. **Isochromosome 17q** 3. **Deletion of 16q**
Where does MB most commonly arise?	**Midline cerebellar vermis** (75%), with the rest in cerebellar hemispheres
What is the DDx for a posterior fossa (PF) mass?	DDx for a PF mass: 1. **MB** 2. **Ependymoma** 3. **Astrocytoma** 4. **Brainstem glioma** 5. **Juvenile pilocytic astrocytoma** 6. **Hemangioblastoma** 7. **Mets**

■ Workup/Staging

What are some common presenting Sx for MB?	HA, n/v, altered mentation due to hydrocephalus, truncal ataxia, head bob, and diplopia (CN VI)
To what are common presenting Sx due in MB?	Obstructive hydrocephalus/↑ICP (HA and vomiting)
What is the "setting-sun" sign?	Downward deviation of gaze from ↑ICP (CNs III, IV, and VI)
List the general workup for a PF mass at presentation.	PF mass workup: H&P (funduscopic exam, CN exam), CBC/CMP, MRI brain/spine, CSF cytology (may not be possible due to herniation risk), and baseline ancillary tests
Is a tumor Bx necessary for Dx? Is a BM Bx necessary?	Per current COG MB protocol **ACNS0331, a tumor Bx is unnecessary;** pts often go straight to surgery. **BM Bx is not part of the standard workup.**
Is there any risk of CSF dissemination with shunt placement for MB?	**No.** There is no risk of CSF dissemination.
What are some important ancillary tests to obtain prior to starting Tx?	Baseline audiometry, IQ testing, TSH, and growth measures
What tests should be obtained on days 10–14 postop?	MRI spine, CSF cytology. (Delay to day 10 to avoid a false+ result from surgical debris.)
When is MRI of the brain done? Of the spine?	<u>MRI brain</u>: preop and 24–48 hrs postop <u>MRI spine</u>: preop or 10–14 days postop
What can be done before Tx to reduce ICP?	Ventricular shunt/drain, steroids, acetazolamide (Diamox)

Is there a risk of CSF dissemination with shunt placement?	**No.** There is no risk of CSF dissemination with shunt placement.
List the T staging according to the modified Chang staging system for MB.	**T1:** ≤3 cm, confined **T2:** >3 cm, partial fill of 4th ventricle, invades 1 adjacent structure **T3a:** invades 2 adjacent structures, complete fill of 4th ventricle **T3b:** extends into brain stem, arises from floor of 4th ventricle, complete fill of 4th ventricle **T4:** extends beyond aqueduct of Sylvius or foramen magnum to involve 3rd ventricle/midbrain/upper cervical cord
List the M staging according to the modified Chang staging system for MB.	**M0:** no mets **M1:** +CSF **M2:** nodular seeding intracranially **M3:** nodule in subarachnoid space in cord **M4:** extraneural spread
Define standard-risk and high-risk MB.	<u>**Standard risk:**</u> >3 yo, GTR/NTR <1.5 cm² residual, and M0 <u>**High risk:**</u> <3 yo or STR >1.5 cm² residual, or M+

■ Treatment/Prognosis

What is the most important prognostic factor at Dx for MB? What are other poor prognostic factors for MB?	**M stage** is the most important prognostic factor. Other poor prognostic factors include male gender, age <3 yrs, and unresectable Dz/STR.
What is the management paradigm for standard-risk MB?	Standard-risk MB management paradigm: max safe resection → RT with concurrent weekly vincristine → adj chemo (8 6-wk cycles of cisplatin/CCNU/vincristine). **RT is CSI to 23.4 Gy → CD1 to PF to 36 Gy, then CD2 to cavity/residual or PF to 55.8 Gy.**
What chemo regimens are typically used for MB?	Initial studies that established the efficacy of reduced-dose CSI (23.4 Gy) with chemo in standard-risk MB used **concurrent vincristine with RT → adj cisplatin/ CCNU/vincristine**. The **CCG A9961** trial recently found similar outcomes when cyclophosphamide was substituted for CCNU. (*Packer R et al., JCO 2006*)
What is the management paradigm for high-risk MB?	High-risk MB management paradigm for pts >3 yo: same as standard risk, but the **CSI dose is 36 Gy;** also, nodular intracranial or spinal mets need to be boosted to 39.6–50.4 Gy depending on location.

What are the RT technique questions being addressed in COG protocol 0331?

In **ACNS0331, standard-risk pts 3–7 yo** are randomized to **CSI to 18 Gy vs. 23.4 Gy.** For the **18 Gy arm, all pts get a PF boost to 23.4 Gy.** All standard-risk pts 3-7 yo undergo a 2nd randomization: CD to **55.8 Gy to PF vs. tumor bed only.** Standard-risk pts >8 yo: 23.4 Gy CSI → randomization to CD to 55.8 Gy to PF vs. tumor bed only.

Is there a role for pre-RT chemo in MB pts >3 yo?

No. In MB pts >3 yo, intensive chemo prior to RT is associated with ↑ RT toxicity, RT Tx delays, and worsened RFS. (German **HIT 91:** *Kortmann RD et al., IJROBP 2000*)

What benefit does proton therapy have in the Tx of MB?

Retrospective data suggests that proton plans have ↓ **dose to the cochlea/temporal lobe compared to IMRT** (0.1%–2% vs. 20%–30%), and virtually no exit dose to the abdomen/chest/heart/pelvis.

Is there a role for hyperfractionated RT to reduce cognitive sequelae of MB Tx?

MSFOP 98, a phase II trial, evaluated hyperfractionated RT in MB and showed promising results. 48 standard-risk pts were treated with CSI 1 Gy bid to 36 Gy → tumor bed boost 1 Gy bid to 68 Gy. **6-yr OS was 78%, and EFS was 75%. Decline in IQ appeared less pronounced than in historical controls.** (*Carrie C et al., JCO 2009*)

How are MB pts simulated?

MB simulation: **prone, neck extended** (so PA spine field does not exit through the mouth), **shoulders positioned inferiorly** (to allow for lat cranial fields)

In CSI, which fields are placed 1st?

Spinal fields are placed 1st (to allow calculation of collimator angle for the cranial field based on spinal field beam divergence).
Cranial fields are placed 2nd (down to C5-6 or as low as possible).

By what angle are the cranial field collimators rotated?

Arctan (one half length of sup spine field/SSD), which matches the cranial field to the spine field divergence

What are the borders of the spine field(s)?

Superior: matched to cranial field
Inferior: S3
Lateral: 1 cm past pedicles (wider in sacrum)

By what angle is the couch kicked and in which direction?

Couch kick for CSI: **arctan (one half length of cranial field/source axis distance); couch kicked toward side treated** to match cranial field divergence

If multiple spinal fields are used, what is the skin gap? At what depth is the match?

With multiple spine fields, the **skin gap = ([0.5 × Length 1 × d]/SSD1) + ([0.5 × Length 2 × d]/SSD2)** where *d* is the depth of the match, which is typically at the ant cord edge.

How is "feathering" done? Why is it used?

At the Johns Hopkins Hospital, 0.5-cm gap shifts/day (for a total 1.5 cm over 3 days). Feathering helps reduce hot and cold spots in plan.

How do field edges and isocenters of respective fields move with feathering?

There are many techniques; however, at the Johns Hopkins Hospital, the following technique is typically used:
  · Cranial fields: isocenter is fixed, lower jaw moves
  Spinal fields: isocenter and inf jaw moves

Where should the isocenter be placed in the cranial field for CSI? What cranial structure should be assessed for adequate coverage?

The isocenter should be placed **behind the lenses** to minimize divergence of beams into the opposite lens; the **cribriform plate** is not optimally visualized on conventional simulation films. A generous margin must be given in this area, or CT contours of the cribriform plate can be outlined to ensure coverage.

What CSI techniques can be employed if the entire spine cannot be included in 1 field?

The practitioner can **increase the SSD or rotate the collimator** using a single field, but if the length is >36–38 cm, then **2 spinal fields** are needed, with the inf field's isocenter placed at the junction (using half-beam block to minimize the cold spot). Match at L1-2, as this is the area where the depth of cord changes the most.

What is Collins law as it pertains to the max length of follow-up needed for pediatric tumors?

Defines period of risk for recurrence (**age at Dx + 9 mo** [gestational period])

■ Toxicity

What are some long-term toxicities of CSI + boost?

↓Growth (↓GH), ↓IQ, ototoxicity, hypopituitarism, and 2nd malignancy

What factors predict for greater decline in IQ after CSI?

Factors for decline in IQ after CSI:
  Age <7 yrs (most important)
  Higher dose (36 Gy vs. 23.4 Gy)
  Higher IQ at baseline
  Female gender

(*Ris MD et al., JCO 2001*)

For how long can the pt's IQ decline after CSI?

>5 yrs. *Hoppe-Hirsch et al.* reviewed 120 MB pts treated with CSI to 36 Gy. At 5 yrs, 58% had an IQ >80. At 10 yrs, only 1% had an IQ >80. (*Childs Nerv Syst 1990*)

What are some important factors influencing IQ scores/neurotoxicity after RT?

Age at Tx with RT (most important), volume and dose of RT, and gender (female > male)

What evidence supports the omission of CSI for anaplastic ependymomas after resection if there is no evidence of neuroaxial involvement?

Multiple retrospective reviews reveal the following: LR is the primary pattern of failure (>90%) regardless of field size; spinal seeding is uncommon without LR; and prophylaxis with CSI or WBRT does not affect survival when compared to local RT.

What is the role of chemo in ependymoma? What is the response rate?

Traditionally chemo is utilized for <3 yo to delay RT and for salvage (CDDP, VP-16, temozolomide, nitrosoureas). The response rate typically is 5%–15%. However, a new prospective study out of St. Jude's Children's Hospital (*Merchant TE et al., Lancet Oncol 2009*) that included many pts <3 yo (78%) treated with maximal safe resection and postoperative conformal RT to 59.4 Gy with 10-mm margin around postop bed, suggests that RT can be given safely and effectively for pts <3 yo. The 7-yr OS was 81%, EFS was 69%, and LC rate was 87.3% (cumulative LF rate is 16.3%). Therefore, young age should not preclude pts to receive high-dose RT after surgery, except for infants <1 yo.

What is the single most important favorable prognostic factor in ependymoma?

Completeness of surgical resection (correlates closely with LC for ependymomas)

What is the difference in 5-yr OS between GTR and STR for ependymomas?

75% vs. 35% (similar for low-grade vs. high-grade ependymomas)

What ependymoma locations are most amenable to GTR? Least?

Spinal (GTR ~100%) > supratentorial (80%) > infratentorial

What is given to children <3 yo after STR for ependymoma?

Chemo is typically used as a bridge Tx. RT is deferred until >3 yo.

What types of chemo are typically used for ependymoma?

Cisplatin, cyclophosphamide, and etoposide are typical chemo agents for ependymoma.

What is the dose and volume of RT to be used if no CSI is given for ependymomas?

Preop GTV + 1–2-cm margin to **54–59.4 Gy** (54 Gy for children <18 mos and >18 mos with GTR)

How is ependymoblastoma treated? What is the total dose to spine lesions vs. cranial lesions?

Treat like medulloblastoma/PNET: **CSI 36 Gy + vincristine** +/− carboplatin, boost to cavity/gross Dz. 45–50.4 Gy if spine and 54–59.4 Gy if cranial → vincristine/Cytoxan/prednisolone 6 wks after RT.

How is infratentorial ependymoma managed?

Infratentorial ependymoma management: **max resection.** At the Johns Hopkins Hospital, regardless of histologic grade, **all get postop RT** to involved fields and a dose of **59.4 Gy.**

How is supratentorial ependymoma managed?

If not anaplastic (i.e., if grades 1–2), observation after max GTR is acceptable.

How is recurrent ependymoma managed?

If no prior RT: surgery → RT
If prior RT: surgery → stereotactic RT or chemo

Which phase II study showed min neurocognitive decrement with conformal/small RT fields?

St. Jude study ACNS0121 (*Merchant TE et al., JCO 2004*): 88 pts, 33 pts with grade 3. 3-yr PFS was 74%. IQ testing was stable after 2 yrs.

What is a major reason infratentorial lesions should get adj RT, regardless of histologic grade?

Difficulty with complete resection due to proximity to 4th ventricle, CNS vessels → higher LR if infratentorial without RT

What study suggested a benefit to hyperfractionation for ependymomas?

POG 9132; better EFS with 1.2 Gy bid to 69.6 Gy

Which recent studies showed a benefit with adj RT after GTR for posterior fossa ependymomas?

Rogers L et al., J Neurosurg 2005: 10-yr OS GTR (67%), GTR/RT (83%)

Merchant TE et al., Lancet Oncol 2009: update from the phase II study **ACNS0121.** All rcv conformal RT to 59.4 Gy for NTR/all sites and grade, and for R0 infratentorial lesions of all histologies. Well-differentiated lesions after GTR were observed. Chemo for STR, then evaluated for surgery and RT. 10-yr OS was 75%, LC was 87%, and EFS was 69%. Median age 2.9 yrs, with 78% of the patients <3 yo.

When is RT used in spinal ependymomas?

When resection is incomplete or anaplastic histology (Kaiser data: *Volpp PB et al., IJROBP 2007*)

What fields/doses are used for spinal ependymomas?

Include 2 vertebral bodies/sacral nerve roots above and below tumor to 45–50.4 Gy (boost if below cord to 54–59.4 Gy)

What molecular profile is associated with poor outcomes in ependymoma?

Overexpression of erbB-2/erbB-4 is associated with poor outcomes in ependymoma.

Do young children or young adults with ependymoma have a worse prognosis?

Children. Age <4 yrs is a poor prognostic factor.

What is the workup for a suspected germ cell tumor?

Suspected germ cell tumor workup: H&P (especially CNs, fundoscopy), MRI brain/spine, basic labs, serum AFP/β-HCG, CSF AFP/β-HCG, and CSF cytology

What AFP levels exclude the Dx of a germinoma?

If an **AFP is >10 ng/mL,** it is not a pure germinoma.

What β-HCG levels exclude the Dx of germinoma?

None are truly exclusive, but if the β-HCG is >50 ng/mL, then it probably is not a germinoma.

What stain definitively confirms the Dx of a germinoma?

Placental alkaline phosphatase staining confirms the Dx of germinoma.

What are the typical MRI findings of pure germinoma? Are there any distinctions on imaging from NGGCTs?

Homogeneous or heterogenous pattern, hypointense T1, hyperintense T2, +Ca, cysts. These are indistinguishable from NGGCTs on imaging.

Historically, how was RT used in the Dx of intracranial germinomas?

Tumors were irradiated with a diagnostic dose of 10–30 Gy. If there was a response, then the Dx was germinoma and RT was continued to a definitive dose of 40–56 Gy. *This is no longer done.*

What staging system is used for intracranial germ cell tumors?

The **medulloblastoma staging** (modified Chang) system is used for staging of intracranial germ cell tumors.

▪ Treatment/Prognosis

What is the most important prognostic factor in germ cell tumors?

Histology is the most important prognostic factor in germ cell tumors.

What is the prognosis of pure germinomas vs. NGGCTs?

The prognosis is **better for germinomas** (5-yr PFS 90% vs. 40%–70%, respectively).

Describe 2 Tx paradigms for localized germinomas.

Tx paradigms for localized germinoma:
  1. Definitive RT
  or
  2. Neoadj chemo → RT (experimental protocol)

Describe the definitive RT technique for localized germinoma.

Whole ventricular radiation therapy (WVRT) to 24 Gy, boost to primary tumor to 45 Gy

For which pineal tumor type is surgery generally *not* done?

Surgery is generally not done for **germinomas.**

What is the RT technique for disseminated germinoma/CSF spread?

CSI to 24 Gy, gross Dz **boost to 45 Gy**

Can chemo replace RT in the Tx of pure germinomas?

No. In a large CNS GCT study (*Balmaceda C et al., JCO 1996*), 45 germinomas were treated with carboplatin/etoposide/bleomycin. 84% had CR, but 48% recurred in 13 mos and 10% of pts died due to Tx toxicity. >90% were salvaged by RT

(ifosfamide/carboplatin/etoposide [ICE] × 3 → involved-field radiation therapy [IFRT] of 24 Gy).

What hypothesis is being tested in the current germinoma study ACNS0232?

ACNS0232 is attempting to determine **if neoadj chemo can help reduce RT doses.**

Describe the RT technique with neoadj chemo for localized germinoma.

Reduced RT doses: WVRT to **19.8 Gy;** boost to **30 Gy**

In germinoma protocols, to what does "occult multifocal germinoma" refer?

Pineal-region tumor and DI

For pts with occult multifocal germinoma, what is the boost volume?

Enhancing tumor (pineal region), infundibular region and the 3rd ventricle

In ACNS0232, what chemo agents are being tested?

Carboplatin, cisplatin, and etoposide are being tested in **ACNS0232.**

With pre-RT chemo, what are the RT doses in the experimental arm of ACNS0232?

In **ACNS0232,** the RT doses depend on the chemo response. **Experimental arm:** induction chemo, cisplatin/etoposide × 2 cycles.
If CR, RT to 30 Gy with IFRT alone.
If <CR, 2 additional cycles of chemo → if CR, give WVRT 21 Gy → boost to 30 Gy.
If <CR after 2 additional cycles, give standard Tx (M0 or M1).

What studies showed that even with CR to chemo, IFRT (without WVRT) may not be sufficient?

SIOP CNS GCT96 (*Calaminus G et al., SIOP Education Book, pp. 109–116*): M0 pts treated with CSI 24 Gy + 16 Gy boost vs. 2 × ICE → IFRT 40 Gy. CRT 5-yr EFS was 85% vs. 91% with RT alone; 5-yr OS was 92% vs. 94%. All CRT failures were within the ventricular system.

What other evidence demonstrates that involved-field RT may not be sufficient for germinomas?

Rogers SJ et al., Lancet Oncol 2005: literature review of 788 pts. There was a greater failure rate in focal RT vs. WBRT or WVRT + boost or CSI + boost (23% vs. 4%–8%). The pattern of relapse was mostly isolated spinal (11%), but there was no difference in WVRT vs. CSI in spinal relapse (3% vs. 1%). Similar findings were found in a **Seoul study** (*Eom KY et al., IJROBP 2008*).

What early studies established the feasibility of RT dose reduction?

German MAKEI 83/86/89 studies (from 50 Gy to 34 Gy)

Describe 2 Tx paradigms for NGGCT.

NGGCT Tx paradigms:
1. **Induction** platinum-based **chemo** 4–6 cycles → **CSI RT 30–36 Gy** (lower dose for CR) → **boost primary to 50.4–54 Gy;** surgery for residual or recurrent Dz
2. Max surgical resection → adj platinum-based chemo; restage; if no neuroaxial involvement, consolidate with IFRT; if +neuroaxial Dz, CSI to 30–36 Gy, boost to 50.4 Gy

When is chemo indicated in the Tx of NGGCTs?

Chemo is **always** indicated for NGGCTs (influences survival).

What is the Tx paradigm for pineoblastoma?

Pineoblastoma Tx paradigm: treat as medulloblastoma (CSI 23–36 Gy + local boost to 54 Gy)

What is the Tx paradigm for pineocytoma?

Pineocytoma Tx paradigm: treat like a low-grade glioma (GTR → observation; STR → consideration of adj RT or observation with Tx at the time of progression [50–54 Gy])

Which study showed that bifocal germinoma can be treated as localized Dz?

Canadian data (*Lafay-Cousin L et al., IJROBP 2006*): chemo and then limited-field RT (WVRT + boost) resulted in a CR.

■ Toxicity

Which recent study showed better QOL with CRT (dose/field reduction) than with RT alone?

Seoul study (*Eom KY et al., IJROBP 2008*), need for hormonal therapy: RT alone 69% vs. CRT 38% (however, all RT alone pts rcv CSI)

What is the long-term rate of RT-induced 2nd CNS malignancies? What type is most common?

5%–10%; usually **glioblastoma multiforme**

What chemo agent should be avoided with brain RT? Why?

6-mercaptopurine. It is associated with **high rates of secondary high-grade gliomas.**

10
Craniopharyngioma
Boris Hristov and Ori Shokek

Background

What is the origin of craniopharyngioma?

Epithelial tumor arising from an incompletely involuted hypophyseal-pharyngeal duct (**Rathke pouch**) from an anatomic region called the **tuber cinerium**

In what region of the brain does it usually arise?

Suprasellar region (most common), sella proper (less common)

Are craniopharyngiomas malignant?

No. They are histologically benign but are problematic due to local progression around critical structures.

Approximately how many cases of craniopharyngioma occur annually in the U.S.?

~300–350 cases/yr of craniopharyngioma in the U.S.

At what ages does craniopharyngioma occur?

Median age 5–10 yrs; higher risk age <20 yrs and >40 yrs (bimodal); one third of cases occur in pts age 0–14 yrs.

What are the 2 histologic subtypes of craniopharyngioma?

Adamantinomatous and squamous

Which subtype is characterized by a solid and cystic pattern?

Adamantinomatous craniopharyngioma has a solid and cystic pattern.

Historically, how has the cyst fluid consistency been described?

"Machine oil" like (very proteinaceous fluid)

What structures do cysts usually abut superiorly?

Tumors/cysts usually abut the 3rd ventricle and the hypothalamus superiorly.

Name the most common presenting signs/Sx of craniopharyngioma.

HA, N/V (i.e., ↑ICP), visual change, diabetes insipidus

What is the most common hormone deficiency at presentation?	At presentation, **GH** is the most common hormone deficiency.
Which type of craniopharyngioma has a better prognosis: calcified or noncalcified?	**Noncalcified** craniopharyngioma has a better prognosis.
Do craniopharyngioma tumors respond rapidly or slowly to RT?	Craniopharyngioma tumors respond **very slowly** to RT.

■ Workup/Staging

What is the workup for a craniopharyngioma?	Craniopharyngioma workup: H&P, basic labs, pituitary panel, and MRI brain
What ancillary studies need to be done before Tx?	Endocrine, audiology, vision, and neuropsychiatric studies
What is the classic appearance of craniopharyngiomas on CT/MRI?	Craniopharyngiomas are **partially calcified and cystic** on CT/MRI.
Is histology absolutely necessary for the Dx of craniopharyngioma?	**No.** A Dx can be made based on radiographic appearance and cyst fluid analysis.
What is the staging of craniopharyngioma?	There is **no formal staging.**

■ Treatment/Prognosis

What is the Tx paradigm for craniopharyngioma?	Craniopharyngioma Tx paradigm: max safe resection, EBRT/intracystic chemo adjuvantly or at recurrence
What surgical approach is typically employed for craniopharyngioma resection?	**Lat pterional approach** (temporal craniotomy)
Is observation ever appropriate after incomplete resection for craniopharyngioma?	**Yes.** Observation is especially appropriate in young pts. Adj and salvage therapy may have similar LC in closely followed pts.
What are the RT doses used for craniopharyngioma?	**54 Gy** with EBRT, **12–14 Gy** with SRS

What volumes are typically irradiated for craniopharyngioma?

GTV is decompressed/postop volume = tumor + cyst wall (cysts decompressed before Tx); PTV is GTV + 1–1.5 cm; **no CTV.**

What % of attempted craniopharyngioma GTRs result in STR?

Depends on location, but overall, **20%–30%** (*Tomita T et al., Childs Nerv Syst 2005*)

Estimate the 10-yr LC with surgery alone vs. surgery + postop RT for craniopharyngioma.

Surgery (GTR + STR) alone ~**42%**; surgery + RT ~**84%** (*Stripp DC et al., IJROBP 2004*)

Estimate the 10-yr LC with adj RT vs. salvage RT.

Both ~83%–84% (*Stripp DC et al., IJROBP 2004*). RT can be deferred for children <5–7 yo after surgery.

In what 3 ways can craniopharyngioma cysts be managed?

Aspiration, radioactive isotope injection, and bleomycin injection

What isotopes have been used for intracystic RT? To what dose?

β-emitting isotopes (yttrium-90, P-32, Rh-186); **200–250 Gy** to the cyst wall

Why is P-32 conjugated to a sugar moiety, and why is it toxic to the brain tissue if it leaks outside the cyst?

It is conjugated to a large sugar molecule **so it stays within the cyst.** It is toxic because the **preservative in the P-32 suspension** (Na benzoate) **is neurotoxic.**

What is the energy and half-life of P-32, and to what depth is it effective?

0.7 MeV, 2 wks. The effective depth is **3–4 mm.**

What are the indications for intralesional cyst management (vs. cyst aspiration)?

Intralesional Tx is an option if the cyst is >50% of total tumor bulk *and* the number of cysts is ≤3.

What intracystic chemo has been used?

Bleomycin typically has been used for intralesional cyst management.

If a pt has worsening visual Sx while getting adj RT, is this likely due to an acute side effect from RT?

No. Acute Sx during RT are likely due to a rapidly enlarging cystic component; therefore, urgent surgical intervention for decompression is indicated (some even advocate serial MRIs during RT).

What is the typical response rate to intralesional brachytherapy?

80%, with stable or visual Sx improvement in 51%. MS is 9 yrs. (*Julow J et al., Acta Neurochir 1985*)

The # of lesions seen in hemangioblastomas correlates with what in terms of etiology?

Single lesion (sporadic, older pts) **vs. multiple lesions** (familial, younger pts)

What hematologic abnormality is present in pts with hemangio-blastomas? Why?

Polycytemia is present because of erythropoietin production by the tumor.

How do hemangio-blastomas cause morbidity if not treated?

Local compression and hemorrhage

What are common Sx of hemangioblastoma at presentation?

HA, hydrocephalus, and imbalance

▪ Workup/Staging

What steps are critical during the workup of a hemangioblastoma?

Thorough **neurologic exam and MRI** (craniospinal); **angiography** to aid in embolization before surgery

What is the typical radiographic appearance of a hemangioblastoma?

Eccentric/peripheral cystic mass (70%) in the posterior fossa

How do hemangio-blastomas appear on MRI?

On MRI, hemangioblastomas are **intensely enhancing.**

▪ Treatment/Prognosis

What are the 2 main Tx approaches for hemangioblastoma?

Surgery (max safe resection is curative) **and SRS**

What are the LC rates of surgery vs. SRS for hemangioblastomas?

Surgery: 50%–80%
SRS: 85%–90% at 2 yrs, 75% at 5 yrs

What is the SRS dose range used for the Tx of hemangioblastomas?

15–21 Gy to 50% IDL

What does the older dose-response data show for fractionated EBRT for the Tx of hemangioblastomas?

It showed **better results with higher doses** (*Smalley SR et al., IJROBP 1990*: better OS with dose >50 Gy; *Sung DI et al., Cancer 1982*: better survival with 40–55 Gy vs. 20–36 Gy).

What are traditionally employed EBRT doses for hemangioblastomas?

50–55 Gy in 1.8 or 2 Gy/fx

For cystic hemangioblastoma lesions, what component does *not* have to be removed during surgery?

If there is a –margin, there is no need to remove the **entire cyst.** In this case, only the mural nodule/tumor should be removed.

When has RT (either SRS or EBRT) been traditionally used in the management of hemangioblastomas?

After recurrence (i.e., after definitive surgery or after STR for recurrence)

For what type of hemangioblastoma lesions is fractionated EBRT a better choice than SRS?

Multiple tumors, larger lesions (>3 cm), and lesions in eloquent regions of the brain

Which hemangio-blastoma pts have a better prognosis after EBRT: VHL+ or VHL− pts?

VHL+ pts have a better prognosis after EBRT. (Princess Margaret Hospital data: *Koh ES et al., IJROBP 2007*)

What is the prognostic significance of a cyst component after SRS for hemangioblastoma?

LC is worse if the tumor is cystic. (Japan data: *Matsunaga S et al., Acta Neurochir 2007*)

What is the median time to recurrence after EBRT for hemangioblastoma?

Hemangioblastomas tend to recur **2–4 yrs** after EBRT.

What is the pattern of failure after EBRT for pts with hemangioblastoma?

Failure is **predominantly local.**

◾ Toxicity

What is the surgical mortality rate of pts treated for hemangioblastoma?

The surgical mortality rate is **10%–20%** in pts treated for hemangioblastoma.

12

Brainstem Glioma

Steven H. Lin and Ori Shokek

Background

What is the prevalence of brainstem gliomas (BSGs) in relation to pediatric CNS tumors overall?

BSGs comprise **10% of pediatric CNS tumors** (<2% of adult CNS tumors).

What is the peak age of presentation for BSGs? What is the gender predilection?

The peak age of BSG presentation is **5–9 yrs. Males** are more commonly affected than females.

What are the 2 classes of BSGs? Where are they most commonly located, and what is the prognosis?

The 2 classes of BSGs are **focal and diffuse.**
<u>Focal</u> (30%): in the **upper midbrain/lower medulla;** best prognosis
<u>Diffuse</u> (70%): in the **pons and upper medulla;** infiltrative and worst prognosis

What BSG histology most commonly involves the medulla? The midbrain?

Glioblastoma multiforme in the medulla; **grade 2 or 3 astrocytoma** in the midbrain

Why does adult BSG tend to have a better prognosis?

Lesions in adults tend to be **mostly low grade.**

What is the median OS of BSG in adults vs. children vs. the elderly?

<u>Adults</u>: 7.3 yrs
<u>Children</u>: 1 yr
<u>The elderly</u>: 11 mos
Overall, the Dz is fatal in >90% of pts.

Workup/Staging

What are some typical clinical findings with diffuse pontine glioma?

Typical findings with diffuse pontine glioma:
1. CN palsy (CNs VI–VII)
2. Ataxia
3. Long tract signs (hyperreflexia, etc.)

What is the typical workup for a child with a suspected BSG?

Suspected BSG workup for a child: H&P, labs, MRI, typically *no* Bx

When should Bx be done for BSG?	When mass lesions have an **unusual MRI appearance or** there is an **atypical clinical course** (either possible benign tumors or an infectious/inflammatory etiology)
How is BSG staged?	There is **no formal staging** of BSG.

■ Treatment/Prognosis

What is the typical Tx paradigm for BSG?	BSG Tx paradigm: steroids/shunts $\to$ RT alone $+/-$ chemo with temozolomide (TMZ)
What type of BSG is amenable to surgical resection $+/-$ adj RT?	**Dorsally exophytic BSGs** have a 10-yr OS with surgery $+/-$ RT in 75% of pts. These are usually juvenile pilocytic astrocytomas (JPAs) with a good prognosis.
What is the typical RT dose for BSGs?	The typical RT dose for BSGs is **54 Gy** in 1.8$-$2 Gy/fx.
What proportion of BSG pts will have stabilization or improvement of Sx after RT?	After RT, **two thirds** of pts will have stabilization or improvement of Sx.
Is there a role for hyperfractionation or dose escalation in BSG?	**No.** Both did not improve survival in multiple Pediatric Oncology Group/Children's Cancer Group (POG/CCG) trials (only better radiographic response at higher doses, however, with greater radionecrosis and long-term steroid dependence).
Is there any benefit with chemo in BSG?	**No.** There is very minimal response with single, combination, or high-dose/stem cell rescue.
Is there a role for TMZ after RT? How about concurrently with RT?	No (*Broniscer A et al., Cancer 2005*). MS is 12 mos. **Concurrent TMZ is being tested** in a COG phase II trial.
Is there a role for brachytherapy or Gamma Knife boost after RT in BSG?	**No.** There is no role for brachytherapy or Gamma Knife boost after RT.
How are tectal plate tumors managed? What is their histology?	Tectal plate tumors are managed with **observation and a ventriculoperitoneal shunt** for obstruction. They are typically **JPAs** (indolent).
What are the major prognostic factors dictating outcome in pts with BSGs?	Diffuse vs. focal, adult vs. child, and histology

What is the survival of pts with diffuse vs. focal BSG lesions?

<u>Diffuse</u>: 12 mos (median)
<u>Focal</u>: 10-yr OS ~50%−70%

What usually causes death in pts with BSGs?

Local expansion usually causes death in pts with BSGs.

▪ Toxicity

What is the RT dose tolerance of the brain stem?

The dose tolerance of the brain stem is **54 Gy** (if fractionated EBRT) and **12 Gy** (if SRS).

13

General Central Nervous System

Steven H. Lin and Anita Mahajan

Background

What is the estimated annual incidence of primary CNS tumors in the U.S.?	**~50,000–55,000 cases/yr** of CNS tumors (per the National Program of Cancer Registries database)
What is the most common intracranial tumor?	**Brain mets** (20%–40% of all cancer pts develop brain mets)
What is the most common type of primary CNS tumor?	**Glioma (~40%)** > **meningioma** (15%–20%)
What % of adult astrocytomas are low grade vs. high grade?	25% low grade vs. 75% high grade
What is the most common histologic type of malignant CNS tumor in children? In adults?	<u>Children</u>: juvenile pilocytic astrocytoma (JPA) (20% <14 yo vs. 12% >14 yo) <u>Adults</u>: glioblastoma
What is the strongest risk factor for developing CNS tumors?	**Ionizing RT** in children (no threshold—glioma, meningioma, nerve sheath)

What CNS tumors are linked to the following?
1. NF-1
2. NF-2
3. Tuberous sclerosis

4. Von Hippel-Lindau
5. Li-Fraumeni
6. Cowden

1. Optic glioma, JPA
2. Bilat acoustic neuroma, spinal ependymoma
3. Subependymal giant cell astrocytoma, retinal hamartoma
4. Hemangioblastoma

5. Glioma
6. Meningioma

7. Gorlin	7. Medulloblastoma
8. Turcot	8. Medulloblastoma, glioblastoma
9. Retinoblastoma (RB)	9. Pineoblastoma
10. Ataxia telangiectasia	10. CNS lymphoma
11. MEN 1	11. Pituitary adenoma

What are the 4 factors used for grading in the WHO brain tumor grading system?

Nuclear **A**typia
Cellularity and **M**itosis
Endothelial proliferation
Necrosis

(Mnemonic: **AMEN**)

What CNS tumors tend to have CSF spread?

Medulloblastomas and other blastomas (except astroblastoma/glioblastoma multiforme [GBM]), CNS lymphoma, choroid plexus carcinomas, germ cell tumors, and mets

What CNS tumors have Flexner-Wintersteiner rosettes?

Pineoblastoma and RB (any PNET)

What CNS tumors have psamomma bodies?

Meningioma and pituitary tumors (uncommon)

What CNS tumor type exhibits Verocay bodies? Schiller-Duval bodies?

Schwannomas exhibit Verocay bodies, and **yolk sac tumors** exhibit Schiller-Duval bodies.

What receptors are commonly overexpressed in gliomas?

EGFR (30%–50% in GBM tumors) **and PDGFR** (non-GBM tumors)

Neural stem cells express which marker? Why are they important?

CD133. Neural stem cells are thought to be **precursors for astrocytomas.**

What gene on chromosome 17 is frequently lost in both low-grade and high-grade gliomas?

The **p53** gene is frequently lost in low- and high-grade gliomas.

What is the genetic mutation in NF-1, and for which sites does it predispose to gliomas?

In NF-1, the genetic mutation is **17q11.2/ neurofibromin.** It predisposes to **optic/intracranial gliomas.**

■ Workup/Staging

What brain region is associated with expressive aphasia?	The **Broca motor area** (dominant/left frontal lobe) is associated with expressive aphasia.
What brain region is associated with receptive aphasia?	The dominant/left temporal lobe at the post end of the lateral sulcus **(Wernicke area)** is associated with receptive aphasia.
Which CN exits on the dorsal side of the brain (midbrain)?	**CN IV** exits on the dorsal side of the brain.
What structure produces CSF?	CSF is produced in the **choroid plexus.**
What structures are in the cavernous sinus?	CNs III, IV, VI, V1, and V2; internal carotid artery
What common defect does tumor involving the cavernous sinus produce?	**CN VI palsy** (no abduction of the lateral rectus)
What components traverse the superior orbital fissure?	CNs III, IV, VI, and V1
What nerve passes through the foramen rotundum?	**V2** passes through the foramen rotundum.
What nerve passes through the foramen ovale?	**V3** passes through the foramen ovale.
What structures pass through the foramen spinosum?	The **middle meningeal artery and vein,** as well as the **nervus spinosus** (branch of CN V3), pass through the foramen spinosum.
Through what structure do CNs VII–VIII traverse?	CNs VII–VIII trasverse through the **internal auditory meatus.**
Through which foramen does CN VII traverse the skull base?	CN VII emerges through the **stylomastoid foramen.**
What passes through the jugular foramen?	**CNs IX–XI** pass through the jugular foramen.
How many spinal nerves are there in the spinal cord?	There are **31 spinal nerves** in the spinal cord (8 cervical, 12 thoracic, 5 lumbar, 5 sacral, and 1 coccygeal).

Where does the cord end? Where does the thecal sac end?	The cord ends at **L3-4 in children** and **L1-2 in adults.** The thecal sac ends at **S2-3 in both children and adults.**
What tumors present with a dural tail sign?	**Meningioma** (60%), also chloroma, lymphoma, and sarcoidosis

▉ Toxicity

Name some acute RT complications in pts receiving RT for CNS tumors.	Alopecia, dermatitis, fatigue, transient worsening of neurologic Sx, n/v, otitis externa, seizures, and edema
What is the timing and mechanism of somnolence syndrome?	**6–12 wks post-RT,** due to transient **demyelination** of axons
What are some late complications of RT to the CNS? What is the timing for these?	Radionecrosis, leukoencephalopathy, retinopathy, cataracts, endocrine deficits, memory loss, learning deficits, and hearing loss; **3 mos to 3 yrs**

14

Low-Grade Glioma

John P. Christodouleas and Shiao Y. Woo

▉ Background

Low-grade gliomas (LGGs) account for what % of all primary brain tumors?	~**15%** of all primary brain tumors are LGGs.
Is there a racial predilection for LGG?	**Yes. Whites** are more commonly affected than blacks (2:1).
What are the 2 classes of LGGs?	Noninfiltrative (WHO I) and infiltrative (WHO II)

What are the histologic subtypes of LGGs?

Histologic subtypes of LGG:
  Grade I: juvenile pilocytic astrocytoma (JPA), sub-ependymal giant cell tumor
  Grade II: diffuse (fibrillary, protoplasmic, gemisto-cytic), pilomyxoid astrocytoma (PMA), pleo-morphic xanthoastrocytoma, oligodendroglioma, oligoastrocytoma

What 4 pathologic features determine glioma grading?

Necrosis
Atypia
Mitotic figures
Endothelial proliferation

(Mnemonic: **NAME** or AMEN)

Which subtype of grade II glioma has the worst prognosis?

The **gemistocytic subtype** tends to de-differentiate and has the worst prognosis. Some prefer to treat it like a high-grade glioma.

Where does JPA most commonly present?

JPA most commonly presents in the **posterior fossa** (80% cerebellar, 20% supratentorial).

What pathologic feature is characteristic of JPA?

Rosenthal fibers are characteristic of JPA.

Where do grade II LGGs most commonly present?

Grade II LGGs most commonly present in the **supratentorium.**

What is the median age of Dx for JPA vs. other LGG?

The median age for **JPA is 10–20 yrs** and for grade II **LGG is 30–40 yrs.**

What genetic change is an important prognostic factor in LGG?

In LGG, **p53 mutation** is an important prognostic factor (poorer survival and time to malignant transfor-mation).

What is the natural Hx of PMA?

PMA tends to occur in **infants** (10−18 mos), mostly in **chiasmatic-hypothalamic regions.** It is an atypical JPA with a higher rate of CSF dissemination and recurrence.

What genetic change is prognostic in oligodendroglioma?

LOH 1p + 19q (50%−70%) is prognostic in oligo-dendroglioma.

What is the characteristic pathologic appearance of oligodendroglioma?

"Fried egg" appearance (round cells with nuclear halo) is characteristic of oligodendroglioma.

Where do most oligodendrogliomas occur in the brain?

Most oligodendrogliomas occur in the **hemispheres** (80%).

Anaplastic transformation from LGG to HGG occurs in what % of pts?

~70%–80% of pts with LGG will undergo anaplastic transformation (based on **EORTC 22845**).

What is the genetic mutation in NF-1, and with what type of gliomas is it associated?

NF-1 is a result of a mutation on the long arm of **chromosome 17** and is associated with **optic/intracranial gliomas.**

What is the genetic mutation in tuberous sclerosis, and with what glioma is it associated?

Tuberous sclerosis is a result of a mutation on **chromosome 9** and is associated with **subependymal giant cell astrocytoma.**

What syndrome is associated with gliomas and GI polyposis?

Turcot syndrome is associated with gliomas and polyposis.

Can you have mitoses in LGGs?

Yes. If the tumor is small, even a single mitosis upgrades it to at least WHO III (anaplastic). However, if the tumor is large, a single mitosis may not upgrade it to a high-grade histology.

With what Sx do LGGs most commonly present?

Seizures (60%−70%, better prognosis) > HA, focal neurologic Sx

■ Workup/Staging

What is the workup for suspected glioma?

Suspected glioma workup: H&P, basic labs, and MRI brain

How should tissue be acquired for Dx?

Tissue should be acquired by **max safe resection** (per the NCCN), otherwise by stereotactic Bx.

What is the typical MRI characteristic seen in LGG?

On MRI, LGGs appear hypodense on T1, are **nonenhancing with gadolinium,** and show +T2 prolongation.

What is the typical MRI appearance of JPA?

Well-circumscribed, cystic mass, intensely enhancing solid mural nodule

What % of nonenhancing lesions are grade III gliomas?

~**30%** are grade III gliomas (65% are LGG).

Is there a need for seizure prophylaxis in pts with LGG?

Yes. Per the American Academy of Neurology, prophylactic anticonvulsants are necessary in pts with a Hx of seizures.

What is the min oligodendroglioma component needed histologically to classify a tumor as a mixed oligoastrocytoma?

According to the most recent WHO classification, there is **no consensus on a standard cutoff** to classify mixed tumors (prior cutoff was 25%).

What feature has been associated with oligodendrogliomas on imaging?	**Calcifications** are a prominent feature on imaging of oligodendrogliomas.
What is suggestive of a malignant tumor on MR spectroscopy?	**Increased choline** (cell membrane marker), **low creatine** (energy metabolite), and **low N-acetyl-aspartate** (a neuronal marker) are suggestive of malignancy on MR spectroscopy.
What is the staging of LGG?	There is **no formal staging** for LGG.

▪ Treatment/Prognosis

What are the 5 negative prognostic factors for LGG as determined by EORTC 22844 and 22845?	Negative prognostic factors per the EORTC index: 1. Age >40 yrs 2. Astrocytoma histology 3. Tumors >6 cm 4. Tumors crossing midline 5. Preop neurologic deficits (*Pignatti F et al., JCO 2002*)
What is the general Tx paradigm used for LGGs?	LGG Tx paradigm: max safe resection → observation for GTR or STR, reserving RT for recurrence.
What adj and salvage chemo regimens are typically used in LGG?	Chemos used in LGG: 1. Temozolomide (TMZ) 2. BCNU/CCNU 3. PCV (procarbazine/CCNU/vincristine)
What RT dose is typically used for LGG?	LGG is commonly treated to **50.4–54 Gy.**
A complete resection can be achieved in what proportion of pts with LGGs?	**Approximately one third** of pts with LGGs have a GTR.
Within what time frame should postop MRI be obtained for pts with LGGs? Why is it needed?	**Postop MRI should be done within 48–72 hrs** of surgery to assess for residual Dz/extent of resection.
In LGG, how are the RT Tx volumes defined, and what margins are typically used?	Initial PTV: preop T2 volume + 0.5–1 cm Boost PTV: postop T1 + 0.5–1 cm Alternatively, postop T2 (or FLAIR) + 2 cm to 54 Gy with 3D-CRT can be used (per **RTOG 9802**).
In what 2 clinical circumstances can adj RT be considered for LGGs?	1. For pts s/p STR/Bx only and with Sx 2. For pts with 3 of 5 high-risk features per the EORTC index (above)

What prospective data support initial observation over adj RT in LGG?

EORTC 22845 randomized 290 LGG pts to surgery alone vs. surgery + adj RT. NTR in 42%, debulking in 20%, and Bx only in 38%. PFS favored adj RT (5-yr PFS 35% vs. 55%, median PFS 3.4 yrs vs. 5.3 yrs), but there was no significant difference in OS (7.2−7.4 yrs). (*Van den Bent MJ et al., Lancet 2005*)

What % of LGG pts undergoing initial observation in EORTC 22845 eventually required salvage RT?

In **EORTC 22845, 65% of pts** in the observation arm rcv subsequent salvage RT.

What proportion of pts do not need salvage RT when observed after surgical resection for LGG?

Per EORTC 22845, approx ⅓ of patients will not require salvage RT.

In EORTC 22845, how did the OS after 1st recurrence compare in the adj vs. observation arms?

Survival after 1st recurrence was better in initially observed pts, most of whom rcv salvage RT. OS after 1st recurrence was **3.4 yrs vs. 1 yr** (SS).

Which study suggested that doses >53 Gy improved outcomes in LGG?

Shaw et al. retrospectively reviewed the outcomes of 126 LGG pts treated +/− varying doses of RT. Pts receiving >53 Gy had an 18% OS advantage at 10 yrs vs. pts receiving <53 Gy (*J Neurosurg 1989*). More recent prospective studies (**EORTC 22844** and the NCCTG LGG study) do not support a benefit of doses above 45−50.4 Gy.

Is there prospective evidence to support dose escalation with adj RT for LGG?

No. Dose escalation in LGG has been evaluated in 2 RCTs, neither of which showed a benefit:
1. **EORTC 22844** randomized 343 pts to adj RT 45 Gy vs. 59.4 Gy. **There was no difference in 5-yr OS (58%–59%) or PFS (47%–50%).** (*Karim AB et al., IJROBP 1996*)
2. INT/NCCTG randomized 203 pts to adj RT 50.4 Gy vs. 64.8 Gy. **There was no difference in 5-yr OS (65%–72%). 92% of failures were in-field.** (*Shaw EG et al., JCO 2002*)

What evidence is there to support observation after GTR or STR for pilocytic astrocytoma in adults?

Brown et al. prospectively followed 20 adult pilocytic astrocytoma pts s/p GTR, STR (6 pts), or Bx (3 pts). **5-yr PFS was 95%.** (*IJROBP 2004*)

Is there a benefit of chemo with RT for LGGs with high-risk features?

This is **controversial. RTOG 9802** stratified pts into low risk (age <40 yrs s/p GTR) and high risk (age >40 yrs or STR/Bx only). Low-risk pts were observed. **High-risk pts were randomized to adj RT alone (54 Gy) vs. RT + PCV × 6.** Outcomes were better in the chemo arm but did not reach SS (5-yr OS: 63% vs. 72%; PFS: 46% vs. 63%). Pts who lived >2 yrs had significantly improved PFS and OS (↓ risk of death by 48%) with chemo, suggesting a possible delayed benefit. (*Shaw EG et al., ASCO abstract 2006*)

In RTOG 9802, what were the 5-yr OS and PFS for low-risk pts observed after GTR?

In **RTOG 9802**, low-risk pts (<40 yo s/p GTR) were observed and had **5-yr OS of 94% and PFS of 50%.** (*Shaw EG et al., ASCO abstract 2006*)

Is there a role for TMZ in the initial Tx of LGG?

Results of 2 trials are **not yet available:**

1. **EORTC 22033** is randomizing high-risk LGG pts (3 of 5 EORTC features) to adj RT vs. adj TMZ. Results have not yet been reported.
2. **RTOG 0424** is a phase II study that enrolled high-risk LGG pts (3 of 5 EORTC features) and treated with adj 54 Gy RT + TMZ. This study is closed to accrual (results pending).

For JPA, what is the estimated 10-yr RFS in pts treated with GTR alone?

10-yr RFS is ~**95%** in JPA pts treated with GTR alone. (*Watson GA et al., Semin Radiat Oncol 2001*)

In pts with oligodendroglioma/mixed oligoden-droglioma, what is the median OS for those +/− LOH for 1p19q?

With LOH 1p19q: median OS ~13 yrs
Without LOH 1p19p: median OS ~9 yrs

(*Jenkins RB et al., Cancer Res 2006*)

■ Toxicity

How does RT affect QOL in the Tx of LGG?

QOL in LGG is impacted by **surgery, RT, chemo, and seizure meds.** Based on the **EORTC 22844** dose escalation study, higher-dose RT was significantly associated with fatigue/malaise and insomnia and ↓ emotional functioning. (*Kiebert GM et al., Eur J Cancer 1998*)

Does RT predispose LGG lesions to malignant transformation?

No. RT is not associated with an ↑ rate of malignant transformation. In **EORTC 22845,** there was a 70% transformation rate in both the adj and observation arms.

What is the commonly used RT dose constraint for the chiasm with fractionated RT vs. SRS?	The chiasm is commonly constrained to **50–54 Gy** in 1.8−2 Gy/fx and **8 Gy** in a single fx.
What is the commonly used RT dose constraint for the inner ear?	The inner ear is commonly constrained to a **mean dose of 30–35 Gy** in 1.8−2 Gy/fx.
What is the commonly used RT dose contraint for the brain stem with SRS?	The brain stem is commonly constrained to **12 Gy** in a single fx.
What is the cause of somnolence syndrome after brain RT?	Somnolence syndrome is thought to be caused by **demyelination.**

15
High-Grade Glioma
Steven H. Lin and Shiao Y. Woo

▌ Background

What % of primary CNS tumors are malignant?	~**40%** of primary brain tumors are considered malignant.
In adults, what is the most common malignant CNS neoplasm?	~**85%** of CNS neoplasms in adults are **glioblastoma multiforme** (GBM), which constitutes 20% of all primary tumors.
What are the WHO classifications for high-grade CNS tumors?	WHO III: anaplastic astrocytoma (AA)/ oligodendroglioma/oligoastrocytoma WHO IV: GBM
What are some common genetic changes seen in malignant brain tumors?	↑ EGFR (50%) and PTEN mutation (30%–40%)
What are the initial genetic changes associated with primary vs. secondary GBM?	Primary: ↑ EGFR/MDM2 amplification/LOH10/ p16 loss Secondary: p53 mutation → low-grade glioma (LGG) → LOH 19q/p16 loss → AA → LOH 10, DCC → 2nd GBM

What % of GBMs are multicentric?	**<5%** of GBMs are multicentric.
What are the 4 pathologic characteristics that define GBM?	Pseudopalisading necrosis, vascular proliferation, ↑ mitotic rate, and pleomorphic nuclei

■ Workup/Staging

What is the Cushing triad, and what does it represent in brain tumors?	HTN, bradycardia, respiratory irregularity. It represents ↑ ICP.
With what Sx do high-grade gliomas (HGGs) most commonly present?	**HA** (especially in the am, 50%), seizures (20%), focal neurologic dysfunction, and mental status change
What are the common imaging characteristics of HGGs on MRI?	Hypodense on T1, **gadolinium enhancing,** T2 enhancing, and +T2 FLAIR (edema)

■ Treatment/Prognosis

What is the MS for LGG vs. HGG?	<u>Low grade</u>: pure oligodendroglioma: 10 yrs; oligoastrocytoma: 7 yrs; anaplastic oligodendroglioma (AO): 5 yrs <u>High grade</u>: AA: 3 yrs; GBM: 14 mos
What are the most important factors used for the RTOG recursive partitioning analysis (RPA) stratification?	Age 50 yrs, histology (AA or GBM), Karnofsky performance status (KPS) of 70, MS changes, and Sx greater or less than 3 mos (*Curran WJ et al., J Natl Cancer Inst 1993*)
What constitutes RPA class III pts?	Age <50 yrs, AA with poor MS, or GBM with good KPS
What defines RPA class VI pts?	Any histology with KPS <70 and altered MS
What is the MS of a pt with RPA class I–II, III–IV vs. V–VI?	MS by RPA class: **Class I–II:** 40–60 mos (3–5 yrs) **Class III–IV:** 11–18 mos (1–1.5 yrs) **Class V–VI:** 5–9 mos
Under what RPA classes can GBM fall?	GBMs fall under **classes III–VI:** **Class III:** <50 yo, KPS 90–100 **Class IV:** <50 yo, KPS <90 or >50 yo, good KPS **Class V:** >50 yo, KPS <70 but no change in MS **Class VI:** KPS <70 and MS change
On what is the current modified RPA based?	**Outcomes with temozolomide** (TMZ) (*Mirimanoff RO, JCO 2006*)

Is there a benefit to radiosurgery boost for HGGs?

No. RTOG 9305 showed no benefit or higher toxicity.

Before the TMZ data, was there any benefit to CRT for HGGs?

Yes. This was shown by evidence from 2 large meta-analyses.

The *MRC Glioma Meta-analysis Trialist Group* showed a small improved median PFS (7.5 mos vs. 6 mos) with chemo, reduced risk of death by 15%, and ↑ 1-yr OS by 6%. There was no RT dose response with less or more than 60 Gy. (*Lancet 2002*)

Fine meta-analysis also showed improved MS 12 mos vs. 9.4 mos. (*Cancer 1993*)

What is the evidence that supports the current gold standard in GBM Tx with TMZ?

EORTC/NCIC data (*Stupp R et al., NEJM 2005* and 5-yr update *Stupp R et al., Lancet Oncol 2009*): 5-yr OS 10% (+ TMZ) vs. 2% (− TMZ)

Which modified RPA class did TMZ + RT not benefit significantly, per *Mirimanoff RO et al., JCO 2006*?

Class V. MS per RPA: class III, 17 mos; class IV, 15 mos; and class V, 10 mos. The only significant benefit of TMZ + RT vs. RT alone was in classes III–IV.

What is the role of MGMT methylation in terms of response to Tx with HGGs?

Greater response to TMZ + RT in those with methylated MGMT (*Hegi ME et al., NEJM 2005; Mirimanoff RO, ASTRO 2007*): 4-yr OS unmethylated (RT alone vs. RT + TMZ): **0% vs. 11%** and methylated **5% vs. 22%**, all SS

What are the options for recurrent GBM?

TMZ alone, re-irradiation to ~36 Gy (*Combs SE et al., BMC Cancer 2007*) +/− TMZ, radiosurgery, brachytherapy (Gliasite), Gliadel, or clinical trial

What is the dose used for Gliasite in GBM? What is the radioisotope used?

60 Gy to 5–10 mm at a dose rate of 50 cGy/hr (*Chan TA, IJROBP 2005*); **I-125**

What are the approved uses of Gliadel?

FDA approval: recurrent Dz with re-resection improved survival advantage 8 mos vs. 6 mos. (*Brem H et al., Lancet 1995*)

In newly diagnosed adj setting: MS was 13.9 mos vs. 11.6 mos. (*Westphal M, Neurooncol 2003*)

What are the general guidelines for RT target volume delineation in HGGs?

Initial volume (46 Gy): GTV1 = T1 + T2/FLAIR, CTV1 = GTV1 + 1.25 cm

Boost volume (14 Gy): GTV2 = T1/tumor bed, CTV2 = GTV2 + 0.75 cm. PTV adds 0.5 cm to CTVs. Postop imaging (with MRI fusion) should be used for target delineation.

Which recent study showed similar survival outcomes with adj RT vs. adj chemo with procarbazine/lomustine/vincristine (PCV) or TMZ in WHO III gliomas (AA)?

German **NOAH-04** study (*Wick W et al., JCO 2009*): same PFS/OS for all arms (RT alone or 2 chemo agents alone). <u>Good predictors</u>: extent of resection, oligo component (oligodendroglioma or oligoastrocytoma), IDH1 mutation, MGMT promoter hypermethylation. <u>Toxicity</u>: grade 3–4 hematologic toxicity was significantly higher for PCV than for TMZ

Which study investigated sequential PCV → RT vs. RT alone in oligodendroglial tumors?

RTOG 9402/INT-0149 (*Cairncross G et al., JCO 2006*): no OS benefit. There was improved PFS with chemo but at significant toxicity cost. 1p19q deletion conferred better outcomes.

Which recent study investigated sequential RT → BCNU vs. RT alone in AA? What did it find?

EORTC 26882 (*Hildebrand J et al., Eur J Cancer 2008*): no OS or PFS difference

What study tested the role of adj PCV after RT in oligodendroglial tumors?

EORTC 26951 (*Van den Bent MJ et al., JCO 2006*): same OS but prolonged PFS. 1p19q deleted pts did better. There was no long-term difference in QOL after PCV.

What ongoing phase III study is investigating the efficacy of combining RT with either TMZ or nitrosourea in anaplastic gliomas?

RTOG 9813 is investigating RT with TMZ or nitrosourea.

What study is investigating the use of upfront TMZ + RT in AO?

RTOG 0131. Pts are treated with neoadj TMZ for 6 mos → TMZ and concurrent RT. An interim report suggests that combination therapy with TMZ + RT is well tolerated and that the response correlates with 1p19q deletion status.

What is the Tx paradigm for gliosarcoma?

Gliosarcoma Tx paradigm: treat like GBM (surgery → RT + TMZ)

What ongoing study is testing dose-intensified TMZ after TMZ + RT?

RTOG 0525. This study is randomizing the pts after TMZ + RT (after a 1-mo break) to TMZ on days 1–21 vs. standard days 1–5 for up to 12 cycles (max) depending on the response.

▌Toxicity

What is the radiographic appearance of radionecrosis?

Central hypodensity, ring enhancement, edema, and low PET avidity (occurs >6 mos post-RT)

What data support prolonged chemo as a way of avoiding/delaying RT without compromising OS or visual function?	*Laithier et al.* prospectively evaluated prolonged chemo (alternating procarbazine/carboplatin, etoposide/cisplatin, and vincristine/cyclophosphamide q3wks). 2nd-line chemo was given at relapse before RT. The objective response rate was 42%, 5-yr OS was 89%, and 5-yr freedom from RT was 61%. (*JCO 2003*)
What is the ongoing Children's Cancer Group (CCG) protocol (A9952) comparing?	**CCG A9952** is comparing **chemo regimens** (carboplatin/vincristine vs. thioguanine/procarbazine/lomustine/vincristine)
When is RT indicated in OPG?	RT is typically used after **chemo options are exhausted,** when there are **progressive Sx,** or when there is **intracranial extension.**
OPGs are typically treated to what RT dose and fractionation?	OPGs are typically treated to **45–54 Gy in 1.8–2 Gy/fx.**
What is the preferred RT technique used to treat OPGs?	Proton therapy has dosimetric advantages, though there is limited clinical data. **FSR** has shown promising results (5-yr PFS 72%) (*Combs SE et al., IJROBP 2005*).
What is the estimated 5-yr OS in OPG?	The estimated 5-yr OS is **89%.** (*Laithier V et al., JCO 2003*)

■ Toxicity

What is the main risk of surgery for OPGs?	**Visual morbidity** is the main surgical risk.
What are common late complications of RT in the Tx of OPGs?	Common late complications of RT include **endocrine dysfunction and vision loss.**
What is the main disadvantage of RT in NF-1 pts?	**High incidence of 2nd CNS tumors** (RR 5.3: *Sharif S et al., JCO 2006*)
What is the RT TD 5/5 dose threshold for developing hypopituitarism?	The hypopituitarism TD 5/5 is **40–45 Gy** (GH levels ↓ 1st, then LH/FSH, then TSH/ACTH.)

17

Primary Central Nervous System Lymphoma

Steven H. Lin and Timothy A. Chan

Background

What are the incidence and median age at Dx of primary central nervous system lymphoma (PCNSL)?

1,000 cases/yr of PCNSL (2% of all CNS tumors); median age **55 yrs (immunocompetent)** vs. **35 yrs (immunocompromised)**

What is the gender predilection, and how does it relate to immunocompetency?

Immunocompetent pts: males > females (2:1)
AIDS pts: 95% males

What risk factors are often associated with CNS lymphoma?

Immunodeficiency (congenital or acquired) and EBV infection

What type of non-Hodgkin lymphoma (NHL) is most often associated with PCNSL?

Diffuse large B-cell lymphoma is most often associated with PCNSL.

What % of PCNSL has ocular involvement?

15% of PCNSL has ocular involvement (vitreous, retina, choroid > optic nerve) that is typically bilat.

What is the most common genetic alteration seen in PCNSL?

The most common genetic alteration in PCNSL is the **gain of chromosome 12** (12p12-14), which corresponds to the amplification of MDM2 to enhance p53 suppression

If the pt presents with ocular lymphoma, what % later develop CNS involvement?

75% of pts who present with ocular lymphoma develop CNS involvement.

With what is orbital lymphoma often associated?

Systemic NHL is often associated with orbital lymphoma.

What % of pts present with isolated spinal cord/meningeal involvement?

<5% of pts present with isolated spinal cord/meningeal involvement—a rare occurrence.

How can the Dx of PCNSL be most definitively established?	Bx brain/globe or CSF sampling
What additional workup is done for pts with suspected PCNSL?	Additional PCNSL workup: H&P with neurology emphasis (include visual/spinal Sx), MRI brain $+/-$ spine, and ocular slitlamp exam. Consider PET/CT and/or testicular US for elderly men (per the NCCN), labs (basic, LDH, HIV, toxoplasmosis, $+/-$ BM Bx), and LP with cytology if such testing would be safe.
What must be ruled out in AIDS pts with multiple brain lesions?	Toxoplasmosis and other opportunistic infections
What are the 5 poor prognostic factors for PCNSL according to the IELSG?	Poor prognostic factors for PCNSL: 1. Age >60 yrs 2. ECOG performance status >1 3. Elevated LDH 4. Elevated CSF protein 5. Deep brain involvement (*Fererri AJ et al., JCO 2003*)
What is the 2-yr OS for pts with 0–1, 2–3, and 4–5 factors?	2-yr OS for these pts is **80%, 50%, and 15%, respectively.** (*Fererri AJ et al., JCO 2003*)
When is PCL more likely to be multifocal?	PCL is more likely to be multifocal when the **pt is immunocompromised** (60%−80% of such pts).

▪ Treatment/Prognosis

What is the management paradigm for a immunocompetent pt with PCNSL?	PCNSL management paradigm: high-dose methotrexate (Mtx) or multiagent chemo. If there is a CR, observe (particularly >60 yrs). Use RT for recurrence.
How does the RT response differ between PCNSL and other types of extranodal NHL?	PCNSL is **very radioresistant** (5-yr OS is 4%). Extranodal NHL response is 90% of the LC rate.
What are other prognostic factors for PCNSL?	Poor response to chemo, AIDS, and multifocality
How did the IELSG determine the prognostic groups that may predict for better survival?	*Fererri AJ et al., JCO 2003:* 378 pts from 1980−1999, **HIV−** with CNS lymphoma. All were treated with various regimens ($+/-$ chemo, $+/-$ RT).

How do survival outcomes differ between CRT and RT alone?	MS is 40 mos (CRT) vs. 12 mos (RT alone). 5-yr OS is 30% (CRT) vs. 5% (RT alone).
What is the outcome of pts with ocular lymphoma?	The outcome of pts with ocular lymphoma is **uniformly fatal.** MS is only 6–18 mos.
If a pt is suspected of harboring PCNSL, why should steroids *not* be started right away before obtaining a Bx?	**Tumor regression (in 90%) with subsequent Bx yielding nondiagnostic results;** Bx 1st → start of steroids (upfront steroids only for unstable pts)
Is cyclophosphamide HCl/doxorubicin/ Oncovin/prednisone (CHOP) effective again PCNSL?	**No.** There is ineffective blood–brain barrier penetration. 3 RCTs, including **RTOG 8806** (*Schultz C et al., JCO 1996*), demonstrated no benefit of CHOP or cyclophosphamide HCl/doxorubicin/ Oncovin/dexamethasone (CHOD).
Which study demonstrated that an RT boost is not beneficial for PCNSL?	**RTOG 8315** (phase II): WBRT 40 Gy → CD to 60 Gy. MS was 11.5 mos. 80% failed in the boost field.
What does the Memorial Sloan Kettering Cancer Center (MSKCC) data (*Abrey LE et al., JCO 2000*) demonstrate on the use of high-dose Mtx + WBRT and the relation of age to developing neurotoxicity?	MSKCC data: phase II, 52 pts. MS was 60 mos. High-dose Mtx × 5 cycles (3.5 g/m²) was alternated with intrathecal Mtx (12 mg) → procarbazine/ vincristine + WBRT 45 Gy → high-dose cytosine arabinoside (Ara-C) (intravenous 3 mg × 2). Of those age >60 yrs, some did not rcv RT. Survival was the same between no RT vs. RT, but DFS was worse if there was no RT. Those >60 yrs who rcv RT had ↑ risk of neurotoxicity (83%) vs. age <60 yrs (6%). With chemo alone, only 1 pt developed neurotoxicity.
In the Abrey study, what was the response rate to pre-RT chemo?	**CR 56%** and PR 33% **(ORR 89%)**
In RTOG 9310, did 36 Gy (1.2 Gy bid) benefit PCNSL pts when compared to 45 Gy (conventional qd) WBRT?	**RTOG 9310** (*Fisher B et al., J Neurooncol 2005*): no difference in control and survival, but worse neurotoxicity (23% vs. 4%); prospective study of Abrey chemo regimen → **45 Gy vs. 36 Gy bid** (if CR to chemo) (63 pts rcv 45 Gy, and 16 pts rcv 36 Gy. MS was 37 mos.)
What study examined the feasibility of observation after CR to high-dose Mtx?	**NABTT 96-07,** phase II study (*Batchlor T et al., JCO 2003*): intravenous high-dose Mtx (8 g/m²) was given every 2 wks until CR or until 8 cycles. Once there was a CR, the pt rcv 2 × high-dose Mtx q2wks and 11 cycles of high-dose Mtx q28days. MS was not reached at 22.8 mos. There was no neurotoxicity. CR was 52%, and PR was 22%.

In pts with failure after high-dose Mtx, what salvage RT regimens/doses are used?	**45 Gy.** Recent Massachusetts General Hospital data suggests **36 Gy WBRT** (*Nguyen PL et al., JCO 2005*). MS s/p RT was 10.9 mos, and overall MS was 30 mos. There was neurotoxicity in 3 pts >60 yrs and in those who rcv >36 Gy (31% vs. 0%).
What is the typical response rate to salvage WBRT for pts failing initial chemo?	CR 37% and PR 37% (*Nguyen PL et al., JCO 2005*)
What critical volumes need to be covered with WBRT?	The **post retina and CNS down to C2** need to be covered.
What volumes are treated with RT if the pt presents with an ocular primary?	WBRT to C2, + bilat orbits with opposed lats to 36 Gy → CD to WBRT + post retina to 45 Gy
What are considered "good-risk" immunocompromised pts with PCNSL?	Non-HIV immunosuppression and HIV+ with CD4 >200
How should AIDS+ PCNSL be treated?	**Trial of toxoplasmosis antibiotics.** If there is no response, consider Bx. Chemo is not well tolerated. Consider intrathecal Mtx. Consider palliative WBRT alone (30−45 Gy). If the pt is severely immunocompromised, consider HAART 1st.
Should CHOP or CHOD chemo be used?	**Neither.** Prospective data has shown no benefit to either regimen before RT (per **RTOG 88-06**).
What is the most active chemo regimen used in PCNSL? Why?	**Mtx.** There is high CNS penetration of Mtx.
What is the 1st intervention in a symptomatic pt after Bx?	The use of **high-dose steroids** is the 1st intervention in a symptomatic pt after Bx.
What was the Tx regimen in RTOG 93-10 (*DeAngelis LM et al., JCO 2002*)? What was the MS?	Intravenous/intrathecal Mtx/vincristine/procarbazine → WBRT to 45 Gy → intravenous cytarabine. MS was **3 yrs.**
Why is chemo not preferred in AIDS-related PCNSL?	Chemo is not preferred in AIDS-related PCNSL b/c **CD4 counts are already low** (usually <50).
What is the Tx paradigm in such severely immunocompromised HIV pts?	Immunocompromised HIV pt Tx paradigm: **WBRT to 36–45 Gy with concurrent HAART**

What options are there for leptomeningeal PCNSL?	Intrathecal Mtx or CSI to 36 Gy with a boost to 45–50 Gy
What is the Tx paradigm for ocular lymphoma?	Ocular lymphoma Tx paradigm: **RT to 36 Gy or intraocular chemo**
What is the rationale for omitting WBRT in the elderly with PCNSL?	**Neurotoxicity** in older pts (*Abrey LE et al., JCO 2000*): 80% of pts >60 yo had neurocognitive defects after 45 Gy; 6% if <60 yo. Some pts >60 yo did not get WBRT and had similar OS (worse DFS with no WBRT, however).
What is the WBRT dose for PCNSL after CR to chemo?	**24–36 Gy.** Consider omitting RT altogether if the pt is >60 yo.
What is the WBRT dose for PCNSL after PR to chemo?	**36–45 Gy** WBRT; focal CD to gross Dz to 45 Gy
What prospective data supports RT omission/ deferral after high-dose chemo (Mtx/Ara-C)?	German data supports RT omission/deferral following high-dose chemo. (*Pels H et al., JCO 2003*; *Jahnke K et al., Ann Oncol 2005*)
What is 1 additional option after RT, especially after PR to initial chemo?	**Consolidation Ara-C** is an additional option after RT.
What is the role of Rituxan in PCNSL? How can it be incorporated, and what studies support its use?	Can be used with Mtx/procarbazine/vincristine) as induction regimen → dose-reduced WBRT to 23.4 Gy if CR (45 Gy if PR) → Ara-C consolidation. MSKCC data (*Shah GD et al., JCO 2007*): 2-yr OS was 67% and two thirds of pts had a CR (these pts were able to rcv reduced-dose RT).
What did RTOG 8315 (*Nelson DF et al., IJROBP 1992*) investigate? What did it show?	**RTOG 8315:** RT alone/dose escalation (40 Gy + 20 Gy boost). There was high LR in the brain at 61% and significant neurotoxicity with higher doses.
Which recent randomized international phase II study investigated the use of induction cytarabine for PCNSL? What did it find?	IELSG (*Ferreri AJ et al., Lancet 2009*): randomized to 4 cycles of Mtx vs. Mtx/cytarabine → WBRT. CR rates were 18% vs. 46% and ORR 40% and 69%, respectively.

For meningiomas, with what are slower growth rates associated?

Slower growth rates are associated with **older pts and calcifications.**

What surgical grading system is used in meningiomas? For what does it predict?

Simpson grade (I/GTR−IV/STR). The Simpson grade predicts for the **likelihood of LR.**

GTR is possible in what % of pts?

80% of pts achieve a GTR surgery.

In what anatomic regions is GTR more difficult to achieve for meningioma resection?

Cavernous sinus, petroclival region, post saggital sinus, and optic nerve

What is the prevalence of grade II–III meningiomas?

6% and 4%, respectively. **90% are grade I.**

Name the histologies associated with WHO grade II–III meningiomas.

Grade II: atypical, clear cell, chordoid
Grade III: anaplastic, rhabdoid, papillary

How is optic sheath meningioma diagnosed?

Optic sheath meningioma is diagnosed clinically/ radiographically by a neuro-ophthalmologist/MRI (*no* Bx).

■ Treatment/Prognosis

What are the Tx paradigms for meningiomas?

Meningioma Tx paradigms:
    If incidental/asymptomatic: observation
    If grade I and symptomatic/progressive:
        surgery +/− RT
    If grade II or III: surgery + RT

For which types of meningioma is RT the primary Tx modality?

Optic nerve sheath and cavernous sinus (inaccessible regions)

When should observation be considered?

Observation should be considered with **incidental/ asymptomatic and stable lesions.**

When is RT utilized after surgery for meningiomas?

RT should be utilized after surgery if there is **recurrent Dz or STR** or if there is **atypical/anaplastic histology or brain invasion.**

What are the 10-yr recurrence rates with surgery alone after either GTR or STR?

10-yr recurrence rates with surgery alone are ~**10% after GTR** and **40% after STR.**

Is there a benefit to upfront RT after STR?	This is **controversial** (upfront control rates are considered equivalent to salvage rates). Data from an ongoing RCT (**EORTC 26-021**) is pending.
What are the RT doses employed for meningiomas?	RT doses are **54 Gy for benign** and **60 Gy for malignant** tumors (PTV = GTV + 1.5 cm).
Is there any RT dose-response data for meningiomas?	**Yes.** *Goldsmith et al.* showed improved PFS with doses >52 Gy. (*J Neurosurg 1994*)
What are typical SRS doses used for meningiomas?	Typical SRS doses range from **12–16 Gy** to 50% IDL at the tumor margin (depending on location/size).
What is the 5-yr LC rate for meningiomas after SRS?	The 5-yr LC rate is **98%.** It is worse in men and if the RT dose is <12 Gy. (*Kullova A et al., J Neurosurg 2007*)
What poor prognostic factors have been identified in pts receiving SRS for meningiomas?	Male gender, conformity index <1.4, and size >10 cc (*DiBiase SJ et al., IJROBP 2004*)
Should the dural tail be covered in the RT field?	**Yes** (if possible). Some studies have shown improved 5-yr DFS. (*DiBiase SJ et al., IJROBP 2004*)

■ Toxicity

What is the surgical complication rate after resection for meningiomas?	After resection, the surgical complication rate is **2%–30%** depending on the location/type; 1%−14% mortality (worse in the elderly).
If observed, pts should get MRIs at what intervals?	At **3 mos, 9 mos, then yearly** if stable (q6mos for 5 yrs at Johns Hopkins Hospital)
What is the toxicity rate for SRS if doses >16 Gy are used?	There is **temporary toxicity in 10%** of pts and **permanent toxicity in 6%** of pts. Perilesional edema is observed in 15%. (*Kullova A et al., J Neurosurg 2007*)
What is the RT dose limitation to the chiasm when SRS is used?	The chiasm should be limited to **8 Gy** with SRS.
How are optic nerve sheath/cavernous sinus meningioma pts followed?	These pts should be followed with **serial MRIs, neuro-ophthalmology exams, and regular endocrinology exams.**

What histologic features are prominent in prolactinomas?	**Calcifications and amyloid deposits** are prominent in prolactinomas.
What immuno-histochemical stains are positive in pituitary adenomas?	Synaptophysin, chromogranin, and hormone-specific stains

▪ Workup/Staging

With what signs/Sx do pts with pituitary tumors present?	Bitemporal hemianopsia, HA, and oculomotor deficits (CNs III–IV, VI, V1–V2)
What is the workup of a pt with a pituitary tumor?	Pituitary tumor workup: H&P (physical: CNs, visual field, endocrinopathy), check of hormone levels, thin-slice MRI, and tissue Dx (transsphenoidal resection)
What is the DDx of a pt with a pituitary mass?	Pituitary tumor, craniopharyngioma, meningioma, glioma, suprasellar germ cell, mets, and benign lesions (cyst, aneurysm, empty sella syndrome)
How do pts with prolactinomas present?	Galactorrhea, amenorrhea, ↓libido, and infertility (PL typically >20–25)
What pituitary tumors have a high recurrence rate after resection?	**TSH-secreting tumors** (risk factors: Hx of thyroid ablation, Hashimoto thyroiditis, prior RT/surgery)
How do nonsecretory tumors commonly present?	Mass effect, visual defect, and hypopituitarism
How do GH-secreting tumors present? ACTH-secreting tumors?	<u>GH</u>: acromegaly, gigantism (kids) <u>ACTH</u>: Cushing Dz
What lab findings are suggestive of a GH adenoma?	**GH >10 (not suppressed by glucose) and elevated IGF-1** are findings that suggest GH adenoma.
What is considered a normal level of PL after RT?	**<25 ng/mL** is a normal level of PL after RT.
What lab abnormalities are noted in Cushing Dz?	High cortisol not suppressed by low-dose dexamethasone and normal or ↑ ACTH
What is Cushing syndrome?	Cushing syndrome is **elevated cortisol due to a variety of causes (e.g., adrenal production, exogenous use).** Pts have low ACTH, unlike in Cushing Dz.

What is the definition of micro-, macro-, and picoadenoma?	Microadenoma: <1 cm Macroadenoma: >1 cm Picoadenoma: <0.3 cm

■ Treatment/Prognosis

What are the two Tx paradigms of choice for the management of pituitary adenomas?	Pituitary adenoma Tx paradigms: 1. Surgical resection if hypersecreting or symptomatic (for nonsecreting tumors) → observation or postop RT 2. Definitive RT alone
What is the Tx paradigm for nonfunctioning pituitary adenomas?	Nonfunctioning pituitary adenoma Tx paradigm: surgery → observation or RT vs. definitive RT alone
What is the hormone normalization rate after surgery for a hyperfunctioning pituitary tumor?	Initially, the hormone normalization rate after surgery is **70%–80%,** but it declines to 30%–40% with time.
What types of surgical resection are used for pituitary tumors, and what are the indications?	Transsphenoidal microsurgery: for microadenomas, decompression, debulking of large tumors, reducing hyperfunctioning tumors Frontal craniotomy: for large tumors with invasion into cavernous sinus, frontal/temporal lobes
Where is the scar located after transsphenoidal resection?	There is **no visible scar.** Transsphenoidal resection is done through the nose or alternatively from behind the upper lip.
What are the LC rates after transsphenoidal resection? Are they better for macroadenomas or microadenomas?	**95%.** LC rates are better for **microadenomas** after surgical resection.
What are some poor prognostic factors after transsphenoidal resection of prolactinoma?	Size >2 cm, high preop PL level, ↑ age, and longer duration of amenorrhea
What are some poor prognostic factors after surgical resection of GH-secreting tumors?	High preop GH and somatomedin C levels, tumors >1 cm, and extrasellar extension
What are the indications for radiotherapy in the Tx of pituitary tumors?	Pituitary tumor indications for radiotherapy: 1. Medically inoperable 2. Persistence of hormone defect after surgery 3. Macroadenoma with STR or decompression 4. Recurrent tumor after surgery

What are the long-term control rates for hormone-secreting tumors after RT?

Best outcomes with RT for GH-secreting tumors (80%) > ACTH (50%–80%) > PL (30%–40%)

What should be done with medical/pharmacologic Tx before initiating RT for pituitary adenomas?

Medical Tx **needs to be D/C** b/c of lower RT sensitivity with concurrent medical Tx. (*Landolt AM et al., J Clin Endocrinol Metab 2000*)

What is the preferred Tx paradigm for prolactinoma?

Prolactinoma Tx paradigm: bromocriptine, but 30% cannot tolerate it due to nausea, HA, and fatigue.

How long does it take for normalization of the PL level to occur after initiating pharmacologic suppression?

Normalization of the PL level takes **1–2 mos** following the initiation of pharmacologic suppression.

What is the typical LC rate with RT for pituitary tumors?

The LC after RT is **>90%** for most pituitary tumors.

What are the typical RT volumes and doses used for pituitary tumors?

Tumor + 1.5–2 cm, IMRT or FSR; **45–50.4 Gy if no gross Dz, 54 Gy for gross Dz**

How long does it typically take for hormone stabilization to occur after Tx with RT?

It takes **yrs** for hormone stabilization after Tx with RT (GH: 50% normalize at 2–5 yrs, 70% after 10 yrs).

What evidence supports at least 45 Gy as the min effective RT dose for pituitary tumor control?

Older Florida data (*McCollough WM et al., IJROBP 1991*): 10-yr LC was 95%.

What are the indications for and the benefits of SRS in the Tx of pituitary adenomas?

SRS is used for **microadenomas** and yields **better control of hormone secretion** (same LC as FSR).

What are the typical SRS doses used for functional vs. nonfunctional tumors?

Functional SRS dose: ~20 Gy
Nonfunctional SRS dose: ~14–16 Gy

What are the differences between LINAC-based and Gamma Knife (GK)-based SRS for pituitary tumors?	With GK, there is **less homogeneous dose to the tumor, more precise setup, and slightly less normal tissue treated** (similar outcomes/conformality can be achieved with LINAC-based SRS, however).
When is FSR preferred instead of SRS for pituitary adenomas?	FSR is preferred **when the pituitary lesion is >3 cm and/or the lesion is <2 mm from the chiasm.**
What pharmacologic agents are used for GH-secreting pituitary adenomas?	Somatostatin, octreotide, and pegvisomant (GH receptor antagonist)
What pharmacologic agents are used for ACTH-secreting pituitary adenomas?	Ketoconazole (best), cyproheptadine (inhibits ACTH secretion), mitotane (↓ cortisol synthesis), RU-486 (blocks glucocorticoid receptor), and metyrapone
What RT doses are used with fractionated EBRT? When is EBRT typically used?	**45–50 Gy (nonfunctioning), 50–54 Gy (functioning).** Fractionated EBRT is typically **used for large adenomas.**

■ Toxicity

What is the RT TD 5/5 dose threshold for developing hypopituitarism?	The TD 5/5 is **40–45 Gy.** GH levels ↓ 1st, then LH/FSH → TSH/ACTH.
What is the tolerance of the optic nerves/chiasm with the use of conventional RT?	With conventional RT, **50–54 Gy** is the tolerance of the optic nerves/chiasm.
What is the TD of the optic nerve to single-fx SRS?	**8 Gy** is the TD of the optic nerve with single-fx SRS.
What are the main benefits of using SRS for pituitary adenomas?	Benefits of SRS include ↓ **neurocognitive sequelae and possible preservation of normal pituitary function** by reducing the dose to the hypothalamus (↑risk of damage to the optic nerve/chiasm).
What is the best way to assess the response to RT in GH-secreting tumors?	The response to RT can be assessed by **monitoring IGF-1 levels.**
What hormone is the 1st to respond/decrease after RT?	**GH** is the 1st hormone to respond/decrease after RT.

What is the operative mortality/complication rate after surgery?	Mortality: 1%–2% Complication rate: 15%–20%
What are the most common surgical complications after resection of pituitary tumors?	**Diabetes insipidus (6%)** → hyponatremia and CSF leak
How long does it take for hormone normal-ization to occur after RT for pituitary tumors?	It takes **mos to yrs** for hormone normalization after RT for pituitary tumors.
What is the most common side effect after RT for pituitary tumors?	For pituitary tumors, **hypopituitarism** is the most common side effect after RT.
Which pituitary pts/ tumor types are prone to increased rates of 2nd malignancies after Tx with RT?	Men with **GH-secreting pituitary adenomas** have increased rates of 2nd malignancies after RT. (*Norberg L et al., Clin Endocrinol 2007*)

20
Primary Spinal Cord Tumor
Boris Hristov and Timothy A. Chan

■ Background

At what level does the spinal cord (SC) end in adults? Newborns?	Adults: L1-2 Newborns: L3-4
What is the filum terminale?	The filum terminale is the **filamentous process that anchors the dural sack inferiorly to the coccyx.**
What is the conus medullaris?	The conus medullaris is the **inf/tapering portion of the SC.**
What % of all primary CNS malignancies arise in the SC?	~**15%** of all primary CNS malignancies arise in the SC.

What is the age range for primary SC tumors?

Primary SC tumors occur in the age range of **10–40 yrs.**

Are most primary SC tumors intra- or extradural?

Intradural. If extradural, SC tumors are most likely to be metastatic, not primary.

Are most primary SC tumors intra- or extramedullary?

Two thirds of primary SC tumors are **extramedullary.**

What are the most common and 2nd most common intradural/ extramedullary primary SC tumors?

Two thirds are **schwannomas,** and one third are **meningiomas.**

What % of primary SC tumors are intramedullary?

10% of primary SC tumors are intramedullary.

What are the most common intramedullary SC tumors, and what age group do they typically affect?

Astrocytomas > ependymomas; **children/young adults** (<30 yo)

What type of tumor typically arises at the filum terminale?

Myxopapillary ependymomas arise at the filum terminale.

From what anatomic portion of the meninges do mengiomas arise?

Meningiomas arise from the **arachnoid layer.**

What is a common age range and location for SC meningiomas?

SC meningiomas most often occur at age **50–70 yrs,** with most presenting in the **thoracic spine.**

What grade is most common for primary SC astrocyomas?

~90% are **low grade**/WHO grades I–II (pilocytic/ fibrillary).

What is the 3rd most common intramedullary SC tumor, and with what syndrome can it be associated?

Hemangioblastoma is the 3rd most common intramedullary SC tumor, with ~25% of cases associated with **von Hippel-Lindau syndrome.**

■ Workup/Staging

What is the most common presenting Sx of primary SC tumors, and over what time frame do Sx present?

Primary SC tumors most commonly present with **pain (75%),** with Sx presenting over **mos to yrs** (long prodrome).

What is particularly important as part of the workup for a SC tumor?

Detailed neurologic exam and SC imaging (MRI or CT myelogram)

What is the difference between astrocytomas and ependymomas on MRI (location/appearance)?

Astrocytoma: eccentric/asymmetric expansion of SC
Ependymoma: central/symmetric expansion of SC

What is the MRI appearance of SC lipomas?

On MRI, SC lipomas appear **bright on T1 without contrast,** and **signal disappears on fat suppression.**

Which primary SC tumors require imaging of the entire craniospinal axis?

Ependymomas, glioblastoma multiforme, and anaplastic astrocytomas

■ Treatment/Prognosis

What is the Tx paradigm for primary SC tumors?

Primary SC tumor Tx paradigm: max resection $+/-$ RT or definitive RT alone

What are the 2 main advantages of upfront surgical resection?

Histologic confirmation and decompression of the cord

After GTR, which meningiomas—spinal or intracranial—have higher rates of recurrence?

Intracranial meningiomas have a 10%−20% recurrence rate, while spinal meningiomas have ~5% recurrence rate.

What is the most important predictor for recurrence for meningiomas/ependymomas?

Extent of resection is the most important predictor for recurrence. There are few recurrences after GTR.

In what % of SC meningioma/ependymoma pts is GTR achievable?

GTR is achievable in **>90%** of pts. (Retrospective series: *Gezen F et al., Spine 1976; Peker S et al., J Neurosurg Sci 2005*)

In what proportion of SC astrocytoma pts is GTR possible?

GTR is possible in **fewer than one third** of pts.

Why is RT controversial for most SC tumors, even after STR?

Most SC tumors are **indolent** (slow growing), and there is **potential for SC toxicity** with RT.

What RT options are available after STR for meningioma/ependymoma?

Standard EB to **50.4 Gy** (1.8 Gy/fx or 1 Gy bid) or stereotactic body RT, 16 Gy to 80% IDL (*Bhatnagar AK et al., Technol Cancer Res Treat 2005*)

What Tx options are available for SC astrocytomas?

<u>Low grade</u>: observe after GTR/50.4 Gy after STR
<u>High grade</u>: 54 Gy

What retrospective studies support use of RT in SC astrocytomas?

Rodrigues GB et al., IJROBP 2000 (Princess Margaret Hospital) and *Abdel-Wahab M et al., IJROBP 2006*: PFS was significantly influenced by RT in low- and intermediate-grade tumors; however, the RT group had fewer complete resections as compared with the surgery alone group (13% vs. 53%; $p = 0.01$).

What data supports the RT dose response for SC ependymomas?

Garcia DM, IJROBP 1985: <40 Gy, 23% OS; >40 Gy, 83% OS
Mayo data (*Shaw EG et al., IJROBP 1986*): 35% LF for <50 Gy vs. 20% for >50 Gy

For what type of SC tumor has adj RT been shown to be beneficial, regardless of extent of resection?

Adj RT has been shown to be beneficial with **myxopapillary ependymoma.**
MDACC data (*Akyurek S et al., J Neurooncol 2006*): +/− 50.4 Gy RT 10-yr LC GTR/STR (55%/0%) vs. GTR + RT/STR + RT (90%/67%), all SS

What RT schedule is often used for high-grade ependymomas +/− CSF spread?

CSI to 36 Gy + boost to 50.4−54 Gy gross Dz

What anatomic region needs to be covered with RT in caudal ependymomas?

The **thecal sac down to S2-3** needs to be covered.

What are the typical sup-inf RT margins for SC tumors?

The typical sup-inf margin required for SC tumors is **3–5 cm.**

■ Toxicity

What is the L'hermitte sign? When does it occur, and to what is it due?

The L'hermitte sign is **shocklike sensations in the extremities upon neck flexion.** It occurs within **2–6 mos of RT** from **demyelination of the nerve tracts.**

When does RT myelopathy occur, and what is the temporal sequence of onset for neurologic deficits?	RT myelopathy occurs **13–29 mos** after RT, with paresthesia → weakness → pain/temperature loss → loss of bowel/bladder function.
Within what time frame do SC astrocytoma pts usually relapse?	Relapse in SC astrocytoma pts usually occurs within **2 yrs** (most in-field).
How long of a follow-up is required after SC ependymoma resection?	**>10 yrs** follow-up is required, as **late recurrences (>12 yrs) have been reported** in 5%–10% of pts.
What region of the SC has traditionally been thought to be most sensitive to RT? Least sensitive?	The **lumbar SC is thought to be most sensitive** to RT, while the **cervical cord is thought to be least sensitive.**

21

Choroid Plexus Carcinoma and Papilloma

Boris Hristov and Timothy A. Chan

Background

What are the most common locations of choroid plexus (CP) tumors in children vs. adults?	Children: Lat ventricles Adults: 4th ventricle
What is the name for the benign CP variant, and how frequent is it? How about the malignant variant?	Benign variant: choroid plexus papilloma (CPP)/ WHO I (60%–80% of cases) Malignant variant: choroid plexus carcinoma (CPC)/WHO III (20%–40% of cases)
What proportion of children present with metastatic Dz at Dx?	**One third** of children present with metastatic Dz, all typically with CPC.

What is the most common age of presentation for these tumors?	70% of pts are **<2 yo.**
What % of CPCs can have CSF seeding? How about CPPs?	**Up to 40%** of CPCs have CSF seeding, but such seeding is **very rare for papillomas.**
What are the 2 most important prognostic/ predictive factors for CP tumors?	Histology (papillomas do better) and extent of resection
What is the 5-yr survival of pts with CPCs and CPPs?	**20%–30%** for carcinomas and **90%–100%** for papillomas
What markers do CPCs often express?	CPCs often express **CEA and CD44.**
What markers do CPPs often express?	CPPs often express **prealbumin and S100.**

■ Workup/Staging

What are the 2 most common Sx at presentation in pts with CP tumors?	Hydrocephalus and HA
What studies need to be performed during the workup for CP tumors?	Craniospinal MRI and CSF cytology

■ Treatment/Prognosis

What is the general Tx paradigm for CP tumors?	CP tumor Tx paradigm: max safe resection (after embolization/chemo, if necessary) +/− chemo (younger pts) and/or RT (if age >3 yrs)
What are the indications for RT in pts with CP tumors?	Age >3 yrs and 1 of the following: carcinoma histology, STR, +CSF/spine Dz (CSI), or recurrent tumors
What is the role of RT in CPPs after STR?	**No RT is necessary upfront,** as only 50% of STR pts require reoperation, surgical salvage is good, and reoperation may not be needed until yrs later. Consider RT if there is a STR after recurrence. (Mayo data: *Krishnan S et al., J Neurooncol 2004*)

What imaging modality is ideal to r/o a bleed?	**CT** is ideal to r/o cerebral bleeds.
What is the gold standard imaging modality for AVMs?	**Angiography** is the gold standard modality for imaging AVMs.
What other imaging modalities can be used for AVMs? What are their advantages?	CT angiography (good vascular detail), MR angiography (good anatomy detail), functional MRI (eloquent areas), and diffusion tensor imaging (for white matter tracts)
What scale is used to evaluate AVM pts for surgery?	**Spetzler-Martin scale/grading system** (totals possible: I–V)
What 3 AVM characteristics in the Spetzler-Martin scale are predictive of surgical outcomes?	AVM characteristics that predict surgical outcome: 1. **Diameter** (<3 cm = 1, 3–6 cm = 2, >6 cm = 3) 2. **Location** (noneloquent area = 0, eloquent area = 1) 3. **Pattern of venous drainage** (superficial = 0, deep = 1)
How does AVM diameter/size scoring correlate with surgical outcomes?	The smaller the AVM diameter/size (<3 cm), the better the outcomes.
What brain areas are considered eloquent?	Eloquent areas include sensorimotor, language, visual, thalamus, hypothalamus, internal capsule, brain stem, cerebellar peduncles, and deep cerebellar nuclei.

▪ Treatment/Prognosis

What are the 3 Tx options for AVMs?	Surgery, radiosurgery, and embolization
What is the goal of Tx with AVMs? Why?	**Complete obliteration** is the goal, since there is **no benefit/↑ risk of bleed** if the obliteration is partial.
Which lesions are most amenable to surgery?	Those with **low (I–III) Spetzler-Martin scores** are most amenable to surgery.
What is frequently done for grade III lesions before surgery?	**Embolization** can be performed for grade III lesions before surgery.
What is the main advantage of surgery?	The main advantages of surgery are **immediate cure and reduction in the risk of hemorrhage.**
For which AVM lesions is radiosurgery (SRS) preferred?	Radiosurgery is preferred for **lesions <3 cm that are located in deep or eloquent regions of the brain.**

What is the main disadvantage of SRS for AVMs?

The main disadvantage of SRS is the **lag time of 1–3 yrs to complete obliteration** (i.e., continued bleeding risk).

How does RT lead to AVM obliteration?

Vascular wall thickening and luminal thrombosis from RT effect result in obliteration of the AVM.

Is the bleeding risk completely eliminated after SRS?

No. It is reduced by ~88% but not eliminated. (*Maruyama K et al., NEJM 2005*)

On what do SRS cure rates for AVMs primarily depend?

Size of AVM: 81%–91% if <3 cm, lower if >3 cm (*Maruyama K et al., NEJM 2005*)

What can be done for high-grade AVMs (IV–V) not amenable for surgery?

Staged SRS (different components targeted at separate sessions) (*Sirin S et al., Neurosurg 2006*)

For which AVMs can embolization be curative?

AVMs <1 cm that are fed by a single artery can be cured by embolization alone.

How are AVMs with feeding artery aneurysms managed?

If the aneurysm is >7 mm in diameter, clip or coil the aneurysm 1st, then treat the AVM. The aneurysm is at greater risk for rupture if the AVM is treated 1st.

What is the ongoing randomized ARUBA trial investigating?

The ARUBA trial is investigating **Tx vs. conservative management** for unruptured AVMs.

What SRS doses are commonly used for AVMs?

Lesions <3 cm: **21–22 Gy** to 50% IDL. If the lesion is in the brain stem, lower the dose to ≤16 Gy.
Lesions >3 cm: **16–18 Gy** to 50% IDL

■ Toxicity

What are the reported rates of permanent weakness or paralysis, aphasia, and hemianopsia for grade I–III AVM pts treated with surgery?

The rate of serious postsurgical complications is **0%–15%** (depending on the series).

What are common early and delayed complications after SRS for AVMs?

Early: seizures, n/v, HA
Delayed: seizures, hemorrhage, radionecrosis/edema, venous congestion

What is the incidence of transient vs. permanent neurologic complications after SRS for AVMs?

Complications after SRS for AVMs are as follows: **transient (5%) vs. permanent (1.4%).**

What is the avg growth rate per yr for ANs?

~1 mm/yr. Growth rates range from 0.5 mm/yr (slow-growing lesions) to 2 mm/yr (fast-growing lesions).

What % of ANs are stable (shrink/do not grow)?

~20%–40% of ANs are considered stable.

Is the size of the tumor at presentation predictive of the tumor's growth rate?

No. Tumor size is generally not predictive of the tumor's growth rate.

Does AN tumor size correlate with hearing loss?

Usually not. The location of the tumor (i.e., intra-canalicular vs. not intracanalicular) is more predictive.

What do brainstem auditory evoked potentials typically show in pts with ANs?

A delay of conduction time on the affected side is seen with auditory evoked potentials.

What imaging study is typically performed for ANs?

Thin-slice (1–1.5 mm) MRI with gadolinium. If NF is suspected, neuraxis MRI is performed.

To what is the "ice cream cone" appearance of ANs on MRI due?

This AN appearance is due to enhancing lesions in the canal (cone) and CPA (ice cream).

What scale is used to grade facial nerve (CN VII) function?

The House-Brackman scale (I [normal] to VI [no movement/spasm/contracture]) is used to assess CN VII function.

Facial nerve Sx are present in what % of AN pts?

~6% of AN pts present with facial nerve Sx.

■ Treatment/Prognosis

What options are available for AN pts?

Observation, surgery, or RT

When is observation appropriate for ANs?

Observation is appropriate with small tumors (<2 cm) or no/slow growth without Sx progression.
Rosenberg SI, Laryngoscope 2002: >40% no growth. Lesions >2 cm were more likely to grow fast.

What follow-up is required for AN pts opting for observation?

Audiometry and MRI scans q6–12 mos are required for pts opting for observation.

What are the 3 surgical approaches available for ANs, and what are the prominent disadvantages/advantages of each?

Retromastoid: may not be able to achieve GTR/good facial nerve preservation
Middle fossa: GTR, facial nerve preservation may not be possible/hearing preservation better
Translabyrinthine: sacrifices hearing/good facial nerve preservation

When is surgery the preferred Tx option for ANs?

Surgery is preferred for **large (>4 cm) symptomatic tumors or recurrence/progression after RT.**

What are the recurrence rates after surgery for ANs?

<1% (German data: *Samii M et al., J Neurosurg 2001*; Johns Hopkins Hospital [JHH] data: *Guerin C et al., Ann Acad Med Singapore 1999*)

What are the overall facial nerve and hearing preservation rates after surgery for ANs?

After surgery for ANs, there is an **80%–90% facial nerve preservation rate** and a **50% hearing preservation rate.**

What are the overall facial nerve and hearing preservation rates after RT for ANs?

After RT for ANs, there is ~**95% facial nerve preservation rate** and ~**65% hearing preservation rate** (possibly higher with FSR).

What are the long-term LC rates after RT for ANs?

Long-term LC after RT for ANs is **90%–97%.** (*Lunsford LD et al., J Neurosurg 2005*; *Combs SE et al., IJROBP 2006*)

What are some commonly employed doses when SRS/Gamma Knife (GK) SRS is used for ANs?

12–13 Gy to 50% IDL is a commonly employed SRS regimen for ANs.

What has the dose trend been for the Tx of ANs with SRS?

The dose was **lowered from 16 Gy to 12–13 Gy.** Pittsburgh and Japanese data showed similar LC rates but less facial weakness and hearing loss with lower doses.

What doses are used with FSR?

Combs SE et al., IJROBP 2005: **50–55 Gy** (in 25–30 Gy/fx) if larger (>2–3 cm) lesions
JHH approach: **25 Gy (500 cGy × 5 fx)** with smaller lesions

What are the hearing preservation rates with FSR?

This is **controversial,** but hearing preservation rates are thought to be better with FSR than with SRS or surgery (**94%** in *Combs SE et al., IJROBP 2005*; **81%** in *Andrews DW et al., IJROBP 2001*).

What recent data suggests better hearing preservation and similar LC rates with lower-dose FSR therapy?

Thomas Jefferson data (*Andrews DW et al., IJROBP 2009*): a lower dose of 46.8 Gy (vs. 50.4 Gy) had 100% LC at 5 yrs with a better hearing preservation rate.

What other RT modalities have been successfully employed in AN?

CyberKnife (*Chang SD et al., J Neurosurg 2005*) and protons (*Weber DC et al., Neurosurg 2003*): worse hearing preservation (not used with tumors >2 cm and if pt can hear well)

Where is the optic disc relative to the macula?	The optic disc is **2 mm medial** to the macula (~1.5 mm in diameter).
What are some of the risk factors for developing ocular melanoma?	UV exposure, white, family Hx of ocular melanoma, and personal Hx of cutaneous melanoma
What is the most common chromosomal abnormality seen in ocular melanoma?	Loss of chromosome 3 and amplification of 8q (50%)
What are the histologic subtypes of ocular melanoma, and which carry the best and worst prognosis?	**Spindle cell (best), epithelioid (worst),** and mixed (if <50% epithelioid histology)
What % of pts with ocular melanoma present with DM at Dx? What is the most common location?	**1%–2%** present with DM. The **liver** is the most common site (5%–20% DM rate over 5 yrs).
What are the different ways melanoma can spread within the globe?	Melanoma can spread <u>intraocularly</u> (through the vitreous, aqueous, or along ciliary vessels/nerves); <u>extraocularly</u> (through the optic nerve, transsclerally, vascular tracking), and through <u>extrascleral extension</u> (10%–15%)
What tumor characteristics predict for DM in ocular melanoma? What is the 5-yr mortality rate in these pts?	Epithelioid histology, large tumors, ant location (ciliary body invasion), monosomy 3, scleral penetration, ↑ mitotic rate, ↑ Ki-67, pleomorphic nucleoli, optic nerve invasion, ↑ MIB-1 index, vascular networks of closed vascular loops, extraocular extension

The 5-yr mortality rate is **55%.** |
| **What is the long-term (>10-yr) DM rate from ocular melanoma?** | **50%** of ocular melanoma pts develop DMs at 15 yrs. |

■ Workup/Staging

How do pts with ocular melanoma normally present?	Most (one third) pts are **asymptomatic.** Ocular melanoma is usually found on routine exam; otherwise, pts detect it themselves due to vision loss, scotoma, flashing lights, or pain (rare).
What is the workup for a pt with suspected ocular melanoma?	Suspected ocular melanoma workup: H&P, CBC (LFTs), ophthalmic/funduscopic/slitlamp exam, visual acuity/visual field testing, US (Kretz A-scan, immersion B-scan), fluorescein angiography, MRI, PET/CT to r/o mets

Is Bx commonly done for ocular melanoma?

No. With Bx, there is a potential for tumor seeding. The Dx is made by exam and imaging.

What are simulation lesions?

Simulation lesions are **lesions that may look like melanoma,** such as nevi, hemangiomas, retinal detachment, age-related disciform lesions, and mets.

What feature does ocular melanoma manifest on standard A-scan US?

An **acoustic "quiet" zone** (central hypoechoic area) vs. mets or hemangiomas (have higher internal reflectivity)

What features do ocular melanomas exhibit on fluorescein angiography?

On fluorescein angiography, ocular melanomas exhibit a **double circulation pattern and fluorescein leakage** (appearing as hot spots).

What is the T staging of choroidal/ciliary body melanoma based on the latest AJCC (2009) staging guidelines?

AJCC staging is based on 4 tumor size categories that depend on tumor diameter and height as follows (Fig. 24.1):
T1: tumor size category 1
T2: tumor size category 2
T3: tumor size category 3
T4: tumor size category 4

For the T staging of choroidal/ciliary body melanomas, what do the designations a–e represent?

a: no ciliary body involvement/extraocular extension
b: +ciliary body involvement
c: no ciliary body/+extraocular extension ≤5 mm
d: +ciliary body/+extraocular extension ≤5 mm
e: +extraocular extension ≥5 mm

Describe the AJCC 7th edition 2009 TNM staging for choroidal/ciliary body melanomas.

Stage I: T1aN0M0
Stage IIA: T1b-dN0M0 or T2aN0M0
Stage IIB: T2bN0M0 or T3aN0M0
Stage IIIA: T2c-d, T3b-c, T4aN0M0
Stage IIIB: T3d, T4b-cN0M0
Stage IIIC: T4d-eN0M0
Stage IV: any TN1M0, any T, any NM1a-c

For the M staging of choroidal/ciliary body melanomas, what do the designations a–c represent?

Ma: largest diameter of met ≤3 cm
Mb: largest diameter of met 3.1–8 cm
Mc: largest diameter of met ≥8 cm

In the Collaborative Ocular Melanoma Study (COMS) staging system, what are COMS small, medium, and large lesions?

COMS staging is based on apical height (AH) and basal diameter (BD):
<u>Small</u>: AH 1–2.5 mm, BD ≤5–16 mm
<u>Medium</u>: AH 2.6–10 mm, BD 6–16 mm
<u>Large</u>: AH ≥10 mm, BD ≥16 mm

What is the randomized phase III study that compared the efficacy of enucleation vs. plaque brachytherapy for medium-sized uveal melanomas?	COMS study (*Report No. 28, Arch Ophthalmol, 2006*): 1,317 pts. There was no difference in all-cause mortality and melanoma-specific mortality. 12-yr OS was 17%–21%.
In the COMS medium trial, what is the 5-yr secondary enucleation rate after plaque brachytherapy? To what is it due?	The 5-yr secondary enucleation rate is **13%** due to **Tx failure or ocular pain from brachytherapy complications.**
What is the standard management for large uveal melanomas?	**Enucleation.** Charged particles (protons) can also be used.
What % of pts present with large uveal melanomas?	**30%** of pts present with large uveal melanomas.
Per the COMS trial, does preop EBRT improve outcomes over enucleation alone for COMS large tumors?	**No.** In the COMS trial, there was no OS or DFS difference between the 2 groups.

■ Toxicity

What are some early and late complications associated with plaque brachytherapy?	<u>Early</u>: pain, bleeding, diplopia, infection, edema <u>Late</u>: **retinopathy (42% at 5 yrs, increasing to 80%–90% thereafter)**, cataracts, keratitis, optic neuropathy
The use of what agent has recently been associated with a lower incidence of macular edema after plaque brachytherapy?	**Triamcinolone** (periocular injections). In an RCT, macular edema rates were 58% in the control group vs. 36% in the triamcinolone arm (SS). (*Horgan N, Ophthalmology 2009*)
What % of pts have loss of ≥6 lines of vision 3 yrs after plaque brachytherapy?	~**50%** of pts have significant vision loss after plaque brachytherapy.
What % of pts have cataracts 5 yrs after plaque brachytherapy?	**83%** of pts develop cataracts after plaque brachytherapy.
How should pts treated with plaque brachytherapy be followed?	Plaque brachytherapy follow-up: H&P, ocular US q3mos × 1 yr, q4mos in 2nd yr, q6mos in 3rd and 4th yrs, then annually; CT C/A/P or liver US q6mos with LFTs (can detect >95% of mets)

Are periodic LFTs alone adequate to r/o liver mets?

No. There is very poor sensitivity (15%), PPV (46%), and NPV (71%), with a specificity of 92%. Adding liver US to LFTs increases the detection rate to 95%. (*Eskelin S et al., Cancer 1999*)

What is the best way to detect liver mets? What is the main disadvantage of this modality?

PET/CT is the best imaging modality for the detection of liver mets. The **cost and availability of such testing** is the main disadvantage.

Thickness (mm)	≤ 3.0	3.1-6.0	6.1-9.0	9.1-12.0	12.1-15.0	15.1-18.0	> 18
> 15					4	4	4
12.1-15.0				3	3	4	4
9.1-12.0		3	3	3	3	3	4
6.1-9.0	2	2	2	2	3	3	4
3.1-6.0	1	1	1	2	2	3	4
≤ 3.0	1	1	1	1	2	2	4

Largest basal diameter (mm)

FIGURE 24.1 Primary ciliary body and choroidal melanomas are classified according to the 4 tumor size categories shown. (*Edge SD, Byrd DR, Compton CC, et al., eds. AJCC cancer staging manual. 7th ed. New York: Springer; 2009, p 549.*)

25

Orbital and Intraocular Primary Eye Lymphomas

Boris Hristov and Roland Engel

■ Background

Under what type of lymphomas are intraocular/orbital lymphomas classified?

Intraocular/orbital lymphomas are classified as **non-Hodgkin lymphomas** (B-cell histology > T-cell histology).

What is the median age of onset? What are the 2 main types of eye lymphoma?

The median age of onset is **50–60 yrs** (females > males). The 2 main types are **intraocular and orbital/ocular adnexa lymphoma.**

What chemo regimens are typically used for high-grade orbital/ocular adnexa lymphomas?

Cyclophosphamide HCl/doxorubicin/Oncovin/ prednisone + Rituxan (**R-CHOP) or** cyclophosphamide/ vincristine/Adriamycin/dexamethasone) **(CVAD)** are typically used for high-grade orbital lymphomas.

What is 1 additional option for refractory/ relapsed Dz?

Radioimmunotherapy (RIT) with Bexxar (I-131) or Zevalin (yttrium-90) is another option for refractory/ relapsed Dz.

What RT technique can be utilized for ant (eyelid, conjunctival) lesions?

Ant orthovoltage or electron fields can be employed for ant eye lesions.

How is lens shielding accomplished with an ant orthovoltage field?

A lead shield is **suspended in the beam** to shield the lens (limits lens dose to 5%–10%).

What are some poor prognostic factors for ocular/orbital lymphomas?

High-grade Dz, advanced Dz (stage IVE), and symptomatic Dz

▪ Toxicity

Above what cumulative dose (standard fractionation) is lens opacification seen?

Lens opacification is seen with doses **>13–16 Gy.**

What toxicities are associated with RIT?

Myelosuppression, myelodysplastic syndrome, and acute myeloid leukemia

What is the min dose to induce cataracts with a single fx vs. multiple fx of RT?

Doses of **2 Gy** (single fx) and **4–5 Gy** (multiple fx) can induce cataracts.

Is cataract induction a stochastic or deterministic late effect? Explain.

Deterministic. There is a threshold and the severity/ latency are dose related.

Which region of the lens is affected most by RT?

The **post subcapsular region of the lens** is affected most by RT.

What is the dose tolerance of the retina/ optic nerves?

The dose tolerance of retina/optic nerves is **50 Gy.**

What is the dose tolerance of the lacrimal glands?

The dose tolerance of the lacrimal apparatus is **26–30 Gy.**

Above what dose can painful keratitis be seen?

Doses **>60 Gy** can cause painful keratitis.

26
Thyroid Ophthalmopathy
John P. Christodouleas and Roland Engel

Background

What causes thyroid ophthalmopathy (TO)?	T-cell lymphocytic infiltration of orbital and periorbital tissues (secondary to autoimmune antibody–mediated reaction against the TSH receptor)
Name 2 conditions associated with TO.	**Graves Dz** and **Hashimoto thyroiditis** are both associated with TO.
What is the end result of untreated TO?	Untreated TO will lead to **fibrosis,** which develops over the course of 2–5 yrs.
What are the signs/Sx of TO?	Exophthalmos, impaired extraocular movements/ diplopia, periorbital edema, and lid retraction. In severe cases, compression of the optic nerves and decreased visual acuity can occur.

Workup/Staging

What does the general workup of TO include?	TO workup: H&P (Hertel exophthalmometer), CBC, CMP, TFTs, and CT/MRI orbit
What is the staging/risk stratification?	There is **no formal staging/risk stratification.** Studies have grouped pts into mild, moderately severe, and severe TO, though the exact definition of these terms varies between studies.

Treatment/Prognosis

What is the general Tx paradigm for TO?	TO Tx paradigm: Treat underlying disorder. For mild Dz, consider observation vs. RT; for moderately severe Dz, consider high-dose steroids vs. RT; and for severe Dz, perform orbital decompression surgery (e.g., for acute visual acuity or color perception changes).
RT should be initiated within how many mos from onset of TO?	RT should be initiated **within 7 mos** of TO onset. Delayed RT is not as effective based on retrospective data.
What are 2 common contraindications to high-dose steroids in pts with TO?	**Optic neuropathy and corneal ulceration** are 2 contraindications to steroids in pts with TO.

What % of pts with OP will subsequently develop a malignant lymphoma?	**5%–25%** will subsequently develop a malignant lymphoma. (*Orcutt JC et al., Br J Ophthalmol 1983; Mittal BB et al., Radiology 1986*)

Does OP affect children, adults, or both?	OP affects **both children and adults.** ~5%–15% are pediatric cases. (*Smitt MC et al., Semin Radiat Oncol 1999*)

Name 5 signs/Sx associated with OP.	Signs/Sx associated with OP: 1. Orbital mass 2. Orbital pain 3. Proptosis 4. Abnl extraocular movements (e.g., diplopia) 5. Decreased visual acuity

▉ Workup/Staging

What is the DDx for an orbital mass?	Rhabdomyosarcoma, OP, malignant orbital lymphoma, thyroid ophthalmopathy, and nodular fasciitis

What is the workup for an orbital mass?	The workup is the same as for a suspected lymphoma, including CT/MRI brain/orbit.

Is there a formal staging system for OP?	**No.** There is **no formal staging system** for OP.

▉ Treatment/Prognosis

What is the initial Tx for OP?	**Steroids** are the mainstay initial Tx for OP. (*Smitt MC et al., Semin Radiat Oncol 1999*)

What are the response rate and long-term control rate with a single steroid course?	<u>Response rate:</u> 80% <u>Long-term control rate:</u> 33% (*Mombaerts I et al., Ophthalmology 1996*)

What is the 2nd-line therapy for OP?	**RT** is the 2nd-line therapy for OP.

What is the most common RT dose/fx schedule for OP?	**20 Gy in 10 fx** is the most commonly employed schedule for OP.

What are the estimated control rates for OP with RT?	Control rates with RT range from **66%–100%.** (*Smitt MC et al., Semin Radiat Oncol 1999*)

What is the standard RT setup for OP?	There is no standard RT setup, as the process may involve any aspect of the orbit. Tx must be individualized.

Can RT be repeated for OP?	**Yes.** RT can be repeated, if necessary.

Toxicity

What are the late side effects of orbital RT?	Cataracts, permanent eye dryness, retinopathy, and optic neuropathy
What is the RT dose limit of the lens?	Try to limit the lens to **<8–10 Gy** depending on the clinical situation.
Diabetic pts are at an increased risk for what complication after orbital RT?	After orbital RT, diabetic pts are at an increased risk for **RT retinopathy.** (*Wakelkamp IM et al., Ophthalmology 2004*)

What is the DDx for a pt with a nasopharyngeal mass?

Carcinoma, lymphoma, melanoma, plasmacytoma, angiofibroma, rhabdomyosarcoma (children), and mets

What % of NPC pts present with palpable LAD?

60%–90% of NPC pts present with palpable LAD.

What % of NPC pts present with bilat LAD?

Up to **50%** of NPC pts present with bilat LAD.

Adenopathy near the mastoid tip is indicative of involvement of which nodal group?

Adenopathy near the mastoid tip is indicative of **retropharyngeal** nodal involvement (node of Rouviere).

Pts with upper level V LAD are most likely to have what kind of H&N primary?

Pts with upper level V LAD are very likely to have **NPC.**

What factors predict for DM in pts with NPC?

Predictors of DM include **lower neck nodal involvement, retropharyngeal LN involvement, and WHO type IIb histology.**

What are the common DM sites for NPC?

Common metastatic sites for NPC include **bones > lungs, liver, and brain.**

What correlates better with DM spread in NPC: N stage or T stage?

Mets correlate better with the **N stage** than the T stage in NPC.

Describe the latest T staging of NPC.

T1: confined to NPX, or tumor extends to oropharynx (OPX) and/or nasal cavity without parapharyngeal extension

T2: tumor with parapharyngeal extension (posterolat infiltration of tumor (i.e., beyond pharyngobasilar fascia)

T3: involves bony structures and/or paranasal sinuses

T4: intracranial extension and/or involvement of CNs, infratemporal fossa, hypopharynx, orbit, or masticator space

Describe the latest N staging of NPC.

N1: unilat nodes ≤6 cm above supraclavicular fossa and/or retropharyngeal LNs ≤7 cm (unilat or bilat)

N2: bilat nodes ≤6 cm above supraclavicular fossa

N3a: LNs >6 cm

N3b: extension to supraclavicular fossa (includes some level IV–V nodes)

How does the latest AJCC 7th edition (2009) staging of NPC differ from previous staging schemes?

According to the latest AJCC staging, T2a lesions are now T1; T2b lesions are now T2; old stage IIA is now stage I; and old stage IIB is now stage II. Retropharyngeal LN involvement is now considered N1 Dz.

What is the T stage of an NPC causing CN involvement?

T4 lesions may involve the CNs. They also may involve the intracranial structures, infratemporal fossa, hypopharynx, orbit, or masticator space.

What is the T stage of an NPC with soft palate involvement alone without parapharyngeal spread?

T1 designates lesions without parapharyngeal extension (may have extension to the OPX/nasal cavity). If there is extension beyond the pharyngobasilar fascia (+parapharynx), then the lesion is T2.

What is the T stage of an NPC with sphenoid sinus involvement?

T3 denotes involvement of bony structures and/or the paranasal sinuses.

What is the T stage of an NPC that is confined to the NPX?

T1 designates lesions confined to the NPX or tumor extending to the OPX and/or nasal cavity without parapharyngeal extension.

What is the NPC nodal staging if a supraclavicular node is involved?

N3b designates LAD in the supraclavicular fossa (**N3a** is a node >6 cm).

What is the NPC nodal staging of a single ipsi node measuring 4 cm?

N1—any # of nodes confined to the ipsi neck <6 cm

What is the NPC nodal staging of bilat nodal Dz, none >6 cm?

N2—bilat nodes, all <6 cm

What are the stage groupings for NPC?

Stage I: T1N0
Stage II: T1-2N1, T2N0
Stage III: T3N0-2, any N2
Stage IVA: T4N0-2
Stage IVB: N3
Stage IVC: M1

■ Treatment/Prognosis

What is the typical Tx paradigm for pts with NPC?

NPC Tx paradigm: **RT alone or CRT** (no surgical indication except for Bx)

What must be done before planning the NPC pt for RT?

Nutrition consult, PEG tube, and dental evaluation are all recommended before RT.

When is surgery indicated in the management of NPC?

Surgery is performed **to Bx the lesion and in cases of elective neck dissection** for persistent Dz after CRT.

What NPC stages can be treated with definitive RT alone (without chemo)?

T1N0. RT alone is controversial for certain T2N0 pts and select pts with N1 Dz due to small retropharyngeal nodal involvement, as these pts were likely not considered N1 pts in the Al-Sarraf study.

What NPC stages should be treated with definitive CRT according to the NCCN guidelines?

T2 or N+ pts should be treated with CRT per the NCCN guidelines.

For early-stage NPC, what are the typical survival and control rates with RT alone?

With RT alone, the 3-yr OS is **70%–100% for stage I–II NPC** and LC rates are ~**70%–80% for T1-T2 lesions.**

What stages of NPC should be treated with concurrent chemoradiotherapy?

Per the **Intergroup 0099 study** (*Al Sarraf M et al., JCO 1998*), all T3-T4 or N+ pts should be considered for CRT. Per **RTOG 0225** (*Lee N et al., JCO 2009*), all pts with ≥T2b (old staging) or T2 (new staging) and N+ Dz should be considered.

What was the CRT regimen used for locally advanced NPC in the Intergroup 0099 (Al-Sarraf) study?

Concurrent chemo with **cisplatin IV 100 mg/m^2 days 1, 22, and 43** and RT to 70 Gy → adj chemo with CDDP/5-FU × 3 cycles

What were the PFS and OS outcomes in the Intergroup 0099 (Al-Sarraf) trial?

In **Intergroup 0099,** 3-yr PFS was 24% vs. 69%, and **3-yr OS was 46% vs. 76%** in favor of CRT over RT alone. B/c of these remarkable results, the study was closed early. This was one of the 1st studies to demonstrate a survival benefit with CRT.

What are the main criticisms of the Intergroup 0099 (Al-Sarraf) study?

Major criticisms of **Intergroup 0099** include the large number (25%) of pts with WHO type I NPC (not typically seen in endemic areas) and the poor results of the RT alone arm. Single-institution studies with RT alone (Princess Margaret Hospital: *Chow E et al., Radiother Oncol 2002*) for locally advanced NPC had better 5-yr DFS (48%) and OS (62%). Other groups (New York University: *Cooper JS et al., IJROBP 2000*) also demonstrated better outcomes with RT alone (3-yr DFS was 43%, and 3-yr OS was 61%).

What are the 3 key confirmatory randomized trials from Asia that demonstrated a benefit with CRT vs. RT alone for locoregionally advanced NPC?

Hong Kong (**NPC-9901:** *Lee AW et al., JCO 2005*): 348 pts, RCT, median follow-up 2.3 yrs; just concurrent cisplatin + RT, no adj chemo; better DFS (72% vs. 62%), LRC (92% vs. 82%), but not DM or OS; greater toxicity in the CRT arm (84% vs. 53%); greater otologic toxicity (28% vs. 13%)

Singapore (**SQNP01:** *Wee J et al., JCO 2005*): 221 pts, RCT, median follow-up 3.2 yrs; used **Al-Sarraf** regimen: better DFS (72% vs. 53%), OS (80% vs. 65%), and DM rate (13% vs. 30%); greater toxicity with CRT; confirmed results of **Intergroup 0099** for endemic NPC

Taiwan (*Lin JC et al., JCO 2003*): 284 pts, median follow-up 5.4 yrs; cisplatin/5-FU + RT vs. RT alone: better PFS (72% vs. 53%) and OS (72% vs. 54%). The subgroup reanalysis (*Lin JC et al., IJROBP 2004*) showed that CRT benefited low-risk "advanced" NPC (LN <6 cm, no SCV) but not high-risk "advanced" pts.

Is there a benefit with the use of induction chemo followed by RT or CRT in NPC?

No. Multiple RCTs in Asia demonstrated no benefit in terms of DFS, OS, or DM with induction chemo.

Is there a benefit with the use of adj chemo after definitive RT or CRT in NPC?

No. Multiple RCTs in Asia and 1 Italian study did not demonstrate a benefit with adj chemo.

Estimate the LC of NPC treated with IMRT to 70 Gy in standard fx.

UCSF data (*Lee N, IJROBP 2004*) suggests LC rates as high as 97% for NPC pts treated with IMRT.

What is the typical IMRT dose painting technique, and what are the corresponding IMRT doses used in the Tx of NPC?

Many institutions (Memorial Sloan Kettering Cancer Center [MSKCC]/RTOG) employ the simultaneous integrated boost technique: **2.12 Gy × 33 = 69.96 Gy** to GTV, **1.8 Gy × 33 = 59.4 Gy** to intermediate-risk areas, and **1.64 Gy × 33 = 54 Gy** to low-risk areas.

How would you support the use of IMRT in NPC?

Better salivary outcomes with IMRT were demonstrated in data from Queen Mary Hospital (*Pow EH et al., IJROBP 2006*): 51 pts, stage II NPC, 2D vs. IMRT. At 2 mos, there was no difference in xerostomia; however, over time, QOL and objective salivary function improved for the IMRT group.

What is the basic workup for SNT tumors?

SNT tumor workup: H&P, labs, CT/MRI head/neck, Bx, and CT C/A/P

Describe the T staging of maxillary tumors per the latest AJCC classification.

T1: confined to sinus, no bone erosion
T2: bone erosion *without* involvement of post wall of maxillary sinus or pterygoid plate
T3: invasion of post wall of max sinus, pterygoid fossa, floor/wall of orbit, ethmoid sinus
T4a: invasion of ant orbital structures, skin of cheek, pterygoid plate, infratemporal fossa, cribriform plate, sphenoid or frontal sinus
T4b: invasion of orbital apex, nasopharynx, clivus, intracranial extension, CN involvement (except V2)

How are the nodes staged for SNT tumors?

N1: single, ipsi, <3 cm
N2a: single, ipsi, 3–6 cm
N2b: multiple, ipsi, ≤6 cm
N2c: bilat or contralat ≤6 cm
N3: >6 cm

How are the overall SNT stage groups broken down (based on TNM)?

Stage I: T1N0
Stage II: T2N0
Stage III: T3N0 or T1-3N1
Stage IVA: T4aN0-2 or T1-3N2
Stage IVB: T4b or N3
Stage IVC: M1

What is the T stage for a maxillary tumor with involvement of the pterygoid plate vs. the pterygoid fossa?

Pterygoid **plate** involvement: **T4a**
Pterygoid **fossa** involvement: **T3**

What are the 2 most important prognostic factors for SNT tumors?

Clinical staging and the relationship of tumor to the Ohngren line

What is the Ohngren line, and why is it important?

The Ohngren line is a theoretic plane that extends **from the medial canthus of the eye to the angle of the mandible.** Tumors anteromedial to this plane have a better prognosis b/c of better surgical resection rates. Tumors superopost to this have deeper invasion, with many being unresectable (due to invasion of the orbit, ethmoids, and pterygopalatine fossa).

For SNT tumors, what factor predicts for nodal mets?

Neck nodal involvement is rare at Dx except **when tumors have progressed to involve the mucosal surfaces** (i.e., oral cavity, maxillary gingiva, or gingivobuccal sulcus).

What neck node groups are generally involved with SNT tumors?	**Level Ib or II, retropharyngeal (1st echelon), and periparotid nodes** are most commonly involved.
What subsite of SNT tumors has the highest rate of nodal mets?	**Maxillary sinus tumors** have the highest rate of nodal mets (10%–15%) of all SNT tumors.
What is the 5-yr OS rate for maxillary/ethmoid sinus tumors (all stages)?	The 5-yr OS rate for all stages of SNT tumors is ~**45%**
What is the 5-yr OS rate for N+ maxillary sinus tumors?	The 5-yr OS rate for N+ maxillary sinus tumors is **<10%.**
What is the 5-yr OS rate for nasal cavity tumors (all stages)?	The 5-yr OS rate for all stages of nasal cavity tumors is ~**60%.**
What is the overall LC rate for SNT tumors?	The overall LC rate is **50%–60%.**

▪ Treatment/Prognosis

How are SNT tumors typically managed?	**Surgical resection and adj RT +/− chemo.** Consider induction chemo in sinonasal undifferentiated carcinomas or in very advanced primary squamous carcinomas.
What type of surgery is necessary to manage a maxillary sinus tumor?	**Partial** (2 walls of maxilla removed) **or total maxillectomy to −margins.** For smaller medial tumors, a medial maxillectomy with a midfacial degloving technique is performed with an incision made under the lip. For larger tumors, access through the nasal crease/upper lip may be necessary. Reconstruction is done with skin grafting and obturator placement.
How are ethmoid sinus tumors managed surgically?	Ethmoid sinus tumors are surgically managed by **craniofacial resection,** requiring access both anteriorly through the sphenoethmoid area (through the nose) and superiorly with a craniotomy (neurosurgery) to address the skull base/dura.
When is orbital exenteration necessary in SNT tumors, and when is it not absolutely necessary?	It is **necessary if periorbital fat or extraocular muscles are involved**. It is **not necessary if there is only bone erosion.**
What are some nonadj indications for radiotherapy in the management of SNT tumors?	For inoperable tumors (medically and technically), early-stage tumors (T1-2N0), to preserve the eye, or preoperatively to downstage tumors before resection

What nerve provides motor innervation to the tongue?	The **hypoglossal nerve** (CN XII) provides motor innervation to the tongue.
Where is the ant-most border of the OC?	The **vermilion border of the lips** is the ant-most border of the OC.
Where is the post-most border of the OC?	The **hard/soft palate border superiorly and the circumvallate papillae inferiorly** are the post-most borders of the OC.
What are some premalignant lesions of the OC, and which type has the greatest propensity to progress to invasive cancer?	**Erythroplakia** (~30% progression rate) **and leukoplakia** (4%–18% progression rate) are premalignant lesions of the OC.
What are some risk factors that predispose to OCC?	Tobacco (smoked or chewed), betel nut consumption, alcohol, poor oral hygiene, and vitamin A deficiency
What are the sup and inf spans of level II–IV LN chains/levels?	<u>Level II</u>: skull base to hyoid <u>Level III</u>: hyoid to bottom of cricoid <u>Level IV</u>: cricoid to clavicles
Where are the level IA–IB nodes located?	Level IA nodes are **submental,** and level IB nodes are **submandibular.**
Where are the level V–VI nodes located?	Level V nodes are in the **post triangle,** and level VI nodes are in the **paratracheal/prelaryngeal region.**
What is the delphian node?	The delphian node is a **midline prelaryngeal level VI node.**
What are some important risk factors for LN mets in OCC?	Increasing DOI, increasing T stage, muscle invasion, and high-grade histology
What is the estimated risk of LN involvement with a T1-T2 primary of the lip, FOM, oral tongue, and buccal mucosa?	The risk of LN involvement is **~5% for the lip, 20% for the oral tongue, and ~10%–20% for the other OC T1-T2 primaries.**
What is the estimated risk of LN involvement with a T3-T4 primary of the lip, FOM, oral tongue, and buccal mucosa?	The risk of LN involvement is **~33% for the lip and ~33%–67% for the other OC T3-T4 primaries.**
What is the nodal met rate for a T1 vs. T2 lesion of the oral tongue?	The nodal met rate is **14% for T1 tongue lesions and 30% for T2 tongue lesions**. (*Lindberg R et al., Cancer 1972*)

What is the overall and stage-by-stage nodal met rate for FOM lesions?

Overall: 20%–30%
T1: 10%
T2: 30%
T3: 45%
T4: >50%

(*Lindberg R et al., Cancer 1972*)

Lesions located where in the OC predispose to bilat LN mets?

Midline and anterolat OC lesions (tongue, FOM) predispose to bilat LN mets.

Which OC cancer has the greatest propensity for LN spread?

Oral tongue cancer has the greatest propensity for LN spread.

What OC subsite is 2nd only to the oral tongue in propensity for nodal spread?

The **alveolar ridge/RMT** has the 2nd highest propensity for LN spread (3rd highest is FOM).

Can ant oral tongue lesions involve other LN levels without involving level I LNs?

Yes. ~13% of ant tongue lesions skip the level I LNs. (*Byers RM et al., Head Neck 1997*)

Which anatomic structure divides the oral tongue from the base of tongue (BOT)?

The **circumvallate papillae** divide the oral tongue from the BOT (per the AJCC). Some use the sulcus terminalis as the border.

What type of tumors arise from the hard palate?

Primarily **minor salivary gland tumors** (adenoid cystic, mucoepidermoid, adenocarcinoma) arise from the hard palate.

What are common sites of DM for cancers of the OC?

Lungs, bones, and liver

What anatomic structure divides the FOM anteriorly into 2 halves?

The **lingual frenulum** divides the FOM anteriorly.

Where is the Wharton duct located, and what gland does it drain?

The Wharton duct **opens at the ant FOM** (midline) and **drains the submandibular gland.**

From where in the OC do most gingival cancers arise?

Most (80%) gingival cancers arise from the **lower gingiva.**

Do most lip cancers arise from the upper or lower lip?

Most (~90%) lip cancers arise from the **lower lip.**

What pathologic features of the OCC primary lesion call for prophylactic/ elective neck management?

Tumor thickness >3 mm, grade III Dz, +LVI, and a recurrent lesion are features that increase the need for prophylactic neck management.

What are the indications for PORT to the ipsi neck in OCC?

>N2a (>3-cm LN) or >2 LN levels, ECE, no neck dissection in high-risk pts, and a DOI (primary) >3mm are indications for PORT.

When should bilat neck irradiation be considered for OC lesions?

Bilat neck RT should be considered for **midline primaries, for ant tongue tumors, and with ipsi LAD.**

When is bilat neck dissection recommended for lesions of the OC?

Bilat neck dissection is recommended with **≥N2c Dz** (bilat or bulky LNs).

For what OC sites is definitive RT preferred and why?

Definitive RT is preferred (over surgery) for **lip commissure, buccal mucosa, and RMT lesions with tonsillar pillar involvement.** There is **better cosmesis with RT** (surgery is too morbid).

What is an adequate surgical margin for OC cancers?

The adequate surgical margin is typically **1 cm** (1.5 cm for the oral tongue).

What are the indications for PORT to the primary site for OC lesions?

+ or close (<2 mm) margin, DOI >2 mm, PNI/ perivascular invasion, and T3-T4 Dz are indications for PORT.

What RT doses are typically used in OCC, and how is RT delivered?

PORT: **54** (–margins) to **66 Gy** (+margins) in 2 Gy/fx
Definitive RT: **54 → 70 Gy** to gross Dz +/− chemo

RT has been typically **delivered via opposed lat fields** (IMRT can now be considered for T3-T4 tumors).

When is brachytherapy indicated for OCC?

Definitive: early (T1-T2) lip/early oral tongue/ FOM lesions—LDR to **66–70 Gy** in 1 Gy/hr
As a supplement: T4 tongue/FOM lesions, 40% of total dose or ~**30 Gy**

For oral tongue lesions, which modality is associated with better LC: LDR or HDR?

Both modalities yield similar results. 5-yr LC was 76%–77% for both HDR and LDR techniques in a phase III comparison. (*Inoue T et al., IJROBP 2001*)

What are the common LDR and HDR doses used with an interstitial implant for OCC?

Low dose rate: 60–70 Gy (40–60 cGy/hr)
High dose rate: 60 Gy (5 Gy bid × 12 fx)

What alternate teletherapy modalities can be employed for superficial OC lesions?

An **intraoral cone** can be employed for superficial OC lesions: orthovoltage (100–250 keV) or electrons (6–12 MeV).

What are the borders of the standard lat fields for oral tongue lesions?

Superior: 1–1.5 cm above dorsum of tongue or 2 cm above tumor
Inferior: thyroid notch
Posterior: spinous process
Anterior: 2 cm ant to tumor

What beam-modifying device is used with standard opposed lat fields for the Tx of OC lesions? What beam energy is typically used?

Wedges (usually 30 degree with heels ant) are typically used with standard fields, and the beam energy is **6 MV.**

How can the lat fields be tilted to spare the contralat parotid gland, and what wedge angle is used if this is done?

The lat fields are tilted **obliquely** away from contralat parotid, and a **15-degree wedge** is typically used if this is done.

Why is a tongue depressor/ bite block used when irradiating the OC?

A tongue depressor is used **to spare the sup OC/hard palate and to surround the lat oral tongue lesion with other mucosa** to minimize any buildup effect on the lat surfaces.

What kind of surgical resection is typically performed for leukoplakia or CIS of the lip?

Vermilionectomy with advancement of the mucosal flap ("lip shave"), which involves simple excision from the vermilion to the orbicularis muscle

When is surgery an option for cancers of the lip?

Surgery is an option **if the lesion involves <30% of the lip, if it is a T1 lesion, or the lesion does *not* involve the oral commissure;** otherwise use RT, typically WLE with primary closure (W-shaped excision) and with a 0.5-cm gross margin.

When is definitive RT used for cancers of the lip?

Definitive RT is used for lip tumors **>2 cm, large lesions (>50% of the lip), upper lip lesions, or if the lesion involves the oral commissure.**

Is elective nodal RT of the neck required for T1-T2 cancers of the lip?

No. Elective nodal RT is not needed b/c the occult nodal positivity rate is only ~5%.

What are the doses used for the Tx of T1-T2 cancers of the lip?

T1: 50 Gy (2.5 Gy × 20)
T2: 60 Gy (2.5 Gy × 24) with 100–250 keV photons or 6–9 MeV electrons + 1-cm bolus

When is PORT indicated for lip cancers?

PORT is indicated for lip cancers in case of **T4 Dz (bone invasion), +margin, extensive PNI, +ECE, ≥2 nodes+, or T3-T4 Dz without dissection of the neck.**

What are the 4 most important risk factors for the development of OPC?

Risk factors for developing OPC:
1. Smoking
2. Alcohol
3. HPV infection (HPV 16)
4. Betel nut consumption

What is the 1st-echelon drainage region for most OPCs?

The 1st-echelon drainage site for most OPCs is the **level II (upper jugulodigastric) nodes.**

Are skipped mets common for OPC?

No. Skipped mets are **extremely rare** in OPC (<1%).

What are the 2 most common histologies encountered in the OPX? Rare histologies?

Most common histologies: squamous cell carcinoma (SCC) (90%), non-Hodgkin lymphoma (10% tonsil, 2% BOT)
Rare histologies: lymphoepithelioma, adenoid cystic carcinoma, plasmacytoma, melanoma, small cell carcinoma, mets

What % of pts with OPC fail locoregionally vs. distantly?

50% of OPC pts fail locally, and **50%** fail distantly.

How prevalent is HPV infection in OPC?

Depending on the series, ~**40%–80%** of OPCs are associated with HPV infection.

Which HPV serotype is most commonly associated with OPC?

HPV 16 is the most common serotype in OPC (80%–90%).

What is a surrogate marker of HPV infection in OPC that can be used as an indirect indication of HPV seropositivity?

The surrogate marker for HPV infection is **p16 staining;** E7 protein inactivates Rb, which upregulates p16.

Which pt population is most likely to present with HPV-related OPC?

Nonsmokers and nondrinkers are most likely to have HPV+ SCC of the OPX.

Do HPV+ or HPV− OPC pts have a better prognosis?

HPV+ OPC pts have a better prognosis. Data from **RTOG 0129** (*Ang KK et al., NEJM 2010*) showed better 3-yr OS (82.4% vs. 57.1%) and risk of death (HR 0.42) for HPV+ pts. Smoking was an independent poor prognostic factor.

What is the hypothesis behind why HPV+ OPC pts have a better prognosis?

HPV+ H&N cancers are **usually in nonsmokers and nondrinkers, so p53 status is usually nonmutated;** p53 mutation (which is common in non–HPV-related H&N cancers) predicts for a poor response to Tx.

■ Workup/Staging

What nerves are responsible for otalgia in cancers of the oral tongue, BOT, and larynx/hypopharynx (HPX)?

Oral tongue: CN V (auriculotemporal) → preauricular area
BOT: CN IX (Jacobson nerve) → tympanic cavity
Larynx/HPX: CN X (Arnold nerve) → postauricular area

What is the most common presentation of OPC?

The most common presentation is a **neck mass,** especially with HPV+ OPC.

What are additional common presenting Sx by OPX subsite?

Base of tongue: sore throat, dysphagia, otalgia, neck mass
Tonsils: sore throat, trismus, otalgia, neck mass
Soft palate: leukoplakia, sore throat with swallowing, trismus/perforation, phonation defect with advanced lesions
Pharyngeal wall: pain/odynophagia, bleeding

Describe the workup for a pt with an OPX mass.

OPX mass workup: H&P (bimanual exam of the floor of mouth), labs, direct laryngoscopy, CT/MRI H&N, tissue Bx (EUA if necessary), and CXR (or CT chest)

If the neck mass Bx is positive, is an additional Bx of the primary lesion necessary?

Yes. A Bx of the primary (or suspected primary) should also be done.

What % of OPC pts have clinically occult nodal mets?

30%–50% of OPC pts have clinically occult nodal mets.

What % of OPC pts present with clinically+ nodes, and what % present with bilat nodal Dz?

~**75%** of OPC pts have clinically+ nodes at presentation, with ~**30%** having bilat Dz (especially if lesions are BOT/midline).

What is the T staging of OPC?

T staging of OPC is similar to other **SOOTH** (salivary, oral cavity, oropharynx, thyroid, hypopharynx) H&N cancers:
T1: ≤2 cm
T2: 2–4 cm
T3: >4 cm
T4a (moderately advanced): invades larynx, deep/extrinsic tongue muscles, medial pterygoid, hard palate, mandible
T4b (very advanced): invades lat pterygoid muscle, pterygoid plate, lat nasopharynx, skull invasion, carotid encasement

What are the typical RT doses used for OPC?

<u>T0-1</u>: **66 Gy**
<u>≥T1</u>: **70 Gy,** or **81.6 Gy** with hyperfractionation

What is the 2-yr LF rate after IMRT alone for early (T1-2N0-1) OPC?

RTOG 00-22 (*Eisbruch A et al., IJROBP 2010*) demonstrated excellent results with accelerated hypofractionated IMRT for early OPC: **2-yr LRF was 9%** (if major deviations, 50%; otherwise 6%, SS).

What were the RT techniques and doses employed in RTOG 00-22?

In **RTOG 00-22** (*Eisbruch A et al., IJROBP 2010*), RT was delivered with accelerated hypofractionated IMRT as follows: 66 Gy in 30 fx (2.2 Gy/fx) to the primary target PTV and 54–60 Gy in 30 fx (1.8–2 Gy/fx) to the secondary target PTV.

How was the N stage established in RTOG 00-22 for eligibility purposes?

For **RTOG 00-22** (*Eisbruch A et al., IJROBP 2010*), **neck staging was clinical** (not from CT); however, pts "upstaged" by CT (e.g., cN1 but N2 after CT) were also eligible.

What did the RTOG 90-03 study demonstrate about the use of altered fractionation in H&N cancers?

RTOG 90-03 (*Fu KK et al., IJROBP 2000*): 1,073 pts with H&N cancers (10% oral cavity [OC], 60% OPX, 13% HPX) with stage III (28%) or stage IV (68%) Dz randomized to (a) conventional 70 Gy qd, (b) 81.6 Gy in 1.2 Gy/fx bid, (c) accelerated with split, and (d) concomitant boost (1.8 Gy/fx qd × 17, with last 12 fx bid with 1.8 Gy am, 1.5 Gy pm to 72 Gy). There was better LC with altered fx (54% vs. 46%) but no OS/DFS benefit. There was worse acute toxicity but no difference in late toxicity.

What randomized studies demonstrated better outcomes with hyperfractionated RT over conventional RT for OPC?

RTOG 90-03 (*Fu KK et al., IJROBP 2000*): See above.

EORTC 22791 (*Horiot JC et al., Radiother Oncol 1992*): 325 pts (all OPX, but no BOT): 70 Gy vs. 80.5 Gy at 1.15 Gy bid. There was better LC (60% vs. 40%) but no OS benefit. LC was best for T3 Dz.

What data showed good LC rates with RT alone for select advanced (stage III–IV) OPCs?

MDACC data (*Garden AS et al., Cancer 2004*): pts with small primaries but stage III–IV Dz by virtue of +LNs; treated with RT alone. There were acceptable 5-yr LF (15%), DM (19%), and OS (64%) rates.

What are 2 important randomized trials that demonstrated the importance of adding chemo to conventionally fractionated RT in OPC?

GORTEC 94-01 (*Calais G et al., JNCI 1999*): 222 pts with stage III–IV OPC randomized to conventional RT alone vs. conventional RT + carboplatin/5-FU, no planned neck dissection for N2-3 Dz. The CRT arm had better 3-yr OS (51% vs. 31%), DFS (30% vs. 15%), and LC (66% vs. 42%); however, there was significantly worse grade 3–4 mucositis and weight loss/feeding tube use in the CRT arm.

Cleveland Clinic data (*Adelstein DJ et al., JCO 2003*): 295 pts with unresectable stage III–IV H&N cancers (15% OC, 55% OPX, 20% HPX), RT alone vs. CRT with cisplatin 100 mg q3wks × 3. 3-yr OS was better in the CRT arm (37% vs. 23%). There also was improved DFS (51% vs. 33%) in the CRT arm.

What are the indications for adding chemo to PORT in H&N cancers, and what are 2 important RCTs that support this?

Pooled analysis suggests **+margin and ECE** as the most important indications.

EORTC 22931 (*Bernier J et al., NEJM 2004*): 334 pts randomized to PORT 66 Gy vs. PORT + cisplatin 100 mg/m^2 on days 1, 22, and 43. Eligibility: ECE, +margin, PNI, LVI, and level 4–5 +N from OCC/OPC. There was better OS, DFS, and 5-yr LC with CRT but ↑ grade 3–4 toxicity.

RTOG 95-01 (*Cooper JS et al., NEJM 2004*): 459 pts randomized to 60–66 Gy PORT vs. PORT + cisplatin 100 mg/m^2 on days 1, 22, and 43. Eligibility: >2 LN, ECE, +margin. There was better DFS (43% vs. 54%) and 2-yr LRC (72% vs. 82%) but only a trend to improvement in OS (57% vs. 63%).

What study demonstrated improvement in OS with the addition of cetuximab (C225) to RT in H&N cancers?

Bonner et al. (*NEJM 2006*): 424 pts with stage III–IV SCC of the OPX, laryngeal cancer (LCX), or HC randomized to RT vs. RT + C225. RT options were conventional to 70 Gy, 1.2 bid to 72–76.8 Gy, or concomitant boost to 72 Gy. There was better 3-yr LRC (47% vs. 34%) and OS (55% vs. 45%) with C225 + RT. Subset analysis showed improvement mostly in OPC and in the altered fractionation RT arms (~50% treated with altered fractionation).

What 2 randomized studies demonstrated a benefit with induction taxane/platinum/5-FU (TPF) chemo → RT or CRT in pts with unresectable H&N cancers?

TAX 324 study (induction chemo → CRT) (*Posner MR et al., NEJM 2007*): 501 pts, unresectable stage III–IV H&N cancers (52% OPX, ~13%–18% OC, larynx, HPX) randomized to induction platinum + 5-FU or TPF → CRT with carboplatin. There was better 3-yr OS (62% vs. 48%), MS (71 mos vs. 30 mos), and LRC (70% vs. 62%) in the TPF arm. Pts in the TPF arm had fewer Tx delays than in the platinum/5-FU arm despite higher myelotoxicity in the TPF arm (98% rcv planned Tx in the TPF arm vs. 90% in the PF arm).

What is the most common type of benign tumor of the salivary gland, and where is it most commonly found?

Pleomorphic adenoma (65%). It is most commonly found in the **parotid glands.**

In addition to pleomorphic adenoma, what are some other benign salivary gland tumors?

Warthin tumor (papillary cystadenoma lymphomatosum), Godwin tumor (benign lymphoepithelial lesion, associated with Sjögren), and monomorphic adenoma (oncocytoma, basal cell)

What is the most common malignant salivary gland tumor, and where is it most commonly found?

Mucoepidermoid carcinoma. It most commonly arises in the **parotid** (most are low grade, but if the tumor is high grade, it needs to be managed with surgery + LND + adj RT).

How are tumors of the salivary gland separated into low vs. intermediate vs. high grade by histology?

Low grade: acinic cell carcinoma
Intermediate grade: mucoepidermoid carcinoma, adenocarcinoma
High grade: adenoid cystic carcinoma, squamous cell carcinoma, carcinoma expleomorphic adenoma (malignant mixed tumor), lymphoepithelioma (mostly Asians), ductal carcinoma

What is the relationship between the gland size and malignant nature of the salivary tumor?

Typically, **the smaller the gland, the more malignant the tumor.**

What is the approximate incidence ratio of benign to malignant tumors in the various salivary glands?

Approximate incidence ratio of benign to malignant tumors:
1. Parotid, ~75:25
2. Submandibular gland, ~50:50
3. Sublingual gland, ~10:90
4. Minor salivary, ~10:90

What is the most common malignant histology arising in the submandibular gland?

Adenoid cystic carcinoma is the most common malignant histology of the submandibular gland.

What is the most common malignant histology arising in the minor salivary glands?

Adenoid cystic carcinoma is the most common malignant histology of the minor salivary glands.

Where are the minor salivary glands found in the H&N?

Minor salivary glands are found in the **mucosal lining of the aerodigestive tract.** Most are in the oral cavity (OC) (85%–90%), with the palate (especially the hard palate) being the #1 site. They can be found in all sites of the OC, nasal cavity, paranasal sinus, oropharynx, and larynx.

What are the risk factors for developing salivary gland tumors?

Ionizing RT, wood dust inhalation, personal Hx of tumor, and family Hx

What is the lymphatic drainage predilection of the parotid, submandibular/sublingual, and minor salivary glands?

Lymphatic drainage predilection:
Parotid: preauricular, periparotid, and intraparotid, with deep intraparotid nodes draining to levels II–III
Submandibular/sublingual: level I–II nodes
Minor salivary: depends on site of involvement, but LNs commonly involved b/c of rich lymphatic network

How does the propensity for cervical LN mets relate to the site of origin of the salivary tumor?

The propensity for LN spread is **greatest for the minor salivary gland > submandibular/sublingual > parotid gland malignancies.**

What is the natural Hx of adenoid cystic carcinoma?

Perineural invasion with skipped lesions and late recurrence with DMs (up to 10–15 yrs with pulmonary mets, earlier for bone or viscera) are common. However, the rates are low for cervical nodal mets (5%–8%).

What % of pts with adenoid cystic carcinoma ultimately go on to develop lung mets?

~**40%** of pts with adenoid cystic carcinoma ultimately develop lung mets.

■ Workup/Staging

What is the most common presentation of parotid gland tumors?

A **painless, solitary mass** is the most common presentation of parotid gland tumors.

For what does a painful growth/mass in the salivary gland predict?

It predicts for **malignancy or an inflammatory etiology/condition.**

What are some other presenting Sx in pts with salivary gland tumors?

Pain, facial weakness from CN VII involvement, rapid growth of mass, skin involvement, neck node, and dysphagia/otalgia from CN IX–XII palsies

What is the DDx for a parotid mass?

Primary tumor, mets, lymphoma, parotitis, sarcoid, cyst, Sjögren, stone, lipoma, hemangioma, and a prominent C1 transverse process

What are the 2 most important factors that predict for nodal mets in salivary gland malignancies?

Grade and size are the 2 most important factors that predict for nodal mets: high grade (50%) vs. intermediate/low grade (<10%) and size (>4 cm: 20% vs. <4 cm: 4%).

What is the typical workup performed for salivary gland tumors?

Salivary gland tumor workup: H&P (CNs/nodes), CBC, CMP, CXR, CT/MRI H&N, and Bx

How should Bx be obtained for pts who present with a salivary gland mass?

Excisional Bx is preferred, though FNA may be adequate (however, the FN rate is 20%).

What does the mnemonic *SOOTH* stand for in terms of T staging of the H&N?

Salivary
Oral cavity
Oropharynx
Thyroid
Hyopharynx

(Mnemonic: **SOOTH**) SOOTH tumors are the H&N tumors with similar size-dependent T staging.

What is the T-staging breakdown for major salivary gland tumors?

T1: ≤2 cm
T2: 2–4 cm
T3: >4 cm (and/or extraglandular extension)
T4(a-b): local invasion of adjacent structures (see below)

What salivary gland tumors are considered T3?

T3 salivary gland tumors are **tumors with extraglandular extension or tumors >4 cm**

What is the distinction between T4a vs. T4b major salivary gland tumors?

T4a: usually still resectable; skin, mandible, ear, facial nerve invasion
T4b: usually unresectable; skull base, pterygoid plate, carotid artery invasion

What is the nodal staging system used for major salivary gland tumors?

Nodal staging is the same as for other H&N sites (except for the nasopharynx):
N1: single, ipsi, <3 cm
N2a: single, ipsi, 3–6 cm
N2b: multiple, ipsi, ≤6 cm
N2c: bilat or contralat ≤6 cm
N3: >6 cm

Per the latest AJCC 7th edition classification, what are the stage groupings for major salivary gland tumors?

Stage I: T1N0
Stage II: T2N0
Stage III: T3N0 or T1-3N1
Stage IVA: T4aN0-1 or T1-4aN2
Stage IVB: T4b any N or any TN3
Stage IVC: any T any NM1

On what is the staging system for the minor salivary gland tumors based?

Staging of the minor salivary gland tumors is based on the **site of origin.**

What are some important prognostic factors in salivary gland tumors?

Size, grade, histology, nodal status, and "named" nerve involvement are important prognostic factors.

What is the 5-yr OS for stage I–IV cancers of the salivary gland?	**Stage I:** 80% **Stage II:** 60% **Stage III:** 50% **Stage IV:** 30%
What is the 5-yr OS of pts who present with facial nerve involvement?	The 5-yr OS is **65% with simple invasion and 10% if pts have nerve dysfunction** (i.e., if symptomatic).

■ Treatment/Prognosis

What is the general management paradigm for benign mixed/ pleomorphic adenoma of the parotid?	Benign mixed/pleomorphic adenoma management paradigm: **WLE, or superficial parotid lobectomy → observation** (even if +margin or with extraglandular extension)
What is the management paradigm for low- to intermediate-grade tumors of the salivary gland?	Low- to intermediate-grade salivary gland tumor management paradigm: **superficial parotidectomy with PORT** for close (<2 mm) or +margin, unresectable Dz, pT3, PNI, capsule rupture, +nodes, or recurrent Dz
What is the management paradigm for high-grade tumors of the salivary gland?	High-grade salivary gland tumor management paradigm: **total parotidectomy** (facial nerve sparing, if possible) **with ipsi LND → PORT or CRT** (RT volumes to encompass perineural pathways to the base of skull if "named" nerve involvement)
What is the management paradigm for adenoid cystic carcinoma with pulmonary mets?	Adenoid cystic carcinoma with pulmonary met management paradigm: **same local therapy as in high-grade tumors** since pulmonary mets have a long natural Hx (*Garden AS et al., IJROBP 1995*)
What is the difference between superficial, total, and radical parotidectomy?	<u>Superficial</u>: en bloc resection of gland superficial to CN VII <u>Total</u>: en bloc resection of entire gland with nerve sparing <u>Radical</u>: en bloc resection of entire gland + CN VII + skin + fascia +/− muscle
What are the indications for LND with salivary gland tumors?	**High grade, large tumors, and a clinically+ neck** are all indications for elective LND.
What are the indications for PORT in the management of salivary gland cancers?	Adj RT is indicated for the following: **high grade (regardless of margin), close/+margin, pT3-T4 Dz, PNI, capsule rupture, tumor spillage, ECE, N2-N3 Dz, unresectable tumor/gross residual Dz, and recurrent tumor**

For what cN0 salivary gland tumors, by histology, does elective nodal RT significantly reduce the incidence of nodal relapse?

Elective nodal RT is more likely to reduce the incidence of nodal relapse in **pts with squamous, undifferentiated, or adenocarcinoma histologies**. (*Chen AM et al., IJROBP 2007*)

When should bilat neck coverage with RT be considered for salivary gland neoplasms?

Whenever there is **multilevel nodal involvement and >50% of removed nodes are involved**; otherwise, the ipsi neck is adequate.

What are some ways to deliver RT/set up the RT fields in the Tx of parotid gland tumors?

RT delivery and setup of RT fields:
1. **AP/PA wedge pairs** (120-degree hinge angle) but difficult setup, exit through OC
2. **Sup/Inf wedge pair** (with 90-degree couch kick), avoids exit through OC but exits through brain
3. **Single direct field with 4:1 mixed energy beam** (80% 15 MeV electron: 20% 6 MV photon) with bolus, electron portal 1 cm larger than the photon field b/c of IDL constriction with depth, higher dose to bone, keep contralat parotid at <30 Gy
4. **IMRT**

What are the PORT doses used in the management of salivary gland tumors?

60 Gy for −margin, **66 Gy** for close/+margin, **70 Gy** for gross residual, and **50–54 Gy** to a low-risk neck

What RT techniques are used in the management of the ipsi neck?

RT techniques for the ipsi neck:
1. Single lat appositional electron field
2. Mixed electron-photon beam technique
3. Half beam block technique

What are the indications for chemo and the agents used for salivary cancer?

The indications for chemo (+/−RT) include **unresectable, recurrent, or metastatic Dz,** and the active regimens are **cisplatin/5-FU or Adr/Cytoxan**

What key retrospective data demonstrated the importance of adding PORT for stage III–IV and high-grade salivary gland tumors?

MSKCC data (*Armstrong JG et al., Arch Otolaryngol Head Neck Surg 1990; Harrison L et al., J Surg Oncol 1990*) showed improved LC and survival.

What is the largest retrospective study demonstrating a benefit of adj RT for malignant salivary gland neoplasms?

Dutch NWHHT study (*Terhaard CHJ et al., IJROBP 2005*): 498 pts. Adj RT significantly improved LC in pts with T3-T4 Dz, a close margin, incomplete resection, bony invasion, and PNI.

What is the best RT modality for managing unresectable salivary gland tumors?

Neutrons (superior LC, with photons showing LC of 25% for inoperable cases). If no access to neutrons, EBRT + implant is a good choice.

What is the key prospective randomized trial that demonstrated superior LC outcomes with the use of neutrons over photons/electrons in the Tx of unresectable salivary gland tumors?

RTOG-MRC trial (*Laramore G et al., IJROBP 1993*): 10-yr LRC was 17% vs. 56% (neutrons), SS. 10-yr OS was 15% vs. 25%, NSS.

How is neutron RT prescribed in the Tx of unresectable salivary gland tumors?

1.2 neutron Gy, 4 times/wk → 19.2 nGy for gross Dz (13.2 nGy for uninvolved nodes)

When is surgical resection alone adequate in the management of recurrent salivary gland tumors?

If tumors are of low/intermediate grade, <3 cm, and there are no other risk features, then surgery alone may suffice.

■ Toxicity

What is Frey syndrome, and from what does it result?

Auriculotemporal nerve syndrome (gustatory sweating or redness and sweating on the cheek area when the pt eats, sees, or thinks about or talks about certain kinds of food). It is a **postop complication of parotidectomy.**

What are some possible Tx sequelae from RT?

Xerostomia and otitis media with partial hearing loss

Above what RT doses can salivary gland function be compromised, resulting in xerostomia?

Usually, doses **>26–30 Gy** result in salivary gland dysfunction/xerostomia.

What is the general follow-up for pts with salivary gland neoplasms?

Per the NCCN, H&P (q1–3mos for yr 1, q2–4mos for yr 2, q4–6mos for yrs 3–5, and q6–12mos thereafter), chest imaging if clinically indicated, and TSH q6–12mos if neck RT

■ Workup/Staging

How do pts with LCX typically present?	Hoarseness, odynophagia/sore throat, otalgia (via the Arnold nerve, CN X), aspiration/choking, and neck mass
What is the typical workup for pts presenting with a possible laryngeal mass?	Possible laryngeal mass workup: H&P (voice change, habits, indirect/direct laryngoscopy), CXR, CT/MRI, PET, basic labs, EUA + triple endoscopy, and Bx of the primary +/− FNA of the neck mass
What does the loss of the laryngeal click on palpation of the thyroid cartilage indicate?	Loss of the laryngeal click on exam indicates **postcricoid extension/involvement.**
What does pain in the thyroid cartilage indicate on exam?	Pain on palpation of the thyroid cartilage indicates **tumor invasion into the thyroid cartilage.**
What imaging device is best to assess for bony or cartilage erosion in pts with LCX?	**CT scan** is best for assessing bony/cartilage erosion.
What is the incidence of nodal involvement for T1, T2, and T3-T4 glottic cancer?	**T1:** 0%–2% **T2:** 2%–7% **T3-T4:** 15%–30%
What is the incidence of nodal involvement for supraglottic lesions according to T stage?	**T1:** 39% **T2:** 42% **T3:** 65% **T4:** 59% (*Lindberg R et al., Cancer 1972*)
What proportion of pts with supraglottic cancer present with unilat vs. bilat nodal Dz?	~**55%** of supraglottic cancer pts present with unilat nodal Dz, and **16%** present with bilat nodal involvement. (*Lindberg R et al., Cancer 1972*)
What % of pts with subglottic cancer present with nodal involvement?	~**20%–50%** of subglottic pts present with nodal Dz (generally the prelaryngeal/delphian, lower jugular, pretracheal, or upper mediastinal nodes).
Describe the T staging for cancers of the supraglottic larynx.	**T1:** 1 subsite **T2:** 1 adjacent subsite or outside supraglottis (base of tongue [BOT], vallecula, pyriform sinus) without fixation of larynx **T3:** cord fixation and/or invasion of postcricoid area or pre-epiglottic tissue **T4a (resectable):** through thyroid cartilage, trachea, soft tissue of neck, deep/intrinsic muscles of tongue, thyroid, esophagus **T4b:** invasion of prevertebral space, mediastinum, carotid

Describe the T staging for cancers of the glottic larynx.

T1: limited to TVCs +/− ant/post commissure involvement with normal mobility (1a, 1 TVC; 1b, both cords)

T2: extends to supra- or subglottis with impaired vocal cord mobility

T3: fixed vocal cords

T4a-b: same as above/for supraglottic lesions

What is the T-staging breakdown for cancers of the subglottic larynx?

T1: tumor limited to subglottis

T2: extension to vocal cords, with normal or impaired mobility

T3: limited to larynx with vocal cord fixation

T4a-b: same as above

Describe the overall stage groupings for LCX.

Stages I–II: T1-2N0
Stage III: T3N0 or N1
Stage IVA: T4a or N2
Stage IVB: T4b or N3
Stage IVC: M1

With what stage of Dz do most pts with HPC present?

Most pts (>80%) present with **stage III or IV Dz** (lesions remain asymptomatic until the advanced stages).

What % of pts with HPC present with DMs?

~**2%–4%** of HPC pts present with DMs. ~20%–30% develop DMs within 2 yrs despite Tx.

With what Sx do most HPC pts present?

Neck mass, sore throat, dysphagia, hoarseness, and otalgia (Arnold nerve/CN X involvement)

What is the typical workup for pts who present with hoarseness?

Hoarseness workup: H&P (check for thyroid click), labs, CT/MRI, PET, neck FNA, EUA + triple endoscopy, and Bx of the primary mass

Describe the T staging of HPC.

T1: <2 cm or 1 subsite

T2: 2–4 cm or >1 subsite

T3: >4 cm or fixation of hemilarynx

T4a: invades thyroid/cricoid cartilage, hyoid bone, thyroid gland, esophagus, or central soft tissue

T4b: invades prevertebral fascia, carotid artery, or mediastinal structures

What is the nodal staging breakdown for HPC?

Same system as used for other H&N cancers (except for nasopharynx):

N1: single, ipsi, <3 cm
N2a: single, ipsi, 3–6 cm
N2b: multiple, ipsi, ≤6 cm
N2c: bilat or contralat ≤6 cm
N3: >6 cm

Describe the overall stage groupings for HPC.

Stages I–II: T1-2N0
Stage III: T3N0 or N1
Stage IVA: T4a or N2
Stage IVB: T4b or N3
Stage IVC: M1

■ Treatment/Prognosis

What does total laryngectomy entail?

It entails the **removal of the hyoid, thyroid and cricoid cartilage, epiglottis, and strap muscle with reconstruction of the pharynx as well as a permanent tracheostomy.**

What structures are removed with a supraglottic laryngectomy?

A supraglottic laryngectomy sacrifices the **FVCs, epiglottis, and aryepiglottic folds.**

What is the preferred surgical option for dysplastic lesions on the glottic larynx?

Mucosal stripping is typically curative for dysplastic lesions. Close follow-up is needed.

What are the Tx options for Tis lesions of the glottic larynx?

Cord stripping/laser excision (need close follow-up; cannot r/o microinvasive Dz) **or definitive RT**

What are the ~5-yr LC rates for glottic CIS with the use of stripping vs. laser vs. RT?

Stripping: 72%
Laser: 83%
RT: 88%–92% (all >95% after salvage)

What are the Tx options for T1-T2 glottic cancer?

Cordectomy (CO_2 laser)/partial laryngectomy, definitive RT alone, or surgery + CRT for +margin, and ECE (based on postop H&N data)

What are the 5-yr control and survival rates after hemilaryngectomy for T1-T2 glottic cancer?

After hemilaryngectomy, the **~5-yr LC is 83%** and the **DFS is 88%** for T1-T2 glottic cancer. (*Scola B et al., Laryngology 1999*)

What is the salvage Tx of choice for glottic lesions after RT failure?

The salvage Tx of choice is **total laryngectomy +/− neck dissection.**

What is the ~5-yr CSS for T1 glottic cancers treated with definitive RT?

The 5-yr CSS with RT is **>90%** (95% with salvage; organ preservation rate is >90%).

What are the advantages and disadvantages of using RT for early glottic cancer?

Advantages: better voice quality, noninvasive, organ preservation
Disadvantages: long Tx duration, RT changes could obscure post-Tx surveillance

What is the voice quality preservation rate for early glottic tumors/pts treated with laser vs. RT?

The Johns Hopkins Hospital data (*Epstein BE et al., Radiology 1990*) suggests **better voice quality after RT** (laser: 31%, RT: 74%, $p = 0.012$).

What are the initial and ultimate (after salvage) LC rates for T2 glottic lesions?

Initial LC is ~70%–90% and **~50%–70% after salvage** for T2 glottic lesions.

What are the currently accepted dose fractionation and total dose Rx for CIS and T1 glottic lesions?

The currently accepted RT doses are **56.25 Gy for CIS** and **63 Gy for T1,** at **2.25 Gy/fx.**

What is the typical RT dose used for T2 glottic lesions?

The typical RT dose for T2 lesions is **70 Gy at 2 Gy/fx** or **65.25 Gy at 2.25 Gy/fx.**

What randomized data/ trial highlighted the importance of hypofractionation for early glottic cancers?

Japanese data (*Yamazaki H et al., IJROBP 2006*): 180 pts, 2 fractionations: 2 Gy/fx (60–66 Gy) vs. 2.25 Gy/fx (56.25–63 Gy). 5-yr LC rate was better with 2.25 Gy/fx (92% vs. 72%). The greater toxicity for the hypofractionation regimen was acute skin erythema (83% vs. 63%).

What RT field sizes/spans are employed for Tis/T1 glottic cancers?

5 × 5 cm opposed lat fields are typically employed (from the upper thyroid notch to the lower border of the cricoid, post border at the ant edge of the vertebral body, and flash skin at the ant border).

What RT planning technique can be used when treating T1 glottic lesions with ant commissure involvement?

Generally, for T1 glottic lesions, **wedges** are used (heel anteriorly, usually 15 degrees) to reduce ant hotspots due to curvature of the neck. However, if there is ant commissure Dz, the wedges can be removed to add hotspots to this region. Alternatively, a bolus/beam spoiler can be added for additional coverage.

What structures must be encompassed by the 95% IDL when irradiating T1 glottic cancer?

The 95% IDL must encompass the **TVCs, the FVCs, and the sup subglottis.**

What RT fields are used for T2 glottic lesions?

This is **controversial** and may depend upon degree of supraglottic/subglottic extension. Most advocate using 6 × 6 cm opposed lat fields; others advocate covering level II–III nodes (2 cm above the angle of the mandible, splitting vertebral body, down to the bottom of the cricoid) to **54 Gy,** with CD to the 5 × 5 cm box covering the larynx to **70 Gy.**

What are the Tx options for early-stage supraglottic LCX?

Supraglottic laryngectomy, transoral laser resection, or definitive RT

What are the 5-yr LC and OS rates for early supraglottic cancers treated with surgery and LND?

The **5-yr LC rate is ~85%,** whereas the **5-yr OS is ~100% for T1 and ~80% for T2** supraglottic lesions.

What are the LC rates for early-stage supraglottic cancers after definitive RT alone?

Retrospective series demonstrate LC rates of **73%– 100% for T1 and 60%–89% for T2 lesions** (e.g., University of Florida and Italian data).

Describe the standard RT fields used in treating supraglottic cancers.

Since 20%–50% of T1-T2 supraglottic cancers have +LNs (occult), necks need to be covered for all pts (levels II–IV). This requires an off-cord CD after 45 Gy and a boost to the post neck to 50 Gy with electron fields.

What definitive RT doses are typically recommended for early-stage supraglottic cancers?

T1 dose: **70 Gy** in 2 Gy/fx

T2 dose: hyperfractionated dosing to **76.8 Gy** in 1.2 Gy/fx or with concomitant boost techniques to **72 Gy** (1.8 Gy in am × 30 fx to 54 Gy to areas of subclinical Dz, and 1.5 Gy in pm for the last 12 days of Tx to boost GTV + 1.5−2 cm to 72 Gy)

What data supports the use of re-irradiation for previously treated early-stage LCX pts?

Massachusetts General Hospital data (*Wang CC et al., IJROBP 1993*): 20 pts treated with 1.6 Gy bid to 65 Gy. 5-yr OS was 93%, and LC was 61% after re-irradiation.

What are the Tx options for pts with advanced LCX?

Total laryngectomy (with adj RT or CRT for +margin, +ECE) or organ preservation with definitive CRT **(RTOG 91-11)** or RT alone (altered fractionation)

What are the Tx options for pts with advanced HPC?

Induction chemo → RT or surgery depending on response for T1-3N+ Dz; total laryngectomy/laryngoesophagectomy (with CRT for +margin, +ECE) for T4 Dz

Describe the standard RT fields used to treat advanced LCX/HPC.

Opposed lateral fields: superiorly to the base of skull to cover the retropharyngeal nodes, anteriorly with 1-cm flash, posteriorly behind the spinous process, inferiorly to the shoulders

Low anterior neck: superiorly match with lat fields (may use half beam block), laterally at two thirds of the clavicular length, inferiorly 1 cm below clavicle (include the stoma, if present)

What is the preferred position of the stoma when utilizing the 3-field technique in the adj setting?

If using a monoisocentric 3-field technique for the postop setting, the isocenter is set above the stoma if the stoma is not being boosted; the stoma will be treated in the low ant neck field. Alternatively, the isocenter is set below the stoma if the stoma is to be boosted (generally to >60 Gy).

What techniques can be employed if the shoulders get in the way of the opposed lat fields when boosting an area of concern in the postop setting?

In this scenario, one can employ either the **caudal tilt technique** (both the couch is tilted away from the gantry by 10 degrees and the gantry is angulated 10 degrees above the horizontal plane) or **IMRT**

What are the typical RT doses used to treat advanced LCX/HPC?

Off-cord at 40–44 Gy, boost with electrons posteriorly to 50 Gy; subclinical Dz to **50–54 Gy;** primary tumor to **70 Gy** (in 2 Gy/fx)

What are the 3 indications for boosting the stoma with PORT?

Indications for boosting the stoma with PORT:
1. Emergency tracheostomy
2. Subglottic extension
3. Ant soft tissue extension

What are some indications for performing an elective neck dissection after definitive RT?

This is controversial, but elective neck dissection should be done for persistent Dz and can be considered with >N2 Dz.

What randomized data/ study compared preop RT to PORT for (predominantly) HPC?

RTOG 73-03 (*Tupchong L et al., IJROBP 1991*): 354 pts, 50 Gy preop vs. 60 Gy postop; 69% of pts had advanced supraglottic or HPC. LC was better with PORT but not OS.

What are the 2 randomized phase III trials that demonstrated a benefit with postop CRT vs. PORT alone for high-risk H&N pts?

EORTC 22931 (*Bernier J et al., NEJM 2004*): 334 pts randomized to PORT 66 Gy vs. PORT + cisplatin 100 mg/m^2 on days 1, 22, and 43. Eligibility: ECE, +margin, PNI, LVI, and level 4–5 +N from oral cavity cancer (OCC)/oropharyngeal cancer (OPC). There was better OS, DFS, and 5-yr LC with CRT but ↑ grade 3–4 toxicity.

RTOG 95-01 (*Cooper JS et al., NEJM 2004*): 459 pts randomized to 60–66 PORT vs. PORT + cisplatin 100 mg/m^2 on days 1, 22, and 43. Eligibility: >2 LNs, ECE, +margin. There was better DFS (43% vs. 54%) and 2-yr LRC (72% vs. 82%) with CRT but only a trend to improvement in OS (57% vs. 63%).

What are the presumed reasons why EORTC 22931 showed an OS benefit while RTOG 9501 did not?

The EORTC trial included more margin+ pts (28% vs. 18%), pts with worse tumor differentiation (19% vs. 7%), more HPX cases (20% vs. 10%), and more pts who started RT 6 wks or later after surgery (32%).

What randomized trials demonstrated a benefit with altered fractionation RT in advanced H&N cancer?

EORTC 22851 (*Horiot JC et al., Radiother Oncol 1997*): 512 pts (all H&N except the HPX) randomized to conventional RT to 70 Gy (7 wks) or 1.6 Gy tid to 72 Gy (5 wks). There was better 5-yr LRC with tid RT (59% vs. 46%) but not OS.

RTOG 9003 (*Fu KK et al., IJROBP 2000*): 1,073 pts (all H&N sites) randomized to (a) standard fx 70 Gy/2 qd; (b) 81.6 Gy/1.2 bid; (c) accelerated with split 67.2 Gy/1.6 bid; and (d) accelerated with concomitant boost 72 Gy/1.8 qd × 17 → 1.8 Gy am + 1.5 Gy pm × 33 fx. All altered fx schemes were better than conventional RT in terms of LRC (54% vs. 46%) but not OS.

▌Toxicity

What are some acute and late toxicities with RT in the Tx of LCX?

Acute: hoarseness, sore throat, odynophagia, skin irritation

Late: laryngeal edema, glottic stenosis, hypothyroidism, xerostomia, L'hermitte syndrome, myelitis, laryngeal necrosis

What are the main late toxicities after organ preservation with concurrent CRT for LCX?

Moderate speech impairment, dysphagia (25% of pts; <5% cannot swallow), and xerostomia (advanced cases)

What are some approximate RT dose constraints for laryngeal edema?

Recent data suggests that the incidence of laryngeal edema ↑ significantly with mean doses ≥**44 Gy.** (*Sanguineti G et al., IJROBP 2007*)

What is the QOL impact of larynx preservation when compared to laryngectomy in the Tx of LCX?

VA data demonstrated better social, emotional, and mental health function with larynx preservation (swallowing and speech function were similar), which suggests that better QOL is not due to preservation of speech but due to freedom from pain, emotional well-being, and less depression.

Hanna et al. demonstrated that pts had worse social functioning, greater sensory disturbance, more use of pain meds, and coughing after total laryngectomy than those treated with CRT. (*Arch Otolaryngol H&N Surg 2004*)

What is the follow-up paradigm for LCX pts?

LCX follow-up paradigm: H&P + laryngoscopy (q1–3mos for yr 1, q2–4mos for yr 2, q4–6mos for yrs 3–5, q6–12 mos if >5 yrs), imaging (for signs/Sx), TSH (if neck is irradiated), speech/hearing evaluation, and smoking cessation

34
Thyroid Cancer
John P. Christodouleas and Vincent J. Lee

▮ Background

Name the 4 anatomic subdivisions/lobes of the thyroid.

Subdivisions/lobes of the thyroid:
1. Right lobe
2. Left lobe
3. Isthmus
4. Pyramidal lobe

In the thyroid follicle, what are the normal functions of the epithelial follicular cells and the parafollicular cells?

Epithelial follicular cells: remove iodide from the blood and use it to **form T3 and T4** thyroid hormones
Parafollicular cells (C cells): lie just outside of the follicle cells and **produce calcitonin**

What is the most common endocrine malignancy?

Thyroid cancer (TCa) is the most common endocrine malignancy.

TCa represents what % of all diagnosed human cancers?

TCa is rare and only represents **1%** of all diagnosed malignancies.

What are the 3 main TCa histologies in decreasing order of frequency?

Main TCa histologies (in decreasing order of frequency): **follicular-epithelial derived** (FED) (~94%) > **medullary** (2%–4%) > **anaplastic** (2%)

What are the 3 subtypes of FED TCa in decreasing order of frequency?

Subtypes of FED TCa (in decreasing order of frequency): **papillary > follicular > Hurthle cell carcinoma**

What is the incidence of papillary TCa in autopsy series?

30%–40% of cases have "microcarcinomas."

What is happening to the incidence of diagnosed papillary TCa?

The incidence of papillary TCa is **increasing** (approximately by 15% over the past 40 yrs).

What is the typical age at Dx for follicular vs. papillary TCa?

Follicular incidence peaks at ~40–60 yrs of age, whereas **papillary peaks at ~30–50 yrs of age.**

Is there a gender predilection for papillary or follicular TCa?

Yes. Both papillary and follicular TCa more commonly affect **females** than males (3:1).

What is the strongest risk factor for papillary TCa?	**RT exposure** to the H&N as a child is the strongest risk factor for papillary TCa. There is no increased risk if exposure is after age 20 yrs. Most papillary cases are sporadic.
Name 4 genetic disorders associated with papillary TCa.	Genetic disorders associated with papillary TCa: 1. Familial polyposis 2. Gardner syndrome 3. Turcot syndrome 4. Familial papillary carcinoma
Name a genetic disorder associated with follicular TCa.	**Cowden syndrome** is associated with follicular TCa.
Medullary TCa arises from what precursor cell?	Medullary TCa arises from the calcitonin-producing **parafollicular C cells.**
Name 2 genetic syndromes associated with medullary TCa.	**MEN 2a** and **MEN 2b** are associated with medullary TCa.
What % of medullary TCa is related to a genetic syndrome?	**~25%** of medullary TCa is related to a genetic syndrome.
Name the nerve that lies in the tracheoesophageal (TE) groove, post to the right/left thyroid lobes.	The **recurrent laryngeal nerve** lies in the TE groove.
What are the primary, secondary, and tertiary lymphatic drainage regions of the thyroid?	<u>Primary</u>: central compartment (level VI), TE groove, delphian nodes <u>Secondary</u>: cervical/supraclavicular nodes <u>Tertiary</u>: sup mediastinal/retropharyngeal nodes

■ Workup/Staging

What % of palpable thyroid nodules are malignant?	Only **5%** of palpable thyroid nodules are malignant.
In a pt with low TSH and a nodule that shows uptake by I-123 or Tc-99 scan, what is the likely Dx?	**Adenomas** commonly present with low TSH and increased uptake on I-123 or Tc-99 scans.
Which FED subtypes are difficult to distinguish from adenomas on FNA?	**Follicular and Hurthle subtypes** are difficult to distinguish from adenomas. Histologically, they show only follicular structures. Papillary TCa shows both papillary and follicular structures that help to distinguish it from adenomas.
What pathologic criteria must be met to make the Dx of Hurthle cell TCa?	The Dx requires **hypercellularity with >75% Hurthle cells** (also referred to as oncocytic cells), which are characterized by abundant eosinophilic granular content.

Which TCa subtype is more likely to present with N+ Dz: papillary or follicular?

Papillary TCa (~**30%** node+) is more likely to spread to LNs than follicular (~10% node+).

Name the 2 major and 3 minor prognostic factors for FED TCa.

Major: age, tumor size
Minor: histology, local tumor extension, LN status

For FED TCa, what sizes distinguish T1, T2, and T3 tumors?

T1: <2 cm (T1a if <1 cm; T1b if >1 cm)
T2: 2–4 cm (limited to thyroid)
T3: >4 cm with only min extrathyroidal extension

What is difference between T4a and T4b TCa lesions?

T4a: local extension but still technically resectable
T4b: unresectable Dz

What is the difference between N1a and N1b in TCa?

N1a: mets to pre/paratracheal nodes, prelaryngeal nodes (level VI)
N1b: mets to cervical neck (levels I–V), upper mediastinal nodes

List the latest AJCC 7th edition stage groupings for papillary and follicular TCa.

Stage I: M0 and age <45 yrs or T1N0 and age ≥45 yrs
Stage II: M1 and age <45 yrs or T2N0 and age ≥45 yrs
Stage III: T3N0 or T1-3N1a and age ≥45 yrs
Stage IVA: T4a or N1b and age ≥45 yrs
Stage IVB: T4b and age ≥45 yrs
Stage IVC: M1 and age ≥45 yrs

Can a pt <45 yo with follicular or papillary TCa have stage III or IV Dz?

No. A pt <45 yo with follicular or papillary TCa cannot have stage III or IV Dz.

What is the delphian node?

The delphian node is a **prelaryngeal node that is often involved in TCa.**

What is unique about the staging of FED TCa?

The staging of FED is **age dependent;** it differs for pts greater or less than 45 yo.

What is the stage of a 37-yo pt with FED TCa and a solitary bone met?

Stage II. If the pt were 65 yo, he or she would be stage IVc.

What is the stage of a 45-yo pt with an unresectable primary FED TCa and no mets?

Stage IVb. If the pt were 44 yo, he or she would be stage I.

What must be done prior to an I-123 or I-131 scan?

TSH stimulation must be done prior to an iodine scan.

What are 2 ways to do TSH stimulation?

TSH stimulation can be accomplished through **thyroid hormone withdrawal or by using recombinant TSH.**

What are some advantages of recombinant TSH stimulation?

Fewer side effects and a shorter period of elevated TSH (theoretically a lower risk of tumor progression)

What are the approved indications for recombinant TSH stimulation?

Recombinant TSH is approved for **follow-up iodide scans** and for the **I-131 Tx of low-risk pts.**

What % of pts with FED TCa will have residual uptake on an iodide scan after thyroidectomy?

~**80%** of pts will have residual uptake after thyroidectomy.

What sites of the body show a physiologic uptake of iodide?

The **salivary glands and the GI tract** show physiologic uptake due to the presence of iodide transporters.

Which FED subtype has a better long-term prognosis: papillary or follicular?

Papillary has a better 10-yr OS at ~93% (vs. 85% for follicular).

Is the presentation and Tx of Hurthle cell carcinoma more similar to that of papillary or follicular TCa?

It is more similar to **follicular TCa;** however, Hurthle cell carcinoma has a slightly higher DM rate and worse prognosis (10-yr OS ~76%).

Estimate the 10-yr OS for pts with localized vs. N+ medullary TCa.

For localized medullary TCa, the 10-yr OS is ~**90%.** If N+, the 10-yr OS is ~**70%.**

What are the stage groupings for anaplastic TCa?

All anaplastic TCa is considered **stage IV.** Stage IVA is resectable, stage IVB is unresectable, and stage IVC is metastatic.

Estimate the MS and the 1-yr OS for pts with anaplastic TCa.

MS is ~**6 mos** and the 1-yr **OS is** ~**20%** for pts with anaplastic TCa.

Does the tall cell variant have a more favorable or unfavorable prognosis when compared to classic papillary TCa?

The tall cell variant has an **unfavorable prognosis** when compared to classic papillary carcinomas.

■ Treatment/Prognosis

Generally, what is Tx paradigm for FED TCa?

FED TCa Tx paradigm: **primary surgery** (even in M1 Dz) → **observation vs. adj Tx**

What are the 3 surgical options in TCa?

Surgical options in TCa:
1. Lobectomy + isthmusectomy
2. Near-total thyroidectomy
3. Total thyroidectomy

What is the difference between near-total and total thyroidectomy?

Near-total is less aggressive around the recurrent laryngeal nerve.

For which pts with papillary TCa is a lobectomy + isthmusectomy adequate?

This is **controversial.** It is a good option for pts with none of the following risk factors: age >45 yrs, tumor >4 cm, aggressive histology variant, prior Hx of RT, DM, N+, local extension, and +margins.

In addition to improved LC, what is another reason to advocate for a total thyroidectomy even in low-risk pts?

It allows for **easier follow-up** with whole-body iodide scans and serum thyroglobulin.

Per NCCN guidelines, what are 4 possible indications for adj Tx after GTR in FED TCa?

Indications for adj Tx after GTR in FED TCa:
1. >1-cm tumor
2. N+ or DM
3. Aggressive histologic subtypes
4. pT4 + papillary histology and age ≥45 yrs

What are the 5 aggressive histologic subtypes of FED TCa that merit consideration of adj Tx?

Aggressive histologic subtypes that merit consideration of adj Tx:
1. Tall cell
2. Columnar cell
3. Insular cell
4. Oxyphilic
5. Poorly differentiated

Generally, what is the adj Tx paradigm for FED TCa?

FED adj Tx paradigm: **long-term TSH suppression alone or with I-131 +/− EBRT**

What are the indications for adj I-131 in addition to TSH suppression for FED TCa?

Suspected or proven residual normal thyroid tissue or residual tumor are indications for adj I-131.

What is the mCi dose range to ablate residual normal thyroid tissue?

30–100 mCi is the dose range to ablate residual normal thyroid tissue.

What is the mCi dose range to ablate a residual FED TCa lesion?

The dose to ablate a FED TCa lesion is **100–200 mCi.**

What are the 4 indications for adj EBRT in addition to TSH suppression and I-131 in TCa?

Indications for adj EBRT in addition to TSH supression and I-131:
1. pT4 papillary and ≥45 yo
2. Gross residual Dz in the neck after I-131
3. Bulky mets after I-131
4. Lesions with inadequate iodide uptake

What 3 regions should be irradiated with EBRT in a pt ≥45 yo with pT4 papillary TCa?

Thyroid bed, bilat necks, and the upper mediastinal nodes

What are the typical EBRT doses (in 2 Gy/fx) for FED TCa?

<u>Gross Dz</u>: 68–70 Gy
<u>Microscopic Dz</u>: 60 Gy
−<u>Nodal basins</u>: 45–50 Gy

Generally, what is the Tx paradigm for medullary TCa?

Medullary TCa Tx paradigm: **definitive surgery and EBRT for palliation**

Generally, what is the Tx paradigm for anaplastic TCa?

Anaplastic TCa Tx paradigm: **max safe resection →** **adj CRT;** promising results with postop cisplatin/ doxorubicin before and after 40 Gy in bid fractionation (*De Crevoisier R et al., IJROBP 2004*)

For which group of anaplastic TCa pts does PORT improve survival?

Per a recent **SEER analysis** (*Chen J et al., Am J Clin Oncol 2008*), PORT improved survival in pts with T4b/extrathyroid extension of Dz but not those with T4b/thyroid-confined or stage IVC/metastatic Dz.

What is the prognosis for pts with locoregional vs. distant recurrence of FED TCa?

The prognosis is **excellent if recurrence is locoregional** (long-term OS is 80%–90%). It is much **worse with distant recurrences.**

■ Toxicity

What are the acute side effects of >100 mCi of I-131?

GI irritation, sialadenitis, and cystitis

What are the 3 most important long-term side effects of >100 mCi of I-131?

Pulmonary fibrosis, oligospermia, and leukemia

What does the follow-up of TCa pts entail?

TCa follow-up: H&P + TSH/thyroglobulin levels at 6 and 12 mos, then annually if no Dz; neck US; TSH-stimulated iodine scans if clinically indicated

What kind of additional imaging can be considered if the I-131 scan is negative but the stimulated thyroglobulin level is elevated?

If the I-131 scan is negative but the stimulated thyroglobulin level is elevated, **PET/CT** can be considered.

What is the max recommended lifetime dose for I-131?

The max recommended lifetime dose is **800–1,000 mCi.**

35

Head and Neck Cancer of Unknown Primary

Boris Hristov and Giuseppe Sanguineti

Background

H&N cancers of an unknown primary represent what % of H&N cancers?	~3%–5% of all H&N cancers are of an unknown primary.
What is the most commonly presumed general site of origin for H&N cancers of an unknown primary?	The **oropharynx** (OPX) is the presumed site of origin for most cases (less common are the nasopharynx [NPX], hypopharynx [HPX], and larynx).
What subsites constitute the OPX?	Soft palate, tonsils, tonsillar pillars, base of tongue (BOT), and pharyngeal walls
What are the 2 most common originating sites/ primary locations if the cancer is presumed to be of oropharyngeal origin?	**Tonsils and BOT.** Up to 80% of presumed oropharyngeal tumors are thought to originate from these 2 sites.
Approximately what % of pts with tonsillar primaries harbor Dz in both tonsils?	~5%–10% of pts with tonsillar primaries harbor Dz in both tonsils.
A primary can be identified in what % of H&N cancers of unknown primary?	A primary site of origin can ultimately be identified in ~**40%** of pts.

Workup/Staging

What is the most common presentation for H&N cancers of an unknown primary?	**Painless upper neck LAD** (IB–III) is the most common presentation.
What is the T staging if no primary H&N site is found after workup?	**T0** (not TX) is the assigned T stage if no primary is found.

189

What % of pts with N1 Dz fail at the primary site after neck dissection alone?

~25% of N1 pts ultimately fail at the primary site after neck dissection alone. However, this can vary from 10%–50%.

What is the approximate overall neck failure rate after neck dissection alone?

The overall neck failure rate is ~15% after neck dissection alone. (*Coster JR et al., IJROBP 1992*)

What is the approximate neck failure rate after neck dissection if there is evidence of ECE?

The approximate neck failure rate after neck dissection alone is ~60% with ECE. (*Coster JR et al., IJROBP 1992*)

What are the indications for PORT in pts with an unknown H&N primary?

≥N2 Dz, ECE/+margin, or neck violation (e.g., after open/excisional Bx)

What do the standard RT fields include in pts with an unknown H&N primary?

The fields generally include **both necks and the mucosal sites at risk** (NPX, OPX, HPX, larynx). Some advocate omission of the HPX/larynx from the RT fields.

What are the historical 5-yr LC and OS rates after definitive RT for pts with an unknown H&N primary?

University of Florida data (*Erkal HS et al., IJROBP 2001*): LC 78% and OS 47%
Danish data (*Grau C et al., Radiother Oncol 2000*): OS 37%

What factors have been traditionally associated with inferior OS after definitive RT for H&N tumors of an unknown primary?

More advanced N stage, ECE, and lower RT doses have been associated with inferior outcomes. (*Erkal HS et al., IJROBP 2001*)

What standard RT fields have been traditionally used for H&N tumors of an unknown primary?

Opposed lats matched with an ant low neck/supraclavicular field (with post neck electron fields after 40–44 Gy)

What are the typical borders of the lat fields used for H&N tumors of an unknown primary?

Anterior: behind OC/hard palate
Superior: to base of skull to include NPX
Posterior: below tragus to post edge of spinous processes
Inferior: sup edge of thyroid cartilage; if level III or IV, inf edge of cricoid to cover larynx (Fig. 35.1)

What RT doses are generally employed?

70 Gy to gross Dz, **60 Gy** to intermediate-risk areas, and **50 Gy** to low-risk areas (all in 2 Gy/fx)

What evidence supports the omission of the larynx/HPX from the standard RT fields?

University of Florida data (*Baker CA et al., Am J Clin Oncol 2005*): larynx-sparing RT is just as effective with less toxicity.

What is the evidence in favor of bilat neck irradiation for H&N tumors of an unknown primary?	**Loyola data** (*Reddy SP et al., IJROBP 1997*): contralat nodal failure is higher (44%) in pts receiving unilat nodal RT (vs. 14% for bilat nodal RT). Also, there is a higher primary emergence rate with unilat RT (44% vs. 8%).
What is the role of IMRT in H&N cancer of an unknown primary?	Recent studies (*Klem ML et al., IJROBP 2008*) have shown **feasibility of IMRT,** and it is **widely utilized.**
What are a few of the advantages of IMRT for H&N tumors of an unknown primary?	**Greater parotid sparing**, **can consider concurrent chemo** (*Klem ML et al., IJROBP 2008*), **can use simultaneous integrated boost dosing** (e.g., $212 \times 33 = 6,996$ cGy, $180 \times 33 = 5,940$ cGy, and $170 \times 33 = 5,610$ cGy)
When is neck dissection entertained after definitive RT for H&N tumors of an unknown primary?	Post-RT neck dissection is considered with **persistence of Dz** (e.g., on PET or clinically). Some still consider it standard for all pts with ≥N2 Dz.
Within what time frame after RT should neck dissection be performed if decided upon upfront (i.e., regardless of response to RT)?	Neck dissection should occur ~**3–4 mos** (and no later than 6 mos) after RT.

▪ Toxicity

What are common acute side effects from RT to the H&N region?	Mucositis, hoarseness, and malnutrition (weight loss)
What are common long-term complications from RT to the H&N region?	Xerostomia, dysphagia, neck scarring and edema (especially if combined with neck dissection), hypothyroidism, and laryngeal dysfunction (aspiration, hoarseness, etc.)
After what dose must the practitioner come "off-cord" when irradiating the post necks with standard fields?	The practitioner must come off-cord **after a dose of 40–44 Gy** (in 2 Gy/fx). Use matching electron fields or IMRT if greater post neck doses are desired.
After RT, when should PET be performed to assess for nodal response?	PET should be performed no sooner than ~**2–3 mos** after RT. (TROG analysis: *Corry J et al., Curr Oncol Rep 2008*)

| What is an ant compartment dissection, and when is it done? | Ant compartment dissection is **selective level VI dissection,** traditionally **performed for thyroid cancers.** |

■ Workup/Staging

| Which 3 H&N sites have the highest rates of clinical nodal positivity? | The **nasopharynx** (NPX) (87%), **base of tongue** (78%), **and tonsil** (76%) have the highest rates of clinical nodal positivity. (*Lindberg R et al., Cancer 1972*) |
| Which 2 H&N sites have the highest rates of retropharyngeal nodal positivity on CT/MRI? | On CT/MRI, **nasopharyngeal and pharyngeal wall primaries** have the highest rates of retropharyngeal involvement (74% and 20%, respectively). (*McLaughlin MP et al., Head Neck 1995*) |

■ Treatment/Prognosis

When is a selective neck dissection appropriate?	When there is a **clinically negative neck but ≥10% risk of subclinical Dz;** otherwise, do at least a modified radical neck dissection (rarely is a radical neck dissection done anymore).
Per NCCN guidelines, when is the omission of elective neck dissection appropriate after RT?	Per the NCCN, elective neck dissection may be omitted **after a complete response of a cN1 neck.**
When is an elective neck dissection necessary after definitive RT?	Elective neck dissection is necessary whenever there is a **partial response/residual Dz after RT (any nodal stage).**
When can an elective neck dissection be omitted for a pt with ≥N2 Dz?	This is **controversial.** The decision may be guided by PET response 10–12 wks after RT. If a CR, elective neck dissection may be left out. However, at some institutions, any pt with ≥N2 Dz would get neck dissection regardless of the response to RT.
What are the indications for adj RT after a neck dissection?	After a neck dissection, adj RT should be used with **≥3 cm +nodes, ≥2 +nodes, if ≥2 nodal levels are involved, with +ECE, or if there is an undissected high-risk nodal area.**
When should chemo be added to PORT in the management of H&N cancers?	Definite indications: +margin, +ECE (category 1 per the NCCN) Additional (weaker) indications: multiple nodes, PNI/LVI, T4a, or OC primary with level IV nodes (could consider chemo or just RT alone)
How should cisplatin be dosed when given with RT for H&N cancers?	The cisplatin dosing with RT is **100 mg/m^2 intravenously on days 1, 22, and 43.**

How did the 2 seminal H&N trials supporting the addition of chemo to RT in the adj setting differ, and what did they show?

EORTC 22931 (*Bernier J et al., NEJM 2004*): 334 pts randomized to PORT 66 Gy vs. PORT + cisplatin 100 mg/m^2 on days 1, 22, and 43. Eligibility: ECE, +margin, PNI, LVI, and level 4–5 +N from OC cancer/OPC. There was better OS, DFS, and 5-yr LC with CRT but ↑ grade 3–4 toxicity.

RTOG 95-01 (*Cooper JS et al., NEJM 2004*): 459 pts randomized to 60–66 PORT vs. PORT + cisplatin 100 mg/m^2 on days 1, 22, and 43. Eligibility: >2 LNs, ECE, +margin. There was better DFS (43% vs. 54%) and 2-yr LRC (72% vs. 82%) but only a trend to improvement in OS (57% vs. 63%).

What are the presumed reasons why EORTC 22931 showed an OS benefit while RTOG 9501 did not?

The EORTC trial included more margin+ pts (28% vs. 18%), more pts with worse tumor differentiation (19% vs. 7%), more hypopharynx cases (20% vs. 10%), and more pts that started RT ≥6 wks after surgery (32%).

What important study compared preop RT to PORT for advanced H&N (mostly hypopharyngeal) cancers?

RTOG 73-03 (*Tupchong L et al., IJROBP 1991*): 354 pts, 50 Gy preop vs. 50–60 Gy postop. LC improved with PORT but not OS. Both LC and OS improved with PORT in OPC pts.

What are the indications for boosting the tracheostomy stoma with PORT?

Indications for boosting the stoma with PORT:
1. Emergency tracheostomy/tracheostomy prior to definitive surgery
2. Subglottic extension
3. Ant soft tissue extension
4. T4 laryngeal tumors

What are the dose recommendations for PORT to the neck and primary?

In 2 Gy/fx: undissected clinically negative area, **50 Gy;** postop (−margin), **60 Gy;** postop (+margin, +ECE), **66 Gy;** gross residual, **70 Gy**

When should the retropharyngeal nodes be covered/irradiated?

Nasopharyngeal, hypopharyngeal, and pharyngeal wall primaries or ≥2 +nodal levels (N2-N3) all merit irradiation of the retropharyngeal nodes.

What are the indications for treating the sup mediastinal nodes in H&N cancer?

T3-T4, hypopharyngeal/thyroid primaries, and involvement of the supraclavicular nodes are indications for treating the sup mediastinal nodes.

What is the inf extent of the RT fields if sup mediastinal nodes are to be treated?

The inf extent encompasses **nodes to the level of the carina or 5 cm below the clavicular heads.**

Overall, what is the 5-yr survival rate for lung cancer pts?

The overall 5-yr survival rate for non–small cell lung cancer (NSCLC) is **15%.**

What are the 3 histologic subtypes of NSCLC in decreasing order of frequency?

Histologic subtypes of NSCLC: **adenocarcinoma** (50%) > **squamous cell carcinoma** (35%) > **large cell** (15%)

In addition to tobacco smoke, what are 3 other environmental exposure risk factors for developing lung cancers?

Environmental exposure risk factors for lung cancer:
1. Radon
2. Asbestos (*Note:* Smoking and asbestos exposures are synergistic in early reports, but more recent studies suggest less than a multiplicative effect.)
3. Occupational exposure (arsenic, bis-chloromethyl ether, hexavalent chromium, mustard gas, nickel, polycyclic aromatic hydrocarbon)

What is the estimated RR for lung cancer in heavy smokers vs. nonsmokers?

Heavy smokers have a 20-fold excess of lung cancer (American Cancer Society [ACS] cohort study).

What is the risk of lung cancer in former smokers compared to current smokers?

The risk of developing lung cancer in former smokers is **around half** (9 times vs. 20 times) that of current smokers (ACS cohort study).

What is the risk of lung cancer from passive smoke exposure?

There is an RR of 1.2–1.3 for developing lung cancer from passive smoke exposure.

Approximately what % of smokers develop lung cancer?

<20% of smokers actually develop lung cancer (in the Carotene and Retinol Efficacy Trial, 10-yr cancer risk was 1%–15%).

What histology subtype of NSCLC is least associated with smoking?

Adenocarcinoma is the histologic subtype that is least associated with smoking.

Name 3 histologic variants of adenocarcinoma of the lung.

Bronchoalveolar, acinar, and papillary

Name 2 variants of large cell cancer of the lung.

Giant cell and clear cell

What is the race and gender predilection for NSCLC?

Blacks have the highest incidence of lung cancer. **Males** also are historically at greater risk, but as females continue to start smoking, the incidence in females is rising.

What is the most common stage at initial presentation?

The most common stage of presentation for lung cancer is **metastatic Dz** (around one third of pts).

What are the most common sites of DMs for lung cancer?

Bone, adrenals, and brain

What are the para-neoplastic syndromes associated with lung cancers?

Hypercalcemia of malignancy due to PTHrP, syndrome of inappropriate secretion of antidiuretic hormone → ↓Na, Cushing, Lambert-Eaton syndrome, and other neurologic disorders

What is the cause of Lambert-Eaton syndrome? Clinically, how can Lambert-Eaton be distinguished from myasthenia gravis?

Lambert-Eaton syndrome is caused by **circulating autoantibodies against presynaptic P/Q calcium channel. Lambert-Eaton strength improves with serial effort,** but not myasthenia gravis.

Which histologic subtypes of lung cancer are associated with peripheral and central locations?

Peripheral: adenocarcinoma
Central: SCC

With which histologic subtypes of lung cancer is thyroid transcription factor-1 (TTF-1) staining associated?

Adenocarcinoma, nonmucinous bronchioalveolar carcinoma, and neuroendocrine tumors (i.e., small cell lung cancer, carcinoid). TFF-1 is rare in SCC. A thyroid cancer primary must be excluded.

In NSCLC, what is the role of CT screening for high-risk pts?

This is **controversial** as of 2010. Lead time bias could be the reason why survival is better. IELCAP (*Henschke CI et al., NEJM 2006*) reported that out of 27,456 pts screened, 74 pts were found to have cancer (0.3% detection) and 86% were stage I. 10-yr survival was 93% in stage I pts who underwent resection at Dx. 10-yr OS was 82% for all pts diagnosed by CT.

What is the single most clinically significant acquired genetic abnormality in NSCLC?

EGFR mutation in exon 19 (in-frame deletion of 4 aa, LREA) **and exon 21** (L858R point mutation); results in a constitutive active receptor.

Among pts with NSCLC, in what particular groups are the EGFR mutations common, and for what do these mutations predict?

In the overall lung cancer population, EGFR mutations are **seen in only ~10%,** but this occurs at high rates (30%–70%) in nonsmokers, adenocarcinomas, and Asians. These mutations **predict for a high response rate to TKIs** (gefitinib, erlotinib) **of ~80%.**

What point mutation in the EGFR gene is associated with TKI resistance?

T790M is the point mutation in the EGFR gene associated with TKI resistance.

What other genetic alteration predicts well for response to TKI?

EGFR amplification (by FISH) is a good predictor for TKI response.

For what does the KRAS mutation or ERCC1 expression predict?

The KRAS mutation or ERCC1 expression predicts for **resistance to platinum-based chemo.**

■ Workup/Staging

What is the initial workup for a pt suspected of having lung cancer?

Lung cancer initial workup: H&P + focus on weight loss >5% over prior 3 mos, Karnofsky performance status (KPS), tobacco Hx, neck exam for N3 Dz, CBC, CMP, CT chest to include adrenals or PET/CT, MRI for paraspinal/sup sulcus tumors, Dx of lung cancer rendered by Bx via transbronchial endoscopic or transthoracic FNA, MRI brain for presumed stages II–III, mediastinoscopy or endobronchial ultrasound (EBUS) for suspected hilar or N2 nodes, PFTs prior to Tx, and smoking cessation counseling

What are the 3 most common presenting Sx of NSCLC?

Dyspnea, cough, and weight loss (others include chest pain and hemoptysis)

What is the sensitivity and specificity of sputum cytology for Dx of lung cancer?

Sensitivity <70%, specificity >90%. Accuracy increases with increasing # of specimens analyzed. At least 3 sputum specimens are recommended for the best accuracy.

What is the sensitivity and specificity of FDG-PET compared to CT for the staging of lung cancers?

PET: sensitivity 83%, specificity 91%
CT: sensitivity 64%, specificity 74%

What is the estimated % of pts who will have false+ N2 nodes based on PET/CT?

~10%–20%. PPV ~80%. +N2 nodes by PET/CT need pathologic confirmation before deferring to potentially curative surgery.

What is the estimated % of pts who will have false− N2 nodes based on PET/CT?

~5%–16%. NPV ~95%. −N2 nodes by PET/CT for clinical T1 lesions may not need mediastinoscopic evaluation (this is controversial).

What is the rate of occult mets from lung cancer detected by FDG-PET?

In many series, the range is ~6%–18%.

If a PET scan is being ordered, should a bone scan be obtained to evaluate for bone mets as well?

No. In NSCLC, PET is just as sensitive as bone scan but more specific. However, consider pathologic confirmation for solitary PET+ lesions given the risk of a false+.

What clinical characteristics are important to focus on to determine the nature of a solitary pulmonary nodule?

Nodule size (and whether there are changes in size in the past 2 yrs), **Hx of smoking, age,** and **nodule margin on CT** (i.e., spiculation)

Stage for stage, which histology has a worse prognosis: adenocarcinoma or SCC? Why?

Adenocarcinoma. It has a **greater propensity to metastasize,** particularly to the brain.

Does large cell carcinoma have a natural Hx and prognosis more similar to SCC or adenocarcinoma?

Large cell carcinoma has a natural Hx and prognosis more similar to **adenocarcinoma.**

Describe the T staging of NSCLC using the AJCC 7th edition (2009) of the TNM stage.

T1: ≤3 cm, surrounded by lung parenchyma (T1a ≤2 cm; T1b 2.1–3 cm)

T2: >3–7 cm, +visceral pleura, >2 cm from carina, +atelectasis to lobe (T2a 3.1–5 cm; T2b 5.1–7 cm)

T3: >7 cm, tumor invading mainstem bronchus <2 cm from carina; invasion to diaphragm, chest wall (CW), pericardium, mediastinal pleura; or associated atelectasis or obstructive pneumonitis of entire lung or satellite nodule in same lobe

T4: any size, invading mediastinum, heart, great vessels, trachea, recurrent laryngeal nerve, esophagus, vertebral body, carina, or with separate tumor nodules in a different ipsi lung

Describe the N staging of NSCLC.

N1: ipsi hilar or peribronchial nodes

N2: ipsi mediastinal or subcarinal nodes

N3: any supraclavicular/scalene nodes or contralat mediastinal/hilar nodes

What is the AJCC 7th edition (2009) of the TNM stage for malignant pleural/pericardial nodules/effusion or opposite lung tumor nodules in NSCLC?

M1a, whereas DM is M1b.

What is considered early-stage NSCLC? Categorize the appropriate TNM stratification.

Stages I and II are considered early-stage NSCLC.
  Stage IA: T1aN0, T1bN0
  Stage IB: T2aN0
  Stage IIA: T2bN0 or T1-2aN1
  Stage IIB: T2bN1 or T3N0

What procedures prior to thoracotomy can be used to evaluate the following nodal stations: (a) left and right stations 2, 4, and 7; (b) stations 5–6?

(a) **Mediastinoscopy** to evaluate left and right stations 2, 4, and 7 **or EBUS** to evaluate left and right stations 2, 3, 4, 7, and 10
(b) **Video-assisted thoracic surgery or ant mediastinotomy** (Chamberlain procedure) for stations 5–6

When should pre-Tx mediastinal nodal assessment be done?

1. To confirm PET or CT +nodes
2. All superior sulcus tumors
3. If T3 or central T1-T2 lesions

What routine PFT results (FEV1 and DLCO) indicate that the pt needs further testing prior to undergoing resection?

If the **FEV1 is <80%** predicted for the age and size of the pt **or the DLCO is <80%** predicted, then the pt may need quantitative lung scans/exercise testing to carefully predict postop pulmonary function.

What is the min absolute FEV1 necessary for pneumonectomy and lobectomy?

Pneumonectomy: >2 L
Lobectomy: >1.5 L

Any <1.5-L pt may be a candidate for wedge resection. The marginal % FEV1 for surgery is 40% of the predicted value.

Which subsets of lung cancer pts are at high risk for surgical morbidity?

Subsets at high risk for surgical morbidity:
1. pCO_2 <45 mm Hg
2. pO_2 <50 mm Hg
3. Preop FEV1 <40% of predicted value
4. Poor exercise tolerance
5. DLCO <50% of predicted value
6. Postop FEV1 <0.71 or <30% of predicted value
7. Cardiac problems (left ventricle ejection fraction <40%, myocardial infarction within 6 mos, arrhythmias)
8. Obesity

What are some factors that predict for postop complications (i.e., mortality, infection)?

Active smoking (6 times higher), poor nutrition, advanced age, and poor lung function. It is advised that pts should quit smoking for at least 4 wks prior to resection and have a nutrition evaluation.

What % of lung cancer pts clinically at stage I are upstaged at surgery?

~5%–25% of stage I lung cancer pts are upstaged at surgery.

In addition to stage, name 3 other poor prognostic factors in lung cancer pts.

Poor prognostic factors in lung cancer:
1. KPS <80%
2. Weight loss >5% in 3 mos
3. Age >60 yrs

■ Treatment/Prognosis

Generally, what is a Tx paradigm for a stage I–II medically operable NSCLC pt?

Stage I–II medically *operable* NSCLC Tx paradigm: surgical resection (lobectomy) + mediastinal LND → adj chemo for stage II

Generally, what is a Tx paradigm for a stage I–II medically inoperable NSCLC pt?

Stage I–II medically *inoperable* NSCLC Tx paradigm: if T1-2N0, consider definitive hypofractionated stereotactic body radiation therapy (SBRT). Otherwise, use definitive conventional RT alone.

Name 3 surgical options to resect a T1-T2 tumor.

Surgical options to resect a T1-T2 tumor:
1. Wedge or segmental resection
2. Lobectomy
3. Pneumonectomy

For a T1N0 NSCLC, what is the estimated LC for wedge/segmental resection vs. lobectomy?

Wedge/segmental LC is **82%.** Lobectomy LC is **94%** (LF 18% vs. 6%) based on RCT **LCSG 921** (*Ginsberg RJ et al., NEJM 1995*). Lobectomy is preferred when feasible.

For a T1N0 NSCLC, what is the estimated LC for wedge/segmental resection +/− intraop brachytherapy?

LC is **97% with brachytherapy** compared to **83% without brachytherapy.** The outcomes may be equivalent to lobectomy. (*Fernando HC et al., J Thorac Cardiovasc Surg 2005*)

What % of stage I NSCLC pts will develop a 2nd primary after definitive surgical resection?

Up to **30%** of pts develop a 2nd primary.

What is the estimated 5-yr OS of completely resected T1-2N0 NSCLC with no adj chemo?

T1N0 ~80%; T2N0 ~68% (*Martini N et al., J Thorac Cardiovasc Surg 1999*)

What is the 5-yr OS, CSS, and MS for pts who refuse any Tx for T1-2N0 NSCLC?

5-yr OS is 6%, CSS is 22%, and MS is 13 mos (*Raz DJ et al., Chest 2007*)

What are the indications for adj chemo after definitive resection for stage I–II NSCLC?

Indications for adj chemo after definitive resection for stage I–II NSCLC:
1. Stage II–IIIA Dz after resection (category 1)
2. N1 Dz (category 1)
3. T2N0, especially if the tumor is >4 cm as per unplanned analysis of **CALGB 9633** (category 2b)

What is the estimated 5-yr OS benefit with adj chemo for pts with completely resected stage I or II NSCLC?

~**5%** at 5 yrs based on **LACE meta-analysis** of recent trials (*Pignon JP et al., JCO 2008*)

What is the total lung V20 dose-volume constraint for RT alone?

The total lung V20 dose-volume constraint is **<37%.** (*NCCN 2010*)

What is the mean lung dose (MLD) constraint for definitive RT to lung cancer?

The MLD constraint is **<20 Gy.** (*NCCN 2010*)

What is the distinction between grade 2 and 3 RTOG pneumonitis?

Grade 2 pneumonitis: symptomatic with the need for steroids

Grade 3 pneumonitis: dyspnea at rest and oxygen supplementation needed

Other grades of pneumonitis include grade 1: asymptomatic, seen only on CT; grade 4: hospitalized and intubated; grade 5: death

What are the heart dose-volume constraints for conventionally fractionated RT?

Heart **V45 <67%** and **V60 <33%.** (*NCCN 2010*)

What is the dose constraint for the brachial plexus with conventional fractionation?

The dose to the brachial plexus should be kept at **<66 Gy.**

What is the rate of brachial plexopathy seen for pts treated with SBRT for early-stage lung cancer?

The recommended max dose to the brachial plexus is **<26 Gy in 3–4 fx** (*Forquer JA et al., Radiother Oncol 2009*). Of the 37 apical tumors out of 253 pts treated, 19% of pts developed grade 2–4 plexopathy. A dose >26 Gy resulted in 46% risk vs. 8% risk if the dose was <26 Gy.

What is the esophageal dose constraint for conventionally fractionated RT?

Ideally, the mean dose of RT to the esophagus should be <34 Gy. Try to minimize the V60 as much as possible (V60 <33%, V55 <66%, ≤45 Gy to the entire esophagus).

What is the max BED for SBRT when treating centrally located tumors?

180–210 Gy with grade 3 pulmonary complications (*Timmerman R et al., JCO 2006*). Keeping the BED ≥100 Gy may be sufficient for LC and may avert toxicities for central lesions.

Is a normal SUVmax of FDG-PET required to be considered a good clinical response in the follow-up of stage I NSCLC pts treated with SBRT?

No. Prospective and retrospective reviews suggest that the SUVmax remains elevated for an extended period after SBRT due to an inflammatory response, but there is no evidence of correlation with recurrence. (*Timmerman R et al., IJROBP 2009; Henderson MA et al., IJROBP 2009*)

What % of pts treated with SBRT for early-stage lung cancer have grade 3–5 toxicities?	**15%** of pts have grade 3–5 toxicities in a review of 15 studies (683 pts). (*Sampson JH et al., Semin Radiat Oncol 2006*)
	In **RTOG 0236**, 16.3% of pts experienced grade 3–4 toxicity but no grade 5 toxicity. (*Timmerman R et al., JAMA 2010*)
What factors predict for grade 3–5 toxicities after SBRT for early lung cancer seen on the Indiana University phase II study?	**Location** (46% hilar/pericentral vs. 17% peripheral) and **tumor size** (GTV >10 cc had 8 times the risk of grade 3–5 toxicity.) (*Timmerman R et al., JCO 2006*)
What are the PFT changes before and after SBRT for early-stage lung cancer?	**Very min** based on an institutional review of 92 pts (*Stephans KL et al., JTO 2009*): mean FEV1 −0.05 (−1.88%), DLCO −2.59% of predicted value; no association with central vs. peripheral location or the dose administered

38

Advanced-Stage (III-IV) Non-Small Cell Lung Cancer

Steven H. Lin and James Welsh

▌Background

What % of pts present with stage IIIA non–small cell lung cancer (NSCLC)?	~**30%** of all NSCLC pts have stage IIIA Dz at presentation.
What % of pts will have occult N2 Dz found at the time of surgery?	**25%** of pts will have occult N2 Dz found at surgery.
After definitive Tx of a primary lung tumor, what is the time period after which it is considered a 2nd primary tumor?	A tumor that develops **≥2 yrs** after definitive Tx of primary lung cancer is likely a 2nd primary. Whenever a recurrence with identical histology occurs at <2 yrs, it is considered a met.

Is there a benefit of altered fractionation of definitive RT for stage III NSCLC?

Yes. Several phase II–III trials have demonstrated this benefit.

RTOG 8311 (*Cox JD et al., J Clin Oncol 1990*): randomized phase I–II, 848 pts with unresectable N2, 1.2 Gy bid to 60, 64.8, 69.6, 74.4, and 79.2 Gy. Favorable pts did better overall, and favorable pts with good performance status that rcv ≥69.6 Gy had significantly better 3-yr OS at 20%.

CHART (*Saunders MI et al., Lancet 1997*): phase III, 563 pts randomized to 54 Gy at 150 tid (450/day) × 12 consecutive days vs. 60 Gy for 6 wks. There was 10% improvement in 3-year absolute survival for CHART compared to standard RT. Severe esophagitis was most common (19% vs. 3%). The trial included many stage I pts. Results were very similar if chemo was added to the standard RT regimen.

ECOG 2597 (*Belani CP et al., JCO 2005*): 141 pts, stage IIIA–B unresectable NSCLC treated with induction carboplatin/Taxol × 2 cycles → definitive RT with either (a) qd RT 64 Gy or (b) HART 1.5 Gy tid × 2.5 wks to 57.6 Gy. The study closed early due to poor accrual. There was a trend to better MS with HART (20.3 mos vs. 14.9 mos, *p* = 0.28). There was ↑ esophagitis with HART.

RT should be limited to what dose if the pt is undergoing preop CRT for Tx of locally advanced NSCLC?

45 Gy. >50 Gy has been shown to have complications of bronchopleural fistula, prolonged air leak with empyema, and prolonged postop ventilation.

Is there data to suggest that a pCR (pN2 → pN0) after induction CRT improves survival in NSCLC pts?

SWOG 8805: phase II study in stage IIIA–B pts receiving induction CRT → surgery. pCR was 22%, with 3-yr OS of 27%. Those with pN0 Dz after induction therapy had MS of 30 mos vs. only 10 mos in those with residual N2 Dz. (*Albain KS et al., J Clin Oncol 1995*)

What is considered bulky, unresectable Dz in NSCLC pts?

Pts with a **histologically involved LN >2 cm on CT, +extranodal involvement, or multistation nodal Dz** (regardless of size)

What is the preferred Tx strategy for pts with stage IIIB T4N0 Dz?

Neoadj chemo or CRT, or definitive CRT. 5-yr OS may approach 25%–30%. R0 resection should be attempted if this is technically feasible.

What is the 5-yr OS of pts with satellite nodules in the same lobe?

5-yr OS is **33%** if pts undergo lobectomy. Careful nodal assessment to exclude N2 Dz must be done.

What is the role of adj platinum-based chemo in NSCLC?

Only postoperatively in stage II–IIIA pts.
LACE meta-analysis for 5 of the adj trials demonstrated 5-yr OS advantage of 5.4%. (*Pignon JP et al., JCO 2008*)

The **CALGB 9633** study demonstrated a trend to survival benefit for stage IB pts with tumors >4 cm in subset analysis. (*Strauss GM et al., JCO 2008*)

Is there data to demonstrate the need for adding RT to adj chemo in pts with completed resected stage IIIA N2 NSCLC?

This **cannot be adequately answered** at this point. **CALGB 9734** attempted to address this question (adj chemo alone vs. chemo → RT), but the trial was closed due to poor accrual (*Perry C et al., Lung Cancer 2007*). There was no difference in DFS or OS.

However, based on retrospective analysis, pts with N2 Dz should be evaluated for chemo → PORT

Does postoperative radiotherapy (PORT) for pts with resectable lung cancers improve outcomes? What subset of pts may benefit from PORT?

Possibly. Based on several randomized trials and meta-analysis, pts with N2 Dz may benefit from PORT. There are ongoing prospective phase III trials testing the role of PORT in pN2 pts.

LCSG 773 (*Weisenburger TH et al., NEJM 1986*): RCT, 210 pts, stage II–IIIA (T3 or N2), margin– resection, randomized to PORT or observation. RT: ≥Co-60 to the mediastinum to 50 Gy on postop day 28 (turned out to be nearly all squamous cell carcinoma). Overall LR was better in PORT (3% vs. 41%), and DFS was better in N2 pts. There was no difference in OS between the arms.

PORT Meta-Analysis Trialist Group, Cochrane database, 2005 (*Burdett S et al., Lung Cancer 2005*): meta-analysis of 10 trials of pts treated after 1965. Suggested OS was a detriment to PORT overall. Subset analysis showed a detriment in resected stage I–II Dz but no adverse effect in N2 Dz.

Criticism: (a) 25% of pts were T1N0; (b) the staging technique is no longer used; (c) the RT technique is no longer used (large fields and fx, high total doses, Co-60 machines); (d) >30% of the meta-analysis relied on a poorly done study using poor techniques/technology (*Dautzenberg B et al., Cancer 1999*) that showed PORT to be detrimental due to a high 5-yr mortality from PORT (31% vs. 8%), mostly due to Tx-related cardiac or respiratory deaths.

SEER analysis (*Lally BE et al., JCO 2006*): 7,465 pts, stage II–III NSCLC from 1988–2002, PORT vs. observation, median follow-up 3.5 yrs. Overall, PORT did not affect OS. However, for the N2 subset, PORT was associated with better OS (HR 0.85) but detrimental for N0-N1.

Reanalysis of the **ANITA trial** (*Douillard JY et al., IJROBP* 2008): RCT of adj cisplatin/vinorelbine vs. observation for IB–IIIA pts after resection. 232 pts rcv PORT. Overall as a group, PORT was detrimental on survival (HR 1.34). In subset analysis based on pN stage, PORT was detrimental for pN0 pts. However, there was improved survival in pN1 Dz in the observation arm but detrimental in the chemo arm. PORT improved survival for both observation and chemo arms in pN2 pts.

Is there an advantage of postop CRT vs. postop RT alone for stage III N2 NSCLC?

No. INT-0115/RTOG 9105/ECOG (*Keller MB et al., NEJM 2000*) tested postop RT vs. CRT in resected stage II or III NSCLC. There was no difference in OS (3.2 yrs) or LC.

What are the anatomic areas targeted with PORT when given for unexpected N2 NSCLC? What is the recommended dose?

Bronchial stump, ipsi hilum, and ipsi mediastinum. The **total dose is 50.4 Gy;** 54–60 Gy for extracapsular extension or microscopic +margin and 60–70 Gy for gross residual Dz (*NCCN 2010*).

What should be the rate of Tx-related deaths (death from intercurrent disease [DID]) following PORT for NSCLC?

Based on old data with old techniques, DID was 20%–30%, mainly due to pulmonary or cardiovascular excess deaths from PORT. New data suggests much lower rates (**2%–3%**).

Penn retrospective (*Machtay M et al., JCO 2001*): 202 pts, Tx with surgery + PORT; 4-yr DID PORT (13.4%), vs. matched controls (10%). If <54 Gy, DID was 2%; but ≥54 Gy, DID was 17%.

ECOG 3590 reanalysis (*Wakelee H et al., Lung Cancer 2005*): 488 pts randomized to PORT vs. PORT + chemo; 50.4 Gy RT. Overall 4-yr DID was 12.9% vs. matched controls at 10.1%.

What were the 2 seminal studies that demonstrated the importance of adding chemo to radiotherapy compared to radiotherapy alone in treating stage IIIA–B NSCLC?

CALGB 8433 "Dillman regimen" (*Dillman RO et al., NEJM 1990*): 155 pts with stage IIIA Dz (T3 or N2) treated with (a) RT alone (60 Gy) or (b) sequential chemo (CDDP/vinblastine) → RT (60 Gy). Sequential CRT improved MS from 10 mos to 14 mos, 2-yr OS from 13% to 26%, and 5-yr OS from 7% to 19%.

RTOG 88-08 (*Sause W et al., Chest 2000*): 458 pts with unresectable NSCLC (stage II–IIIB) randomized to 3 arms: 2 Gy qd/60 Gy alone (arm 1); 1.2 bid/69.6 Gy alone (arm 2); or sequential chemo (CDDP/vinblastine) + 60 Gy RT (arm 3). There was improved MS in arm 3 with sequential chemo → RT (13.2 mos) compared with conventional RT (11.4 mos) or bid RT (12 mos).

Which important randomized studies demonstrated the superiority of concurrent CRT over sequential CRT for unresectable or medically inoperable stage II–III NSCLC?

West Japan Lung Cancer Study Group (*Furuse K et al., JCO 1999*): 320 stage II–III pts randomized to sequential vs. concurrent CRT. Concurrent arm: CDDP/vindesine/MMC split-course RT (28 Gy × 2). Sequential arm: same chemo → RT (56 Gy conventional, nonsplit course). There was better OS and PFS in pts with concurrent CRT. MS was 16.5 mos vs. 13.3 mos (SS); 5-yr OS was 15.8% vs. 8.9% (SS).

RTOG 9410 (*Curran W et al., ASCO 2003*): 610 pts randomized to 3 arms: sequential (Dillman regimen with RT to 63 Gy) (arm 1); concurrent CRT (to 63 Gy) (arm 2); and concurrent hyperfractionated RT (1.2 bid/69.6 Gy) + chemo (arm 3). Chemo was CDDP/vinblastine (except etoposide/cisplatin [EP] for arm 3). Definitive concurrent CRT (arm 2) had a better outcome in MS (17 mos) vs. 14.6 mos (arm 1) or 15.2 mos (arm 3) or 4-yr OS (21% vs. 12% vs. 12%). However, there was ↑ toxicity in the concurrent CRT arm.

Which chemo regimen allows a full dose, and which would need to be dose reduced during the course of concurrent CRT?

EP or cisplatin/vinblastine allows a full dose to be administered with RT. **Carboplatin/Taxol, gemcitabine, or vinorelbine requires a significant dose reduction** during RT administration.

Is there a benefit of adding induction chemo → CRT for pts with unresectable stage IIIA–B NSCLC?

No. There was initial enthusiasm in 2 small randomized studies that suggested benefit, but 2 prospective studies (**LAMP and CALGB 39801** trials) demonstrated no benefit to neoadj chemo. Definitive CRT is still the standard.

LAMP trial (*Belani CP et al., JCO 2005*): randomized phase II, 276 pts with stage IIIA–B NSCLC randomized to arm 1: chemo × 2 cycles → 63 Gy RT (Dillman regimen); arm 2: induction chemo × 2 cycles → concurrent CRT (63 Gy); and arm 3: concurrent CRT → consolidation chemo × 2 cycles. Chemo was carboplatin/Taxol. Arm 3 (concurrent CRT) had a better outcome, where MS was 16.3 mos vs. 13 mos (arm 1) or 12.7 mos (arm 2).

CALGB 39801 (*Vokes E et al., JCO 2007*): randomized phase III trial, enrolled 366 pts with unresectable stage IIIA–B randomized to arm 1: CRT vs. arm 2: induction chemo × 2 cycles → CRT. Chemo was carboplatin/Taxol. There was no difference in MS or OS. MS 12 mos (CRT) vs. 14 mos (induction) (p = NS), 2-yr OS 29% vs. 31% (p = NS). Upfront chemo ↑ grade 3–4 heme toxicity.

Is there a benefit of dose escalation in locally advanced NSCLC?

Yes. Dose escalation improves LC and probably translates to better survival.

RTOG 73-01: RCT testing 40 Gy split vs. 40 Gy continuous vs. 50 Gy continuous vs. 60 Gy continuous. The 60 Gy continuous had the best survival. 60 Gy became standard b/c of this trial, and since then 55–66 Gy is standard.

RTOG 93-11: dose escalation without chemo to 70.9 Gy, 77.4 Gy, 83.8 Gy, and 90.3 Gy. The 90.3 Gy is too toxic, but 77.4 Gy and 83.8 Gy is safe if V20 is 25%–36% and <25%, respectively. LC 50% to 78%, with LF in elective nodal areas <8%.

Michigan dose escalation (*Kong FM et al., IJROBP 2005*): 106 pts, stage I–III NSCLC, treated with 63–103 Gy in 2.1 Gy/fx with 3D-CRT; primary tumor + LN + ≥1 cm; no chemo in 81%. MS was 19 mos. MVA showed that the RT dose was the only predictor of better survival.

The safety of 74 Gy + chemo has been demonstrated in a number of phase I–II trials: **RTOG 0117** (74 Gy + chemo), **NCCTG 0028** (74 Gy + chemo), and UNC phase I–II (74 Gy + chemo is safe).

Intergroup Trial (**RTOG 0617/NCCTG N0628/ CALGB 30609/ECOG R0617**): RCT phase III comparison of 60 Gy vs. 74 Gy CRT with concurrent and consolidation carboplatin/Taxol +/– cetuximab in stage IIIA–B NSCLC. This trial is accruing.

What is the role of endobronchial/ intraluminal brachy-therapy for palliation for lung cancer?

Various fractionation schemes (15 Gy × 2 or 8–10 Gy × 1, prescribed to 0.5 cm) have been used in prior irradiated pts with endobronchial Dz causing Sx. Sx relief can be seen in 80% of pts. Complications included fatal hemoptysis (5%–10%), bronchoesophogeal fistula (2%), and bronchial edema (1%).

MDACC published a series of 81 previously irradi-ated lung cancer pts who were treated with palliative HDR endobronchial brachytherapy, 15 Gy × 2, 6 mm depth, over 2 wks. Response was seen in 84%. Pts with excellent response had better survival (MS 13.3 mos) vs. those with poor response (MS 5.4 mos) (*p* = 0.01). 2 fatal complications were due to fistula and trache-omalacia. (*Delclos ME et al., Radiology 1996*).

What fractionation scheme is optimal for pts with lung cancers treated with palliative RT for Sx such as hemoptysis, cough, pain, and shortness of breath?	**Conventional fractionation is probably no better than hypofractionation.** In a Norwegian RCT, *Sundstrom S et al.* tested 30 Gy in 10 fx vs. 17 Gy in 2 fx (1 wk apart) vs. 10 Gy in 1 fx. All achieved equivalent palliation. (*JCO 2007*)

■ Toxicity

What is the typical follow-up schedule of pts treated for lung cancer?	Typical lung cancer follow-up: H&P, CT chest with contrast q4–6mos for yrs 1–2, then noncontrast CT chest annually yrs 3–5, and continued smoking cessation counseling (*NCCN 2010*)
What are the expected acute and late toxicities of RT for lung cancer?	<u>Acute</u>: Skin reaction, fatigue, dysphagia, odynophagia, cough <u>Subacute and late</u>: RT pneumonitis, lung fibrosis, brachial plexopathy, L'hermitte syndrome, RT myelitis, esophageal fibrosis/stricture, pericarditis, 2nd cancers
What are the signs and Sx of RT pneumonitis, and how is it managed?	RT pneumonitis is a subacute reaction that begins as early as 3–6 mos after RT. Typically, Sx include **chest pain, shortness of breath, fever, and hypoxia.** CT scan shows ground glass changes within the RT port. Check oxygenation and supplement if necessary. **If symptomatic, treat with prednisone 1 mg/kg/day for at least 3 wks with a very slow taper. Bactrim can be used for PCP prophylaxis.**
What is total lung V20 dose-volume constraint for RT alone and concurrent CRT in definitive lung cancer Tx?	<u>NCCN 2010</u>: V20 <37% <u>MDACC</u>: RT alone → V20: <40%; CRT → V20: <35% (based on *Lee HK et al., IJROBP 2003*)
What is mean lung dose (MLD) constraint for definitive RT to lung cancer?	MLD is **<15 Gy;** max is **≤20 Gy.**
What is the heart RT dose-volume constraint for RT alone and concurrent CRT?	<u>NCCN 2010</u>: V40 <100%, V45 <67%, V60 <33% <u>MDACC</u>: RT alone→ V40: <50%; CRT → V40: <40%
What is the dose constraint for the brachial plexus?	The dose constraint is **1 cc below 60 Gy;** the max dose point should be <66 Gy.

Once SCLC has been diagnosed in a pt who presents with a large hilar mass, what further workup is necessary besides the basic H&P and labs?

LDH levels, CT C/A/P +/− PET, **MRI brain,** bone scan if PET is not done, **BM Bx** (for pts with elevated LDH), thoracentesis with cytopathologic exam for pts with pleural effusion, and smoking cessation counseling

What % of pts with SCLC at the time of Dx present with brain mets, BM involvement, and bone mets?

Brain mets: 10%–15% (30% are asymptomatic)
BM involvement: 5%–10%
Bone mets: 30%

What is the latest AJCC system for staging SCLC?

The same as for non-SCLC, but this system is not commonly used.

How is SCLC most commonly staged?

SCLC is staged using the **International Association of Lung Cancer system,** which is a modification of the Veterans Administration Lung Cancer Study Group (VALCSG) system. There are 2 stages: limited and extensive. Tumors are staged according to whether the Dz can be encompassed within an RT port. Limited stage Dz is typically confined to the ipsi hemithorax, without malignant pleural effusion, contralat Dz, or mets; other presentations are usually extensive stage.

What % of pts present with limited-stage SCLC?

~**33%** of pts present with limited-stage SCLC.

What are some adverse prognostic factors in SCLC?

Poor performance status (PS); weight loss (>5% in prior 6 mos); ↑LDH; male gender; endocrine paraneoplastic syndromes (controversial), variant, or of mixed cell type; metastatic Dz

What is the MS of untreated limited-stage and extensive-stage SCLC?

~**12 wks** for limited stage and ~**6 wks** for extensive stage, based on a VALCSG trial comparing cyclophosphamide to placebo.

What is the MS for pts with limited- vs. extensive-stage SCLC?

Limited stage: 19–23 mos (*Turrisi AT et al., NEJM 1999*)
Extensive stage: 5–7 mos (*Slotman B et al., NEJM 2007*)

What is the long-term survival rate in limited-stage SCLC treated with a combined modality?

~**20%–30%** long-term survival (5-yr OS)

What additional workup should be considered for pts with carcinoid tumors of the lung?

Consider **octreotide scan.**

■ Treatment/Prognosis

What is the Tx paradigm for pts with extensive-stage SCLC?	Extensive-stage SCLC Tx paradigm: **multiagent chemo regimen including etoposide/cisplatin (EP) or Cytoxan/Adriamycin/vincristine (CAV).** Consider consolidation RT to the thorax for pts who achieve a CR to distant Dz after initial chemo. (*Jeremic B et al., JCO 1999*)
What are some important poor prognostic factors for limited stage SCLC?	Karnofsky PS <70, weight loss, ↑LDH
What is the Tx paradigm for pts with limited-stage SCLC?	Limited-stage SCLC Tx paradigm: 4 cycles of EP **chemo (etoposide [120 mg/m², days 1–3] + cisplatin [60 mg/m², day 1, q3wks]) + concurrent RT (only 1 cycle is concurrent). Current standard RT regimen is based on INT-0096: 45 Gy in 1.5 Gy bid × 30 fx.**
How should a tumor characterized as a high-grade neuroendocrine carcinoma, or as large cell neuroendocrine carcinoma, be managed?	Treat per non-SCLC guidelines. (*NCCN 2010*)
How should a pt with a carcinoid tumor of the lung be managed?	**Surgery is 1ˢᵗ line if it is resectable.** Some centers will treat atypical carcinoid per the SCLC paradigm (nonsurgical). Per *NCCN 2010:* 1. Stage I–III typical carcinoid tumor can be observed after R0 resection. 2. For unresectable or medically inoperable stage III typical carcinoid tumors, RT alone is recommended. 3. For atypical carcinoid tumors, resected stage I can be observed. However, for resected stage II–IIIa tumors, chemo (EP) and RT adjuvantly is recommended.
How should stage IIIB–IV or unresectable carcinoid of the lung be managed?	**Systemic therapy (EP),** or octreotide if octreotide scan positive or symptomatic from paraneoplastic syndrome (*NCCN 2010*)
What is the benefit of smoking cessation prior to Tx in pts with limited-stage SCLC?	↓**Toxicity and** ↑**survival,** based on a retrospective review (*Videtic GMM et al., IJROBP 2003*)

Is there a role for definitive surgical resection in SCLC pts?

This is **controversial** and not standard. Retrospective studies suggest that with modern staging, T1-2N0 SCLC pts have reasonable outcomes with surgery and adj platinum-based chemo. The situation is uncommon (~5% of cases). (*Brock MV et al., J Thorac Cardiovasc Surg 2005*)

A JCOG phase II study tested surgical resection for stage I–IIIA SCLC → EP chemo. 5-yr OS was 69%, 38%, and 40%, respectively. Currently, RCTs in Europe and Japan are testing surgical management.

What is the recommended adj Tx for SCLC if the mediastinal nodes are found to be involved after attempted surgical resection?

Concurrent CRT directed at the MN (*NCCN 2010*); if node–, adj chemo alone

What additional chemo agents, when added to EP, have been shown to modestly improve the survival of pts with extensive-stage SCLC?

Ifosfamide or cyclophosphamide + an anthracycline have been shown to modestly improve survival.

What are some salvage chemo agents used at the time of recurrence for SCLC?

Oral topoiseromase I inhibitors are standard for post-chemo failure. (Topotecan was tested in RCTs showing doubling of survival [26 wks vs. 14 wks] compared with supportive care; irinotecan as a single agent was not tested.) The old combo chemo of CAV can be used (if EP is used as 1st line). Paclitaxel, docetaxel, vinorelbine, and gemcitabine as single agents are not standard since activity is low against SCLC.

What is the role of PCI in limited-stage SCLC? Is there an OS benefit with it?

Auperin meta-analysis of 7 RCTs (*NEJM 1999*) compared PCI vs. no PCI after CR following induction chemo +/− RT and no evidence of brain mets before randomization. There was ↓ 3-yr incidence of brain mets (33% vs. 59%) and **5.4%** better 3-yr OS (20.7% vs. 15.3%) and improved DFS. There was a trend to a better outcome with ↑ doses and RT <4 mos from the start of chemo.

What PCI dose is now standard for limited-stage SCLC?

25 Gy in 10 fx is now the standard dose for PCI for limited-stage SCLC. (**RTOG 0212-Intergroup:** *Le Pechoux C et al., Lancet Oncol 2009*)

For pts with limited-stage SCLC, what PCI doses were compared in RTOG 0212?

Standard doses (25 Gy in 10 fx) **vs. higher doses** (36 Gy in either 18 fx qd or 24 fx bid). There was **no difference in the 2-yr incidence of brain mets,** but there was an **OS and chest relapse advantage for the standard arm** (42% vs. 37%, $p = 0.05$) due to greater cancer-related mortality in the high-dose group. (*Le Pechoux C et al., Lancet Oncol 2009*)

What is the effect of PCI timing after the initiation of chemo for SCLC?

Based on **Auperin meta-analysis**, there was a decrease in risk of brain mets with earlier PCI (<4–6 mos vs. >6 mos) without an effect on risk of death.

Is there data demonstrating greater neuropsychologic complications after PCI for SCLC?

No. The data actually demonstrate no difference with or without PCI in a randomized trial addressing the question of neuropsychologic changes after PCI (*Arrigada et al., JNCI 1995*). Most pts (97%) actually have abnl neuropsychologic testing after chemo and before PCI, without a difference after PCI (*Komaki R et al., IJROBP 1995*).

What seminal study demonstrated a survival benefit with PCI in pts with extensive-stage SCLC with any response to chemo? What are some main criticisms of this study?

EORTC 08993 RCT (*Slotman BJ et al., NEJM 2007*): 286 pts with extensive-stage SCLC treated with chemo; primary endpoint was time to symptomatic brain mets; pts randomized to +/− PCI after *any* response to chemo; most PCI pts given 20 Gy in 5 fx. PCI lowered the risk of symptomatic mets and improved DFS and OS (5.4 mos –PCI vs. 6.7 mos +PCI). 1-yr OS nearly doubled (13% –PCI vs. 27% +PCI).

Criticisms: There was no pre-Tx MRI. The RT group was more likely to rcv chemo at the time of extracranial progression (68% vs. 45%). Only about half (59%) of pts in the control group rcv WBRT for intracranial progression of Dz.

What was the greatest QOL alteration after PCI in the EORTC trial for extensive-stage SCLC?

3-mo QOL assessment showed that the largest negative impact of PCI was **fatigue and hair loss.** Worsening role, emotional, and cognitive function were also seen after PCI. (*Slotman BJ et al., JCO 2009*)

What is the current recommendation for PCI in pts with SCLC?

Limited or extensive stage, CR/PR after chemo +/− RT, +/− MRI brain, PS of ECOG 0–2, within 3–6 wks of last cycle of chemo, 25 Gy in 10 fx. In pts with less than a CR, PCI is at the discretion of the treating physician.

What chest RT volumes are used to treat limited-stage SCLC?

Classic fields: gross tumor, ipsi hilum, bilat MN from thoracic inlet (1st rib) down to 5 cm below the carina. CTV = GTV + 1.5 cm (and elective hilum and MN regions + 8 mm), PTV = CTV + 1 cm.

CALGB 30610/RTOG 0538: **3D-CRT or IMRT allowed. CTV** needs to include **GTV** plus potential occult Dz defined as (a) ipsi hilum (level 10 LN) and (b) N2-N3 levels from the top of the aortic arch down to 3 cm below the carina encompassing levels 3, 4R, 4L, and 7 (and levels 5–6 for left-sided tumors). These areas are treated electively except for the supraclavicular fossa. **PTV** is CTV + 0.5 cm if daily setup imaging is used and if **ITV** assessment is done during simulation and the planning process (either breath-hold or 4D-CT imaging). If a free-breathing non-ITV approach is used (non–4D-CT simulation), the PTV is CTV + 1.5 cm (sup-inf direction) and 1.0 cm in the axial direction. If a breath-holding non-ITV, PTV is CTV + 1.0 cm (sup-inf direction) and 0.5 cm in the axial direction.

What thoracic RT field arrangements are used for treating limited-stage SCLC?

IMRT if V20 <30% and FEV1 >1 L. Otherwise, minimize contralat lung exposure with AP/PA to 15 Gy (1.5 Gy bid × 5 days) with oblique field CD to 45 Gy (AP/PA in am and obliques for pm sessions).

In SCLC pts with SVCO, cord compression, or brain mets, what regimen is preferred as upfront palliative Tx: RT or chemo?

In a chemo-naive pt presenting with SVCO, RCTs have shown a similar symptomatic response rate with chemo compared with RT. But in a chemo-refractory pt, RT is the preferred regimen. In pts with cord compression/brain mets, RT is standard (in both chemo-naive and chemo-refractory pts).

How is palliative RT delivered for SVCO syndrome in pts with SCLC?

Generally, **a few large fx upfront (3–4 Gy × 2–3) → more definitive dosing in conventional fractionation** (qd or bid regimen)

What fractionation scheme is optimal for pts with lung cancers treated with palliative RT for Sx such as hemoptysis, cough, pain, and shortness of breath?

Conventional is probably no better than hypo-fractionation. In a Norwegian RCT, *Sundstrom et al.* tested 30 Gy in 10 fx vs. 17 Gy in 2 fx (1 wk apart) vs. 10 Gy for 1 fx. All achieved similar levels of palliation. (*JCO 2007*)

■ Toxicity

What is the recommended follow-up schedule for SCLC pts?

SCLC follow-up schedule: H&P, CT chest, and labs at each visit (visits q2–3mos for yr 1, q3–4mos for yrs 2–3, q4–6mos yrs 4–5, then annually). PET scan should be considered whenever CT findings suggest recurrence or mets.

What is the total lung V20 dose-volume constraint for RT alone and concurrent CRT in definitive lung cancer Tx?

RT alone: V20 <40%
CRT: V20 <35%

(*NCCN 2010*)

What is the recommended mean lung dose (MLD) constraint with definitive RT for lung cancer?

MLD is **<15 Gy** ideally but not >20 Gy.

What is the max cord dose allowed with the Turrisi bid regimen?

With the Turrisi bid regimen, the max cord dose is **36 Gy.**

What is the main toxicity associated with using bid RT as done in the Turrisi regimen?

Grade 3 acute **esophagitis:** 27% (bid) vs. 11% (qd). Other toxicities (myelosuppression, nausea) were the same as the qd regimen.

What is the distinction between grade 2 and 3 pneumonitis (per the RTOG)?

Grade 3 pneumonitis: dyspnea at rest or oxygen supplementation needed
Grade 2 pneumonitis: symptomatic and not requiring oxygenation

What is the heart dose-volume constraint for RT alone vs. concurrent CRT?

RT alone: V40 <50%
CRT: V40 <40%

According to **RTOG 0538,** the following limits are also acceptable: 60 Gy less than one third, 45 Gy less than two thirds, and 45 Gy <100%.

What is the esophageal dose-volume constraint for RT alone vs. concurrent CRT?

RT alone: V60 <50%
CRT: V55 <50% (ideally, keep the mean dose to <34 Gy per **RTOG 0538**)

40

Thymoma and Thymic Carcinoma

Steven H. Lin and Melenda D. Jeter

▮ Background

What is the embryonic derivation of the thymus?	The embryonic derivation of the thymus is the **3rd pharyngeal pouch.**
Where is the thymus located, and what is its function?	The thymus is in the **ant mediastinum** (MN), **involved in the processing and maturation of T lymphocytes to recognize foreign antigens from "self" antigens.**
What structures are located in the ant, middle, and post MN?	<u>Anterior</u>: LNs, thymus, mesenchymal tissues <u>Middle</u>: heart and great vessels, trachea, esophagus, most mediastinal LNs, vagus and phrenic nerves <u>Posterior</u>: paraspinal tissues, sympathetic and peripheral nerves
What proportion of tumors of the MN are malignant?	**One third** of mediastinal tumors are malignant.
How prevalent is thymoma relative to other mediastinal tumors?	Thymoma comprises **20% of all mediastinal tumors** but **50% of all ant mediastinal tumors.**
What is the median age and gender predilection for thymomas?	The median age for thymomas is **40–60 yrs.** There is **no gender predilection** (male = female).
Are thymomas common in children?	**No.** Thymomas are extremely rare in children, but if present they are extremely aggressive with poor survival.
Pathologically, what is the most important defining feature of thymomas?	Coexistence of nonneoplastic lymphoid cells with **neoplastic epithelial cells** (spindle to polygonal types)
How do thymic carcinomas differ from thymomas?	**Much less prevalent** (<1% of thymic tumors), **very aggressive,** with **poorer survival** (5-yr OS 30%–50%)

What are the WHO designations of thymomas vs. thymic carcinomas?	WHO type is based on **shape** and the **lymphocyte/epithelial ratio.** WHO type A–AB: benign thymoma, medullary, spindle cell WHO type B1–B3: malignant thymoma, lymphocytic, cortical, epithelial WHO type C: highly malignant, thymic carcinoma, clear cell/sarcomatoid types
What is the LN metastatic rate of thymomas vs. thymic carcinomas?	Thymoma: ~1%–2% Thymic carcinoma: ~30% (Kondo & Monden review of 1,320 pts with thymic tumors [*Ann Thorac Surg 2003*])
What is the hematogenous dissemination of thymomas vs. thymic carcinomas?	Thymoma: ~1% (mostly to lung) Thymic carcinoma: 12% (lung > bone, liver)

■ Workup/Staging

What is the DDx of a mediastinal mass by location in the ant, middle, and post MN?	Anterior: thymoma, thymic carcinoma, carcinoid, germ cell tumors, lymphomas (Mnemonic **TTT**: **T**hymoma, **T**eratoma, **T**errible lymphoma) Middle: cysts > lymphoma, teratomas > sarcomas (osteosarcoma, fibrosarcoma, angiosarcoma, rhabdomyosarcoma of the heart), granuloma Posterior: neurogenic tumors (PNET, schwannoma, neurofibroma, neuroblastoma, ganglioneuroma), pheochromocytoma
What clinical presentations are common for pts with mediastinal tumors?	50% are diagnosed incidentally on imaging studies. Sx are caused by a mass effect resulting in **cough, shortness of breath, pain, stridor, Horner, superior vena cava** (SVC) **syndrome, HTN (catecholamine), myasthenia gravis** (MG) (thymoma)
How do pts with thymomas or thymic carcinomas usually present?	50% are incidental findings; but if there are Sx, they reflect either **locally advanced Dz, metastatic sequalae, or paraneoplastic disorders** (in 50%–60% of thymomas but hardly seen in thymic carcinomas).
What paraneoplastic disorders are commonly seen in thymomas?	**MG** (35%–50% of cases), **red cell aplasia** (5%), **immune deficiency syndromes** like hypogammaglobulinemia (5%), autoimmune disorders (collagen vascular, dermatologic, endocrine, renal Dz), and **other malignancies** (lymphomas, GI/breast carcinomas, Kaposi sarcoma)

Is adj radiotherapy necessary for a stage II thymoma after complete resection?

This is **controversial.** It initially was recommended based on a classic review (*Curran W et al., JCO 1988*) in 103 pts with thymomas, finding that pts without PORT had ↑LR (6 of 19 pts for stage II) vs. no LR in PORT (0 of 1 pt for stage II, 0 of 4 pts for stage III). More recent data out of the Massachusetts General Hospital (*Mangi A et al., Ann Thorac Surg 2002*) and Japan (*Haniuda M et al., Ann Surg 1996*) showed that PORT may not be necessary after complete resection for stage II pts. *Haniuda et al.* did demonstrate that stage II thymoma with macroscopic adherence to the pleura did benefit from PORT (LR 36% vs. 0%), but PORT was not useful for microscopic invasion of the pleura or pericardium.

Meta-analysis (*Korst RJ et al., Ann Thorac Surg 2009*): 1981–2008 systematic review of 13 studies, 592 pts, ~42% had surgery + PORT. The LR rate did not benefit from PORT for stage II–III thymoma (OR 0.87 for both stage II–III, $p = 0.69$).

Forquer JA et al., IJROBP 2009: 901 pts, SEER data 1973–2005; 92% thymoma, 8% TC; localized Dz in 274 pts, regional Dz in 626 pts. 5-yr OS benefited from surgery + PORT for regional Dz (76% vs. 66%, $p = 0.01$); for localized Dz, surgery alone was more favorable (98% vs. 91% [PORT], $p = 0.03$).

Current recommendation for adj RT for stage II–III thymoma: +/close margin (<1 mm), gross fibrous adhesion to pleura, or ↑ WHO grade (B3) tumors (*Wright CD et al., Hem Onc 2008*)

What should the postop target volume include?

The postop target volume should include the **entire bed of resection and any involved organs.** It is imperative to have a preop CT scan available to help delineate tumor bed volumes. Also, information from operative and pathology reports may help determine areas that might have had adherent, invasive Dz.

When should postop CRT be considered for the management of thymic malignancies?

Per *NCCN 2010*, thymoma with gross residual Dz or thymic carcinoma with R1-R2 resection

What are some management approaches for unresectable thymic tumors?

Management approaches for unresectable thymic tumors:
1. RT only
2. Induction chemo → surgery → RT
3. Preop RT

What are the results of definitive RT for unresectable thymic tumors?

RT can be used as sole modality, with **5-yr OS 50%–87%.** Surgery should be done whenever possible, however, since resectability is still the most important prognostic factor.

Given the good response rates seen with platinum-based chemo, what is the current preferred Tx paradigm for unresectable thymic malignancy?

Unresectable thymic malignancy Tx paradigm:
1. **Chemo → RT (no surgery)** (*Loehrer PJ et al., JCO 1997*). Cisplatin/doxorubicin/cyclophosphamide (PAC) 2–4 cycles → RT to ≥54 Gy to primary + regional LN. 5-yr OS was 53%.
2. **Chemo → surgery (if possible) → PORT** (MDACC: *Shin DM et al., Ann Int Med 1998*). 3 cycles induction chemo (Cytoxan/Adriamycin/cisplatin [CAP] + prednisone) → max surgery → RT. 7-yr follow-up showed 100% OS and 73% DFS.

What are the 1ˢᵗ-line combination chemo regimens used for the management of thymic malignancies?

CAP +/− prednisone; VP-16/ifosfamide/cisplatin (VIP); cisplatin/VP-16 (EP); carboplatin/Taxol; cisplatin/Adriamycin/vincristine/Cytoxan (ADOC); Cytoxan/Adriamycin/vincristine/prednisone (CHOP)

What are the typical response rates with induction chemo for the management of thymic malignancies?

Typical response rates with induction chemo are **50%–60%.**

What is the most common approach for the management of thymic carcinomas?

If possible, **max surgery → CRT postoperatively.** If inoperable, consider induction therapy with chemo, RT, or combination CRT.

What are the RT doses used for the postop management of thymomas?

Depends on the extent of resection:
   If R0: 45–54 Gy
   If R1: 55–60 Gy
   If R2: 60–70 Gy

What are the RT volumes utilized for high-risk resected thymomas?

Treat at-risk subclinical sites in the surgical bed and LN regions. The entire MN or SCV does not need to be covered unless indicated.

What RT doses can be used for the preop management of unresectable thymomas?

24–30 Gy with chemo → surgery → the consideration for more RT depending on resection status

■ Toxicity

What is the follow-up for pts who have had a complete resection of a thymoma?

Completely resected thymoma follow-up: H&P + annual CT chest

Is 5 yrs of follow-up sufficient for a pt treated for thymomas?

No. Late recurrences can occur at >10 yrs. Pts need lifelong follow-up.

What are the expected early and late toxicities after adj RT for the management of thymic tumors?

Early: skin reaction, fatigue, dysphagia/
  odynophagia, cough
Late: RT pneumonitis/fibrosis, pericarditis, esophageal stricture, myelitis

What are the dose limiting structures and dose limits when the MN is irradiated?

Lung: RT alone → V20 <40%; CRT → V20
  <35%. For DVH analysis, keep V5 <40%,
  V20 <30%, and V30 <8% (*NCCN 2010*).
Heart: V40 <50% (V40 <40% if CRT)
Spinal cord: ≤45 Gy
Esophagus: Ideally, the mean dose of RT to the
  esophagus should be <34 Gy. Try to minimize
  the V60 as much as possible (V60 <33%, V50
  <50%, ≤45 Gy to the entire esophagus, max
  dose point <70 Gy).

41
Pleural Mesothelioma
Steven H. Lin and M. Kara Bucci

■ Background

In what body sites does mesothelioma arise?

Mesothelioma commonly arises in the **pleura** but also occurs in the **peritoneum, pericardium, and tunica vaginalis testis.**

What is the most common cause of mesothelioma?

The highest risk factor for developing mesothelioma is **asbestos exposure** (amphiboles [rodlike] > chrysotile [serpentine form]). Asbestos is commonly found in insulation material, brake pads, and shipyards.

What is the major difference between the incidence of mesothelioma in the U.S. vs. the developing world?

B/c of early adoption of asbestos regulations, the incidence of **mesothelioma in the U.S. peaked in 2004 and has subsequently declined.** The incidence **has not yet peaked in the developing world** and is not expected for the next 10–20 yrs.

What is the estimated latency between asbestos exposure and mesothelioma?

The estimated latency between asbestos exposure and mesothelioma is **20–40 yrs.** (*Lanphear BP & Buncher CR, J Occup Med 1992*)

Approximately how many cases of malignant mesothelioma are diagnosed in the U.S. annually?

~**2,500–3,000 cases/yr** of malignant mesothelioma in the U.S. (*MMWR, CDC 2009*)

What % of mesothelioma cases are related to asbestos exposure?

~70%–80% of cases have documented asbestos exposure.

What is lifetime risk of mesothelioma for someone with an occupational asbestos exposure Hx?

The lifetime risk with asbestos exposure ~**10%.**

Does smoking cause mesothelioma?

No. Smoking alone is not associated with mesothelioma, but smoking increases the risk associated with asbestos exposure.

Is there a gender predilection for mesothelioma?

Yes. Males are more commonly affected than females, likely related to occupational exposure differences.

At what age does the incidence of mesothelioma peak?

The **incidence does not peak.** It continuously increases with age.

What are the 3 most common histopathologic subtypes of mesothelioma in decreasing order of frequency?

Histopathologic subtypes of mesothelioma: **epithelioid** (40%) > **mixed or biphasic** (35%) > **sarcomatous or mesenchymal** (25%)

What are some common genetic changes seen in mesothelioma?

Loss of tumor suppressor genes p16, p14, and NF-2 are common genetic changes in mesothelioma.

▉ Workup/Staging

What are the 2 most common initial presenting Sx of mesothelioma?

Dyspnea and nonpleuritic chest pain

What is a common presentation of mesothelioma?

Recurrent pleural effusion and/or pleural thickening found incidentally on CXR

What should be present for the initial workup of a pleural-based mass seen on CXR?

Pleural-based mass initial workup: H&P, CBC, CMP, serum soluble mesothelin-related peptide and osteopontin levels (optional), CT chest + contrast, thoracentesis for cytology, and pleural Bx. Consider talc pleurodesis or a pleural catheter for management of effusion.

What is the preferred manner for pleural Bx in the workup of possible mesothelioma?

Video-assisted thorascopic surgery (VATS) (preferred), open Bx, or CT-guided core Bx

What additional workup should be done with a Dx of malignant mesothelioma?

Malignant mesothelioma workup: CT C/A/P + contrast, PET/CT, and MRI chest to determine if there is chest wall (CW) or diaphragmatic invasion. Consider mediastinoscopy or endobronchial US for suspicious nodes. Consider laparoscopy to r/o transdiaphragmatic extension. Use VATS to r/o contralat Dz, if necessary. PFTs are done to assess lung function.

How does malignant mesothelioma appear on a CT of the thoracic chest?

On CT of the thoracic chest, malignant mesothelioma appears as **pleural thickening with involvement of interlobar fissures/atelectasis, with possible pleural plaques and calcification.**

What is the DDx of tumors of the pleura?

Primary tumors (benign or malignant), or more commonly, **metastatic Dz.** Malignant tumors include mesothelioma, sarcomas, and mets.

What is the diagnostic yield of mesothelioma from the fluid cytology of the pleural effusion?

Fairly poor, only ~**23%.** Often, cytology finds atypical mesothelial cells only.

With a needle Bx, what entity is often confused with mesothelioma?

Adenocarcinoma (metastatic) is often confused with mesothelioma.

What pathologic features distinguish mesothelioma from adenocarcinoma?

Mesothelioma is negative for periodic acid-Schiff stain, mucicarmine stain, carcinoembryonic antigen, and Leu-M1. It is positive for calretinin, vimentin, WT1, and cytokeratin.

In mesothelioma, electron microscopy reveals that cells have long microvilli, in contrast to adenocarcinomas, which have short microvilli.

What biomarker is elevated in mesothelioma?

SRMP and osteopontin in serum. It may be elevated in >80% of pts.

What is the AJCC 7th edition (2009) T staging of mesothelioma?

Tis: CIS

T1a: limited to ipsi parietal pleura, *no* visceral pleural involvement

T1b: +ipsi parietal pleura and focal involvement of visceral pleura

T2: involves ipsi pleural surfaces with at least 1 of the following: (a) confluent visceral pleural tumor, (b) invasion of diaphragmatic muscle, or (c) invasion of lung parenchyma

T3: involves any ipsi pleural surfaces with at least 1 of the following: (a) invasion of endothoracic fascia, (b) invasion into mediastinal fat, (c) solitary focus of tumor invading soft tissues of CW, and (d) nontransmural involvement of pericardium

T4: involves any ipsi pleural surfaces with at least 1 of the following: (a) diffuse or multifocal invasion of soft tissues of CW, (b) any rib involvement, (c) invasion through diaphragm to peritoneum, (d) invasion of any mediastinal organs, (e) direct extension to contralat pleura, (f) invasion into spine, (g) extension to internal surface of pericardium, (h) pericardial effusion with +cytology, (i) invasion of myocardium, and (j) invasion of brachial plexus

Describe the N staging of mesothelioma.

N1: mets involving bronchopulmonary or hilar nodes

N2: mets to ipsi mediastinum (MN) or to subcarinal or internal mammary nodes

N3: mets to contralat MN, internal mammary nodes, or hilar LNs, or to ipsi or contralat supraclavicular nodes

Describe the overall stage groupings for mesothelioma.

Stage IA: T1aN0
Stage IB: T1bN0
Stage II: T2N0
Stage III: T1-2N1-2 or T3N0-2
Stage IV: T4 or N3 or M1

Which histologic subtype has a worse prognosis?

The **sarcomatous** type has the worse prognosis.

Name the 4 EORTC poor prognostic factors for mesothelioma.

EORTC poor prognostic factors for mesothelioma:
1. WBC >8.3 × 10^9/dL
2. Performance status (PS) 1–2
3. Sarcomatous histology
4. Male gender

What are the estimated 1- and 2-yr OS rates for EORTC low- and high-risk mesothelioma?	Low risk: 1-yr OS 40%; 2-yr OS 14% High risk: 1-yr OS 12%; 2-yr OS 0%
What is the overall MS seen in mesothelioma?	Overall, MS is **4–12 mos.**
Is death from mesothelioma usually due to local progression or DM?	Death is usually due to **local progression** resulting in respiratory failure or infection.

■ Treatment/Prognosis

What is the Tx paradigm for resectable mesothelioma?	Resectable mesothelioma Tx paradigm: 1. Extrapleural pneumonectomy (EPP) → chemo → hemithorax RT *or* 2. Neoadj chemo → EPP → hemithorax RT
What is the Tx paradigm for unresectable mesothelioma?	Unresectable mesothelioma Tx paradigm: **combination chemo**
What are the typical recommended postop RT doses after resection for mesothelioma?	−Margin: 50 Gy Close/+ margin: 54–60 Gy Gross Dz: >60 Gy (if possible)
What are the chemos of choice for the Tx of mesothelioma?	Preferred Tx includes the **combination chemo of choice incorporated into trimodality regimens** utilizing antifolate agents such as pemetrexed (Alimta)/cisplatin or gemcitabine/cisplatin. Pemetrexed/cisplatin is based on an RCT (*Vogelzang NJ et al., JCO 2003*) of unresectable mesothelioma pts to cisplatin vs. pemetrexed/cisplatin. There was improved response rate (17% vs. 41%) and survival (9 mos vs. 12 mos) with pemetrexed/cisplatin. This trial led to FDA approval for use in unresectable Dz. Cisplatin/gemcitabine is based on several phase II studies.
What % of mesothelioma pts are surgically resectable at Dx?	**<5%** of pts are surgically resectable at Dx.
What TNM stage of Dz determines surgical resectability using EPP for mesothelioma?	**T1-3N0-1.** Therefore, mediastinoscopy to r/o N2-N3 Dz will be important.

What clinical factors are important to consider for proper pt selection for EPP?

Factors important for proper EPP pt selection:
1. PS 0–1
2. Predicted postop FEV1 >1.0 L
3. PaO_2 >65 mm Hg (on room air)
4. $PaCO_2$ <45 mm Hg (on room air)
5. Ejection fraction >40%
6. Mean pulmonary arterial pressure <30 mm Hg
7. Epithelial histology
8. No T4, N2-N3, or M1 Dz
9. Able to tolerate trimodality therapy

What is removed with an EPP for mesothelioma?

Parietal pleura, lung, mediastinal nodes, pericardium, and ipsi diaphragm, with a graft to prevent herniation of abdominal contents through the diaphragmatic defect. Mediastinal nodal dissection should be done.

When is a decortication/ pleurectomy a preferred procedure over EPP in a pt with mesothelioma?

Decortation/pleurectomy is preferred over EPP in pts with **more advanced Dz** (↑ nodal Dz, areas of local invasion), **mixed histology,** and **medically high-risk pts.** Periop mortality is 2%–5%.

What is the mortality rate of EPP? What is the MS for mesothelioma after EPP?

The mortality rate of EPP ranges from **4%–31%** and depends largely on the experience of the center and preop selection. MS in most series is **4–20 mos.**

What study supports adj RT after EPP for mesothelioma?

MSKCC phase II trial with hemithorax RT to 54 Gy after EPP improved LC and OS compared to historical controls (*Rusch V et al., IJROBP 2003*). 2-yr OS was 33%. MS was 34 mos for stages I–II and 10 mos for later stages.

What study supports the role of trimodality therapy for mesothelioma?

Harvard retrospective review (*Sugerbaker D et al., J Thorac Cardiovc Surg 1999*) of 183 pts treated with EPP + adj chemo (Cytoxan/Adriamycin/cisplatin [CAP] or carboplatin/Taxol) + RT → adj chemo. Overall MS was 19 mos; 5-yr OS was 15%. The suggested long-term survival in the most favorable subgroup of 2-yr OS was 68%, 5-yr OS was 46%, and MS was 21 mos. 3 factors predicted for best outcomes: epithelial histology, negative resection margin, and negative extrapleural nodes.

Name 2 RT techniques used for adj Tx of mesothelioma after EPP.

AP/PA or IMRT to 45–54 Gy, with a boost to 60 Gy for a close/ + margin

Describe conventional RT field borders for adj RT Tx of mesothelioma after EPP.

Superior: T1
Lateral: skin
Medial: if right-sided, ipsi edge of vertebral body or 1.5 cm beyond edge of vertebral body if MN is positive for Dz; if left-sided, 1.5 cm into ipsi edge of vertebral body
Inferior: L2

Need to block critical structures such as the heart and liver and supplement blocked areas with electrons.

For **right-sided** tumors, the abdominal block is present throughout with electron supplementation at 1.53 Gy/fx (+scatter).

For **left-sided** tumors, the kidney is blocked throughout, and the heart block is present after 19.8 Gy. The spinal cord is blocked after 41.4 Gy by shifting the medial border to the ipsi edge of the vertebral body.

Include scars with bolus in the field and boost if necessary.

How is IMRT delivered for the adj Tx of mesothelioma?

MDACC experience (*Ahamad A et al., IJROBP 2003, 2004*), using 13–27 fields with 8–11 angles, with ~100 segments/field. Target volume was the entire hemithorax, all surgical clips, all sites of instrumentation, and the ipsi MN; initial dose to 45–50 Gy, with a boost to 60 Gy for a close/+margin. 2-yr survival was 62%, and 3-yr DFS was 45% for LN–, epithelioid histology. 5 pts with stage I Dz had 3-yr DFS of 100%.

Under what circumstances should pts be spared the morbidity of an EPP?

Subhistologies of sarcomatous or mixed type, involvement of the mediastinal LNs, large tumor burden, extension to extracapsular sites. These are all poor preop factors that have very poor DFS and OS and may not benefit from EPP. Palliative procedures should be considered.

If the pt is not a good candidate for EPP, pleurectomy or decortication has been advocated by some investigators. What does the procedure entail, and what are the outcomes of the procedure?

Decortication or pleurectomy involves **stripping of the pleura from the apex of the lung to the diaphragm, removing pericardium and parietal pleura**. MS is **6.7–21 mos.**

What is often recommended after a decortication/ pleurectomy procedure for mesothelioma?

B/c of the high LR rate, **adj RT is advocated** (*Gupta V et al., IJROBP 2005*). 125 pts were treated with pleurectomy → interstitial RT or EBRT at MSKCC. MS was 13.5 mos; 2-yr OS was 23%. Those with epithelial-type or earlier-stage Dz did better. Pts receiving <40 Gy, those with left-sided Dz, those with use of an implant, or those with a nonepithelioid histology did worse. LC rate was 40%. However, there were increased rates of toxicity (12 pts with pneumonitis, 8 pts with pericarditis). 2 pts died from grade 5 toxicity within 1 mo of Tx.

What is a palliative surgical procedure to consider for the management of poor-risk mesothelioma?

Pleurodesis with talc can be considered as palliative care with poor-risk mesothelioma.

What is the Tx paradigm for unresectable mesothelioma (stage III or IV)?

Unresectable mesothelioma Tx paradigm: chemo with cisplatinum/pemetrexed or cisplatinum/gemcitabine

What is the role of RT in unresectable mesothelioma Dz?

Palliative RT is used only for temporary pain relief. Use either 30 Gy in 10 fx or 20 Gy in 5 fx. In retrospective studies, the 2 regimens gave similar palliation.

What RT doses are used for palliation of chest pain associated with skin nodules in the CW?

Daily doses ≥4 Gy appear more efficacious than fx dose <4 Gy, for a total dose of 20–40 Gy.

What is the role of RT after invasive procedures for mesothelioma? What study evaluated the role of prophylactic RT, and what were the results?

Historically, RT was given to areas of invasive procedure to avoid needle tract seeding with tumor. RT was **7 Gy × 3, for a total of 21 Gy.** However, *O'Rourke et al.* (*Radiother Oncol 2007*) showed in a randomized trial that **prophylactic RT to drain sites did not statistically reduce the rate of seeding**. However, b/c recurrence is morbid and this is easy to do, it is still generally done.

■ Toxicity

What is the estimated contralat lung V20 associated with the development of fatal pneumonitis in the Tx of mesothelioma?

RR was 42 for fatal pneumonitis if the V20 was >7% in the contralat intact lung based on a retrospective review from MDACC. (*Rice DC et al., Ann Thorac Surg 2007*)

What are the dose-volume constraints for the contralat lung in RT for mesothelioma?

In the remaining lung, with the V20 <20% (preferably <10%), **mean lung dose ≤8.5 Gy, V5 <50%.**

What is the dose constraint for the liver? Heart? Spinal cord? Esophagus? Kidney?

Liver: V30 <30%
Heart: V40 <50%
Spinal cord: V45 <10%, no volume >50 Gy
Esophagus: V55 <30%
Kidney: V15 <20%

PART VI Breast

42

General Breast Cancer

John P. Christodouleas and Richard C. Zellars

Background

What are the 3 most commonly diagnosed cancers in women in decreasing order of incidence?

Most commonly diagnosed cancers in women: breast > lung >colorectal

What are the 3 most common causes of cancer death in women in decreasing order of incidence?

Most common causes of cancer death in women: lung > breast > colorectal

Approximately how many women are diagnosed with invasive and noninvasive breast cancer, and how many will die of breast cancer annually?

<u>Incidence</u>: ~180,000 invasive breast cancers and ~65,000 noninvasive breast cancers annually.
<u>Mortality</u>: ~40,000

What is median age of Dx for invasive breast cancer?

The median age for invasive breast cancer is **61 yrs.**

What race has the highest rate of breast cancer Dx? What race has the highest rate of breast cancer mortality?

<u>Highest Dx</u>: whites
<u>Highest mortality</u>: blacks

For women born in the U.S. in 2009, approximately what % will be diagnosed with breast cancer in their lifetimes?

~**12%** (1 in 8) of U.S. women born in 2009 will be diagnosed with breast cancer.

In the U.S. in 2009, was the incidence of breast cancer Dx increasing or decreasing?

The incidence of Dx was **increasing.**

In the U.S. in 2009, was the incidence of breast cancer mortality increasing or decreasing?

The incidence of mortality was **decreasing.**

What are the 2 most common hereditary mutations that predispose to breast cancer?

BRCA1 and BRCA2 are the most common mutations.

What ethnic ancestry is associated with the highest risk of carrying a BRCA1/BRCA2 mutation?

Ashknazi Jewish ancestry. As many as 1 in 40 Ashknazi Jews may have a BRCA1 or BRCA2 mutation.

Mutations in which gene, BRCA1 or BRCA2, confer a higher risk of ovarian cancer?

Both BRCA1 and BRCA2 are associated with increased risk of ovarian cancer, but risks are higher with **BRCA1** (40%–60% lifetime risk) compared to BRCA2 (10% lifetime risk).

How does familial breast cancer status and pt age affect breast tumor doubling time?

Pts with familial breast cancer and young age have a shorter tumor doubling time, so consider shortening screening intervals for these pts.

Is HRT with estrogen and progestin associated with an increased or decreased risk of breast cancer?

HRT with estrogen and progestin is associated with an **increased** RR of 1.7.

Separate the following factors into ones that increase or decrease the risk of breast cancer: younger age at menarche, younger age at menopause, nulliparity, prolonged breast-feeding, use of HRT.

Increase risk: younger age at menarche, nulliparity, use of HRT
Decrease risk: younger age at menopause, prolonged breast-feeding

Estimate the annual risk of a contralat breast cancer in pts with a personal Hx of breast cancer.

Premenopausal: 1%/yr
Postmenopausal: 0.5%/yr

What is the definition of menopause?

Menopause criteria for amenorrhea not related to Tx should include (a) bilat oophorectomy, (b) age ≥60 yrs, and (c) age <60 yrs and amenorrheic for ≥12 mos.
If Tx-related amenorrhea, menopausal status must be maintained either from (a) oophorectomy or (b) serial measurements of FSH or estrogen at menopausal levels.

What are the screening recommendations for normal-risk women age 20–40 yrs and women >40 yrs?

For normal-risk women age 20–40 yrs: clinical breast exam every 1–3 yrs and periodic breast exam.

For normal risk women age 40–49 yrs: recommendations are currently controversial, as the U.S. Preventive Services Task Force no longer recommends mammogram for this age group. However, the ACS and ACR still recommend mammograms every 1–2 yrs for this age group and annually for women age ≥50 yrs.

For a woman with prior RT exposure to the breast, when should screening begin for breast cancer and how?

Screening should begin 10 yrs after RT or at age 40 yrs, whichever comes 1st. Screen with an annual mammogram and clinical breast exams every 6–12 mos.

When should a woman be screened for breast cancer using MRI?

Per the American Cancer Society guidelines (2007), screen women who have ~20%–25% or greater lifetime risk of breast cancer based on 1 of many available risk models (e.g., *Tyler J et al., Stat Med 2004*). This does *not* include women with dense breast tissue.

According to *NCCN 2010*, what are the clinical indications and applications of dedicated breast MRI testing?

Clinical indications/application of dedicated breast MRI testing (*NCCN 2010*):
1. Determine multifocality or multicentricity of Dz in the breast.
2. Screening for contralat breast lesions in a newly diagnosed breast cancer pt.
3. Breast cancer evaluation before and after neoadj therapy to define response to Tx and assess breast conservation therapy eligibility.
4. To detect additional Dz in a mammographically dense breast.
5. To detect primary Dz in pts with +axillary LNs with unknown primary or Paget Dz of the nipple.
6. Since false+ findings on MRI are common, all lesions need to be sampled to r/o benign lesions.

Name the 5 rare histologic types of breast cancer that have a more favorable overall prognosis than invasive ductal/lobular carcinoma.

Rare types of breast cancer with a more favorable prognosis:
1. Tubular
2. Mucinous
3. Medullary
4. Cribriform
5. Invasive papillary

Name the 1 rare histologic type of breast cancer that has a less favorable overall prognosis than invasive ductal/lobular carcinoma.

Micropapillary carcinoma has a less favorable overall prognosis.

What is the Oncotype DX, and which breast cancer pts are eligible for its use?

Oncotype DX analyzes a panel of 21 genes within a breast cancer tumor to estimate risk of any recurrence **for early-stage, estrogen receptor (ER)+, node– breast cancer. NSABP B20** suggested that Oncotype DX may quantify benefit of chemo in this subgroup. The TAILORx trial is prospectively evaluating this hypothesis. Other genetic panels for women not eligible for Oncotype DX are being developed.

What are the 5 subtypes of the tissue microarray classification system for breast cancer? Which 2 subtypes carry poor prognoses?

Subtypes of the tissue microarray classification system:
1. Luminal A (↑ER expressing, ↓proliferation)
2. Luminal B (↑ER expressing, ↓proliferation)
3. HER2 overexpressing
4. Normal-like
5. Basal type (ER/progesterone receptor (PR)/HER2N−)

Basal and luminal B carry relatively poor prognoses.

What are phyllodes tumors of the breast, and what is the most important factor that determines risk of recurrence?

Phyllodes tumors are rare tumors containing both stromal and epithelial elements. Although the subtypes range from benign to malignant, the most important prognostic factor for recurrence is a clear margin after resection.

■ Workup/Staging

What is the workup for a breast lesion seen on mammogram?

Breast lesion workup: H&P (inquire about family Hx of breast and ovarian cancer, previous abnl mammogram, Hx of atypical ductal or lobular hyperplasia), CBC, CMP, bilat digital mammogram, spot compression views of abnl lesion, and stereotactic Bx of lesion

In a pt with T1-T2 breast cancer and a clinically– axilla, what is rate of pathologic axillary involvement?

The rate of pathologic axillary involvement is ~**30%.**

In a breast cancer pt with clinically+ axilla, what is chance that the axilla is negative upon dissection?

There is ~**25%** chance that the axilla is negative.

What are the 5 regional LN stations in breast cancer?

Regional LN stations in breast cancer:
  Station I: nodes inf/lat to pectoralis minor muscle
  Station II: nodes deep to pectoralis minor
  Station III: nodes sup/med to pectoralis minor
  Station IV: supraclavicular nodes
  Station V: internal mammary (IM) nodes

Infraclavicular nodes typically refer to the level III axillary nodes by radiation oncology.

What is the AJCC T staging for invasive breast cancer according to the AJCC 7th edition (2009)?

Tis: in situ (ductal CIS, lobular CIS, or isolated Paget)
T1mi: microinvasion ≤1 mm
T1a: >0.1–0.5 cm
T1b: >0.5–1 cm
T1c: >1–2 cm
T2: >2–5 cm
T3: >5 cm
T4a: extension to chest wall, not including pectoralis muscle
T4b: edema (including peau d'orange) or ulceration of skin of breast, or satellite nodules confined to same breast
T4c: both T4a and T4b
T4d: inflammatory carcinoma

(*Note:* T classification is the same whether it is based on clinical judgment or pathologic assessment. In general, pathologic determination should take precedence for determination of T size.)

Does involvement of breast cancer to the dermis alone qualify as T4 Dz?

No. Involvement of the skin by breast cancer qualifies as T4 only if there is ulceration or skin nodules.

What is the AJCC clinical N staging for invasive breast cancer according to the AJCC 7th edition (2009)?

N1: movable ipsi axillary LN
N2a: ipsi axillary LNs fixed to one another
N2b: clinically apparent IM node in absence of clinically evident axillary nodes
N3a: ipsi infraclavicular LNs
N3b: ipsi IM and axillary nodes
N3c: ipsi supraclavicular nodes

What is the AJCC pathologic N staging for invasive breast cancer according to the AJCC 7th edition (2009)?

pN(i–): negative by immunohistochemistry (IHC)
pN(i+): positive by IHC only, but no cluster >0.2 mm (aka isolated tumor cell clusters)
pN0(mol–): negative by RT-PCR
pN0(mol+): positive by RT-PCR only
pN1mi: all nodal mets >0.2 mm but <2 mm
pN1a: 1–3 axillary LNs involved
pN1b: IM node detected by sentinel LND, but not clinically apparent
pN1c: 1–3 axillary nodes and IM node detected by sentinel LND, but not clinically apparent
pN2a: 4–9 axillary LNs involved (tumor deposit at least >2.0 mm)
pN2b: clinically apparent IM nodes in the absence of axillary LN mets
pN3a: >10 axillary LN or mets to infraclavicular (axillary level III) LNs
pN3b: clinically apparent IM node in the presence of axillary nodes; or ≥3 axillary LNs and IM node detected by sentinel LND, but not clinically apparent
pN3c: ipsi supraclavicular node

What is the most common clinical presentation of LCIS?	LCIS most commonly presents as an **incidental finding.** LCIS typically does not result in mammographic or clinical abnormalities.
What is the rate of progression at 10 yrs of DCIS to invasive Dz if left untreated?	~**30%** of DCIS progress to invasive Dz at 10 yrs if left untreated. (*Page DL et al., Cancer 1995*)
For a pt with LCIS, what is the risk of the pt to be diagnosed with invasive Dz by 10 yrs?	A pt with LCIS has an ~**7%** risk of developing invasive cancer at 10 yrs (~**1%/yr**), but approximately half of invasive Dz occurs at the contralat breast, suggesting that LCIS is probably just a marker for propensity to form invasive Dz. (*Chuba PJ et al., J Clin Oncol 2005*)
What % of pts with LCIS who subsequently develop invasive Dz develop invasive lobular cancers?	Only **25%–50%** of subsequent cancers are invasive lobular cancers (i.e., though LCIS is a proliferative lesion of the lobules, it is mostly a marker for subsequent ductal proliferative lesions).
For a pt with LCIS, what is the risk of invasive Dz in the ipsi breast vs. the contralat breast?	For a pt with LCIS, the risk of subsequent invasive Dz is **equal in both breasts.**
How many pathologic grades are there for DCIS?	There are 3 pathologic grades for DCIS: low, intermediate, and high.
What % of DCIS are estrogen receptor (ER)+?	**75%–85%** of DCIS cases are ER+.
Which subtype of LCIS has the worst prognosis?	Of LCIS subtypes, **pleomorphic** LCIS has the worst prognosis.

▓ Workup/Staging

What is the initial workup after a DCIS Dx?	DCIS workup: H&P (with emphasis on risk of hereditary breast cancer), diagnostic bilat mammogram, assessment of ER status, +/− genetic counseling
Is an axillary dissection needed for DCIS?	**No.** An axillary dissection is not needed for DCIS. However, per *NCCN 2010,* consider if (a) the pt is undergoing mastectomy for Tx or (b) if the location of lumpectomy will compromise future sentinel Bx should it be necessary.
What is the T stage for DCIS?	DCIS has its own designation: **Tis.**
What is the definition of DCIS with microinvasion, and what is the significance for workup?	DCIS with microinvasion refers to invasion ≤**1 mm** in size. If microinvasion is present, then a sentinel **LN Bx is indicated, as the LN+** rate is ~**4%–8%**.

For a pt with DCIS, if there is <1-mm margin at excision, what is the rate of residual Dz at the time of re-excision?

For a pt with DCIS and a <1-mm margin at excision, **~30% will have residual Dz at re-excision.** Notably, low- and intermediate-grade DCIS is more likely to grow in a discontinuous pattern (*Faverly DR et al., Semin Diagn Pathol 1994*). B/c of this, margin status may be, paradoxically, more important in these lesions. In these discontinuous type lesions, gaps of uninvolved tissue between DCIS are typically small (<5 mm in 80% of cases).

For a pt with DCIS, in which situation would re-excision not be indicated with a margin <1 mm?

If a pt with DCIS has an **excisional margin <1 mm at the fibroglandular border** of the breast (skin or chest wall), then re-excision is not indicated.

■ Treatment/Prognosis

What is the Tx paradigm for unifocal DCIS?

There are 2 Tx paradigms for unifocal DCIS:
1. Lumpectomy + PORT +/− tamoxifen (if ER+)
2. Mastectomy

What must be done after lumpectomy for DCIS to ensure that all the Dz has been removed?

Post-excision mammography to ensure that all the microcalcifications are removed. **Specimen radiograph** is done after lumpectomy to ensure that the calcifications are removed.

For a pt with DCIS, what is rate of LR after mastectomy alone?

For a pt with DCIS, the rate of LR after mastectomy is **~2% at 10 yrs.**

What are considered adequate surgical margins in pts receiving breast conservation surgery for DCIS?

A systematic review of published trials in DCIS with breast conservation therapy (BCT) involving 4,660 pts found that a **2-mm margin** was superior to a margin <2 mm (OR 0.53), without any LC benefit in margins >2 mm. (*Dunne C et al., J Clin Oncol 2009*)

What are the contraindications for BCT for DCIS?

Contraindications for BCT for DCIS: multifocal Dz, persistently +margins, cosmetic limitations, inability to get postop RT (pregnancy or prior RT).

For a pt with DCIS treated with lumpectomy, what is the impact of PORT on ipsi breast recurrence (invasive and noninvasive) and OS?

For DCIS treated with lumpectomy, PORT **reduces LR by 50%, but there is no evidence for OS benefit.**

Is there a benefit of mastectomy over BCT for DCIS?

This is **undetermined.** No prospective study has directly compared mastectomy vs. BCT for DCIS. However, in the **NSABP B06** study, 78 pts were found to have DCIS after final pathology review. The LF rate was 2% for mastectomy, 9% for lumpectomy + RT, and 43% with lumpectomy alone (*Fisher B et al., JSO 1991*).

Name 4 prospective studies that support the addition of RT after lumpectomy in pts with DCIS.

Prospective studies that show LC benefit after lumpectomy in DCIS:
1. **NSABP B17** (*Fisher B et al., Sem Oncol 2001*)
2. **EORTC 10853** (*Bijker N et al., J Clin Oncol 2006*)
3. **UKCCCR** (*Houghton J et al., Lancet 2003*)
4. **SweDCIS** (*Holmber L et al., J Clin Oncol 2008*)

Describe the Tx arms and the invasive and noninvasive LR outcomes in NSABP B17 and EORTC 10853.

In **NSABP B17,** 818 DCIS pts with −margins (no cells at inked margin) treated with lumpectomy were randomized to 50 Gy ipsi RT or no RT. At 10 yrs, the overall ipsilateral breast tumor recurrence (IBTR) rate was 30.8% vs. 14.9% in favor of RT. Both the invasive and noninvasive recurrence rate was approximately halved by RT.

In **EORTC 10853,** 1,010 DCIS pts with −margins (no cells at ink) were randomized to lumpectomy vs. lumpectomy + whole breast RT at 50 Gy. RT reduced LF from 16% to 9%. Half of all recurrences were invasive.

For a pt with ER+ DCIS, is there a benefit to tamoxifen in addition to lumpectomy + RT? What studies support this?

The evidence for the benefit of adj tamoxifen in addition to lumpectomy + RT is **mixed.**

NSABP B24 compared lumpectomy + RT +/− tamoxifen and found that at 7 yrs, the addition of tamoxifen significantly decreased IBTR (8% vs. 11%). The benefit was seen with respect to invasive recurrences but not noninvasive recurrences. CBTR was also reduced with tamoxifen (2.3% vs 4.9%) (*Fisher B et al., Semin Oncol 2001*). 2 caveats about this trial are that −margins were not required (the inclusion of margin+ or margin unknown pts may have exaggerated the benefit of tamoxifen) and that index lesions were not tested for ER status at the time, though subsequent analyses have attempted to address this.

Another randomized trial by the UKCCCR (*Houghton J et al., Lancet 2003*) did not show a benefit with the addition of tamoxifen with respect to either invasive or noninvasive recurrences. Differences between these studies may be due to the age of cohorts, as **NSABP B24** enrolled generally younger women, and younger age at Dx was shown to be associated with higher IBTR rates in the B24 report. In B24, 30% of pts were <50 yo. In UKCCCR, 10% of pts were <50 yo. ER status has not been compared between the 2 studies. In addition, the design of the UKCCCR trial (2 × 2 factorial design) and institutional choice in participating in 2 × 2 design or only 1 of the randomizations may have created imbalances in the Tx arms. In summary, it is controversial which subgroups of DCIS pts treated with lumpectomy truly benefit from adj tamoxifen, but **in current practice, ER+ DCIS pts are offered adj tamoxifen.**

For a pt with DCIS, what is the effect of adj tamoxifen on contralateral breast tumor recurrence (CBTR)?

NSABP B24 showed that the addition of tamoxifen to BCT in DCIS pts significantly reduced CBTR as the 1st site of recurrence from 4.9% to 2.3% at 7 yrs.

For a pt with ER− DCIS, is there benefit to adj tamoxifen after lumpectomy + RT?

No. Retrospective analysis of **NSABP B24** showed that the benefit of adj tamoxifen was limited to ER+ pts. (*Allred DC et al., Br Cancer Res Treat 2002*)

For a pt with ER+ DCIS, does adj tamoxifen obviate the benefit of RT after lumpectomy? What study evaluated this?

RT is still beneficial for pts with DCIS treated with lumpectomy even with adj tamoxifen. UKCCCR was a 2 × 2 factorial study looking at the benefit of RT and tamoxifen in DCIS pts after lumpectomy. After a median follow-up >4 yrs, RT reduced IBTR in women given adj tamoxifen (6% vs. 18%). (*Houghton J et al., Lancet 2003*)

For a pt with DCIS, name some risk factors associated with LR and which is most important.

Risk factors for LR in a pt with DCIS:
1. Decreased margin width (most important)
2. Increased size of tumor
3. High grade
4. Young age (≤40 yrs)
5. Comedo necrosis
6. Multifocality

For a pt with DCIS treated with lumpectomy + PORT (no tamoxifen), estimate the risk of LR if the pt had a negative surgical margin vs. a positive surgical margin.

For a pt with DCIS treated with lumpectomy + PORT (no tamoxifen), LR at 14 yrs is ~**13% if a −margin vs. 26% if a +margin.**

What is the purpose of the Van Nuys Prognostic Classification, and what are its limitations?

The purpose of the Van Nuys Prognostic Classification system is meant to identify DCIS pts who are at low risk for recurrence after RT alone using width of margins, size, grade, and age. The system was developed retrospectively and has not been validated in prospective studies or in different retrospective data sets. (*Silverstein MJ et al., Am J Surg 2003*)

Do all DCIS pts require PORT?

This is **controversial.** Some data suggest that all women with DCIS need PORT. To date, the prospective randomized trials have failed to identify a subset of DCIS pts who can safely omit adj RT. The Van Nuys investigators have published retrospective data showing low IBTR rates in a subset of selected DCIS pts using special surgical and pathologic techniques. Other groups have not been able to reproduce these results. However, recent unpublished data from the ECOG suggest that recurrence is low without PORT for low- to intermediate-grade DCIS excised to widely −margin (5–10 mm). For high-grade Dz +/− comedo necrosis, PORT is necessary.

The DFCI trial was a prospective study that enrolled women with DCIS after surgery to >1-cm margin, grade 1–2 Dz, to undergo observation. Accrual was halted after 5 yr IBTR reached 12%, meeting early stopping rules of excessive failures. The trial, however, assessed mammographic size (rather than pathologic size) as an entry criteria, did not allow tamoxifen, and included women with "predominant grade 1 or 2 Dz," implying that higher-grade components may have been present in some cases. Nonetheless, the results of the trial are in keeping with the body of literature in general. (*Wong J et al., J Clin Oncol 2006*)

ECOG E5194 (*Hughes LL et al., J Clin Oncol 2009*): prospective study, 711 pts with either low- to intermediate-risk (low/intermediate-grade Dz, ≤2.5 cm) or high-risk (high grade, ≤1 cm) DCIS were excised to >3-mm margins. All nonpalpable Dz was ≥3 mm. No PORT. Tamoxifen was taken by 31%. Accrual to the low/intermediate-grade group was separate from the high-grade cohort. The majority had 5–10-mm margins. 606 pts were in the low/intermediate group, and 105 pts (stopped due to poor accrual) were in the high-grade group. Median follow-up was 6.2 yrs, median age was 60 yrs. *Results:* Low/intermediate-grade cohort: 5-yr and 7-yr IBTR was 6.1% and 10.5%; CBTR was 3.7% and 4.8%. For the high-grade cohort: 5-yr and 7-yr IBTR was 15.3% and 18%; CBTR was 3.9% and 7.4%. There was 50% recurrence with invasive Dz. These results clearly support PORT in even the smallest high-grade DCIS pts, but longer follow-up is warranted to determine whether omission of RT is appropriate for the low-risk groups. Retrospective data sets have demonstrated that with longer follow-up, lower-grade DCIS pts have similar IBTR rates as higher-grade pts.

RTOG 98-04: RCT with the same selection criteria as the ECOG study randomized 636 pts to RT vs. no RT. Results are pending.

What whole breast dose and boost dose is used for a pt with DCIS after lumpectomy?

For DCIS, the whole breast dose is 46–50 Gy with a lumpectomy bed boost to a total of 60–66 Gy. The role of boost in DCIS is controversial. The practice is extrapolated from results of the EORTC and Lyon boost trials for invasive cancers, but there have been no prospective trials of the role of boost in DCIS pts. ~44% of pts from **B24** were given a boost, mainly for +margins.

What is the Tx paradigm for LCIS?

LCIS Tx paradigm: For pure LCIS after lumpectomy, pts can be observed +/− risk reduction procedures. Occurrence of invasive Dz after LCIS is low and is often in the contralat breast. In addition, invasive Dz after LCIS is generally relatively favorable, and deaths subsequently are rare. The exception may be pleomorphic LCIS, though data are limited.

For a pt with LCIS, what are 2 options to reduce the risk of development of an invasive cancer?

Options to reduce the risk of development of an invasive cancer:
1. Antiestrogen therapy with tamoxifen or raloxifene (raloxifene only if postmenopausal) (**NSABP P1 trial**)
2. Bilat mastectomy +/− reconstruction if there is a risk of hereditary breast cancer

What is the management for a woman with LCIS detected on percutaneous core needle Bx?

LCIS does not result in mammographic or physical exam findings; as such, pure LCIS on core needle Bx should typically prompt an open Bx to identify the reason for the abnl mammographic findings that prompted the initial Bx.

Is LCIS associated with invasive cancer a contraindication for BCT?

No. Current literature supports the safety of BCT in the presence of coexisting LCIS in the specimen, and no special effort needs to be made to obtain −margins on LCIS.

For a pt with LCIS, what is the benefit of primary tamoxifen?

For a pt with LCIS, tamoxifen halves the risk of invasive recurrence in either breast. (*Fisher B et al., Lancet 1999*)

In a pt with DCIS or invasive Dz, what is the most common contraindication for adj tamoxifen therapy?

In a pt with DCIS or invasive Dz, the most common contraindication for adj tamoxifen therapy is **Hx of stroke or other coagulopathy.**

What is the workup for invasive breast cancer?

Invasive breast cancer workup: H&P (inquire about family Hx of breast or ovarian cancer, Hx of atypical ductal or lobular hyperplasia), CBC, CMP, bilat mammogram, estrogen receptor (ER)/progesterone receptor/HER2 status, and β-HCG (if premenopausal). If stage >IIA, then bone scan. Otherwise, imaging for suspicious Hx, physical, or lab findings.

List the subsets of stage I breast cancers (T1mic–T1a-c).

T1mic: ≤ 0.1cm;
T1a: >0.1 but ≤0.5 cm
T1b: >0.5 cm but ≤1 cm
T1c: >1 cm but ≤2 cm

All stage I tumors are node–.

What is the TNM staging for stage II breast cancers?

T2N0, T1-2N1, T3N0

T2 has tumors >2 cm but ≤5 cm; N1 has 1–3 +nodes. T3 has tumors >5 cm.

How are pN1(i+) and pN1mi defined for the involvement of breast cancer cells in the axillary LNs?

Based on the **size of micrometastasis.**
<u>pN1(i+)</u>: isolated tumor cells (ITCs) that are immunohistochemistry or hematoxylin and eosin (H&E) positive but ≤0.2 mm
<u>pN1mi</u>: mets >0.2 mm and/or >200 cells but ≤2 mm

Are pN1(i+) counted for the total number of positive involved LNs?

No. ITCs in LNs are not excluded from a total +node count for purposes of N classification.

What % of breast cancer pts are diagnosed with stage I–II Dz?

~**75%** of breast cancer pts are diagnosed with stage I–II Dz. (*Osteen RT & Karnell LH, Cancer 1994*)

What is the T stage for Paget Dz of the breast?

The T stage for Paget Dz is **Tis**, but only if it is *not* associated with an underlying noninvasive (i.e., DCIS and/or lobular carcinoma in situ) or invasive cancers.

How should Paget Dz associated with an underlying breast cancer be staged?

Per the AJCC 7th edition (2009), Paget associated with underlying breast cancer should be staged **according to the T stage of the underlying cancer** (Tis, T1, etc.).

■ Treatment/Prognosis

What are the management options for early-stage breast cancers?

Early-stage breast cancer management options:
1. Modified radical mastectomy +/− chemo +/− RT
2. Breast conservation therapy (BCT = BCS + RT) +/− chemo

Consider endocrine therapy for all women with ER+ tumors (even for T1a tumors) for risk reduction and to diminish the small risk of Dz recurrence.

When should adj chemo be utilized in the management of early-stage breast cancers?	Adj chemo is recommended for **tumors >1 cm** and **T1b tumors that are ER– +/– HER2.** As well, it can be considered for **0.6–1-cm tumors that are grade 2 or 3 or +LVI.** For ER+ tumors with ≥T1c Dz (including T2–T3), consider using Oncotype DX to determine the risk score for the benefit of chemo. However, the benefits of chemo are not certain for pts >70 yrs of age.
What systemic therapy is recommended for pts with ER+ tumors that are <1 cm?	**Endocrine therapy** would be the recommended systemic therapy without chemo.
What are some general principles of administering adj endocrine therapy?	General principles for administration of adj endocrine therapy: 1. If the pt is premenopausal, tamoxifen (20 mg/day) is given for 5 yrs. If the pt remains premenopausal, therapy ends. However, if the pt becomes postmenopausal, aromatase inhibitors (AIs) × 5 yrs are added. 2. If the pt is postmenopausal, AI × 5 yrs or tamoxifen × 2–3 yrs or 4.5–6 yrs → AI × 5 yrs is recommended. 3. Tamoxifen × 5 yrs is given for any pts who are intolerant, refuse, or have contraindications for AIs. (*NCCN 2010*)
What are the contraindications for the use of AIs?	Premenopausal status or the use of HRT in postmenopausal women
What are the major side effects of tamoxifen and AIs?	Tamoxifen: small increase in blood clots, strokes, uterine cancer, and cataracts Aromatase inhibitors: bone loss and osteoporosis, joint pain and stiffness, and hypercholesterolemia. Bone mineral density should be monitored. Consider bisphosphonates or statin drugs to counter the effects.
When should paclitaxel (T) be added to Adriamycin/cyclophosphamide (AC) chemo?	T should be added for node+ pts. AC × 4 cycles can be used alone for >1 cm, –node tumors. AC followed by T should be administered in a dose-dense fashion (q2wks), or AC q3wks → weekly T × 12 wks. Drug doses: Adr, 60 mg/m^2 intravenously day 1; cyclophosphamide, 600 mg/m^2 intravenously day 1; T, 175–225 mg/m^2 by 3-hr intravenous infusion day 1 q21days, or 80 mg/m^2 by 1-hr intravenous infusion weekly × 12 wks.

What systemic therapies are recommended for HER2+ tumors?

Systemic therapies for HER+ tumors:

1. If the tumor is <5 mm and a –node, just give endocrine therapy (if ER+).
2. If the tumor is 0.6–1 cm and a –node, consider combination chemo +/– trastuzumab (Herceptin).
3. If the tumor is >1 cm, add combination chemo with Herceptin.
4. Combination chemo + Herceptin is recommended for all node+ pts. The preferred combination chemo with Herceptin is **Taxotere/carboplatin/Herceptin** (TCH): Taxotere (75 mg/m^2 intravenously day 1), carboplatin (AUC 6 intravenously day 1), q21days × 6 cycles, and Herceptin (4 mg/kg on wk 1 → 2 mg/kg × 17 wks → 6 mg/kg q3wks until 1 yr elapses). B/c of synergistic cardiotoxicity of traditional AC-TH, TCH is preferred.

How should trastuzumab (Herceptin) be used in the management of early-stage breast cancers?

Trastuzumab can be used **in pts with HER2+ tumors >1 cm.** T1a-T1b tumors that are node– have a good prognosis even with HER2 amplification. This cohort is not well studied in randomized trials; therefore, the potential long-term cardiac morbidity risks with uncertain Dz control benefits should be weighed *before* using trastuzumab.

If trastuzumab is added to the Tx of BCT for early-stage breast cancers, how is it administered?

Trastuzumab is added **after completion of Adr-based chemo, but it can be administered with Taxol or Taxotere at 4 mg/kg with the 1st dose of Taxol.** Trastuzumab is given on a weekly basis (2 mg/kg) for 1 yr and can be given concurrently with RT. If capecitabine is added as an RT sensitizer, trastuzumab can also be given concurrently.

What data supports BCT (lumpectomy + radiotherapy) having equivalent survival outcomes to mastectomy +/– LND?

Several large randomized trials (**NSABP B06, Milan III, Ontario, Royal Marsdan, EORTC 10801**) support this, but B06 has the longest (20-yr) follow-up data. Recent Oxford meta-analysis summarizes the data and survival outcomes:

NSABP B06 (*Fisher et al., NEJM 2002*): 1,851 stage I–II pts randomized to (a) total mastectomy, (b) lumpectomy alone, or (c) lumpectomy + RT (50 Gy). 20-yr follow-up results showed that there was no difference in DFS, OS, or DM. The 20-yr ipsilateral breast tumor recurrence (IBTR) rate was 14% with BCS + RT vs. 39% in BCS alone (25% absolute risk reduction).

EBCTCG Oxford meta-analysis (*EBCTCG Collaborators, Lancet 2005*): 7,300 women enrolled in 10 trials for BCS +/− RT. The 5-yr LR risk reduction was 19% (7% in RT vs. 26% in BCS alone). The 15-yr breast cancer mortality was reduced by 5.4% (30.5% vs. 35.9%) with RT. The 15-yr overall mortality risk was reduced by 5.3% (35.2% vs. 40.5%), all highly significant (*p* = 0.005). So for every 4 women prevented to have LR, 1 woman is saved (4:1 ratio).

What % of pts are eligible for BCT for early-stage breast cancers ?

In early-stage breast cancers, **75%–80%** of pts are eligible for BCT. (*Morrow M et al., Cancer 2006*)

What is the relative rate of BCT for invasive lobular carcinoma (ILC) compared with IDC?

The rate of breast conservation is **lower for ILC than IDC** due to the propensity for multifocality (*Fisher ER et al., Cancer 1975*). The rate is ~75% vs. ~80% for IDC (*Morrow M et al., Cancer 2006*).

What are some absolute contraindications for BCT for pts with early-stage breast cancer?

Absolute contraindications for BCT in early-stage breast cancer:
1. Prior RT exposure
2. Multicentricity
3. Diffuse microcalcifications
4. 1st or 2nd trimester of pregnancy
5. Persistently +margin

(*Note:* The 1st 4 contraindications are from BCT guidelines: *Winchester DP & Cox JD, CA Cancer J Clin 1992.*)

What are some relative contraindications for BCT in pts with early-stage breast cancer?

Relative contraindications for BCT in early-stage breast cancer:
1. Ratio of tumor to breast size (suboptimal cosmetic outcome)
2. Locally advanced Dz (but can consider BCT for larger tumors after neoadj chemo)
3. Collagen vascular Dz (especially scleroderma, mixed connective tissue Dz, or CREST syndrome (**C**alcinosis, **R**aynaud, **E**sophageal dysfunction, **S**clerodactyly, **T**elangiectasia)
4. Pregnancy (can possibly delay RT until after delivery)

Is nodal involvement a contraindication for BCT?

No. The extent of nodal involvement may only affect the extent of nodal irradiation, though this is still controversial. With between 1 and 3 nodes, consider breast and axillary irradiation. If >4 nodes are involved, consider comprehensive nodal irradiation.

Is there a contraindication for BCT in pts with a positive family Hx of breast cancer?

No. There is no evidence that demonstrates increased ipsi or contralat breast cancers in pts with a positive family Hx after BCT. (*Vlastos G et al., Ann Surg Oncol 2007*)

Are BRCA mutations a contraindication for BCT?

No. Though *Pierce LJ et al.* reported that the IBTR rate may be higher in BRCA1/BRCA2 mutation carriers compared to wild-type individuals (HR 1.99, $p = 0.04$), this difference becomes indistinguishable after oophorectomy in BRCA carriers. Contralateral breast tumor recurrence (CBTR) is also much higher (10-yr/15-yr recurrence risk is 26%/39% in carriers vs. 3%/7% in wild-type individuals) and is substantially reduced with tamoxifen (HR 0.31) or tamoxifen + oophorectomy (HR 0.13). However, the CBTR rate is still significantly higher in mutation carriers treated with oophorectomy compared to controls. (*JCO 2006*)

What is the typical whole breast RT dose, and what data supports the use of a tumor bed boost?

Typically, the dose is **45–50 Gy** to the whole breast. EORTC and French studies have demonstrated an improved LR rate with a 10–16 Gy boost.

EORTC boost trial (*Bartelink et al., JCO 2007*): 5,318 women with BCT, 10-yr update: 50 Gy vs. 50 Gy + 16 Gy boost (surgical margin [SM]–) or + 26 Gy boost (SM+). 10-yr LF: 6.2% + boost vs. 10.2% – boost. Absolute benefit was greatest in women <50 b/c they have a higher risk of LR (24% – boost vs. 13.5% + boost for women <40 yo), but **proportional benefits were seen across all age groups.**

Lyon boost trial (*Romestaing et al., JCO 1997*): 1,024 pts, 50 Gy vs. 50 Gy + 10 Gy boost. At 3-yr follow-up, LF was reduced in the boost arm (3.6% vs. 4.5%).

In general, a boost of 10–16 Gy should be considered for pts at higher risk for LR (age <50 yrs, positive axillary nodes, +LVI, or close SMs). This can be administered with brachytherapy, electrons, or external photons.

Is there a need for a higher tumor boost dose in pts with incomplete tumor excision after BCS?

No. In the EORTC boost trial, 251 pts with microscopically incomplete tumor excision were randomized to low (10 Gy) vs. high (26 Gy) boost. With median follow-up of 11.3 yrs, there was no difference in LC or survival. There was significantly more fibrosis in the high-dose arm. (*Poortmans PM et al., Radiother Oncol 2009*)

Can RT be used in the Tx of axillary nodes in place of surgery if axillary nodal dissection is not performed?

Possibly. This is based on the results of **NSABP B04.**
NSABP B04 (*Fisher B et al., NEJM 2002*): randomized trial in 2 subsets of pts. Subset 1 included 1,079 pts with clinically– nodes randomized to 3 arms: (a) radical mastectomy, (b) simple mastectomy alone (+ axillary nodal dissection if clinically+ later), and (c) simple mastectomy + nodal RT. Subset 2 included 586 pts with clinically+ nodes randomized to 2 arms: (a) radical mastectomy vs. (b) simple mastectomy – axillary dissection but postop RT; no adj chemo.
Results: At 25-yr follow-up, there were no differences in LF, DFS, or OS in any of the groups.
Caveat: Approximately one third of pts who should not have had a nodal dissection had some nodes removed. Thus, the results of the study may be questioned.

What is the next step in the management for a pt who undergoes a lumpectomy with a focal +margin?

This is **controversial.** Most would advocate taking the pt back to surgery for re-excision, which may diminish the 10-yr risk of LR to baseline levels (initial SM–: 7%, SM+: 12%; SM close: 14%; re-excision SM–: 7%, re-excision persistent SM+: 13%, re-excision persistent SM close: 21%). (*Freedman G et al., IJROBP 1999*)

Is there a subset of women whose LR risk may not be substantially influenced by margin positivity after BCS?

Possibly. There are data to suggest that the effect of margin positivity on LR **may be dependent on age <40 yrs.** In an analysis of 1,752 pts, 193 were SM+. Overall 10-yr LRR was 6.9% (SM–) vs. 12.2% (SM+). 5-yr LRR for pts ≤40 yo was 8.4% (SM–) and 37% (SM+) ($p = 0.005$); for pts >40 yo, the LRR was 2.6% (SM–) and 2.2% (SM+). (*Jobsen JJ et al., IJROBP 2003*)

Should women with T1-2N0 invasive breast cancer treated with mastectomy to a +margin be treated with adj RT to the chest wall (CW) as well?

In a **British Columbia retrospective study** (*Truong PT et al., IJROBP 2004*), out of 2,570 women with early-stage breast cancer treated with mastectomy, 94 pts had a +margin. About half (41 pts) were treated with postmastectomy radiation therapy (PMRT). B/c of the small numbers, there was a trend to improvement with PMRT in pts ≤50 yrs, T2 tumor, grade III, and LVI. In pts without these features, there was no LR without PMRT.

Which is a more important factor to determine LR, margin status, or node positivity?

Margin status is more important to determine LR, whereas nodal positivity is more predictive of distant recurrence and OS. Margin status in relation to LR may be related to nodal positivity. *Besana-Ciani I & Greenall MJ* (*Int Semin Surg Oncol 2008*) showed that in 773 pts treated with BCT, LR was 12% in SM– vs. 28% in SM+ node– pts, but LR was equivalent (12% and 18%) in node+ pts. This may be due to the fact that margin status in node+ pts does not dictate prognosis as much as in node– pts.

What is EIC, and does it have prognostic significance in the recurrence risk of pts treated with BCT?

EIC (extensive intraductal component) is defined as **DCIS comprising 25% of the tumor mass with DCIS and foci of DCIS separate from the invasive Dz.** DCIS with focal microinvasive Dz areas of invasion also fits this category. **Yes, but it is largely dependent on SM status.** From studies mainly out of **JCRT,** EIC is only prognostic for LF if the margin status is considered. **If there is a close or +margin, EIC is associated with a high risk of recurrence.** (*Gage I et al., Cancer 1996*)

What data suggests that results of BCT can be further improved with the use of tamoxifen?

NSABP B21 (*Fisher B et al., JCO 2002*): 1,009 pts with ≤1-cm tumors s/p lumpectomy randomized to 3 arms: (a) tamoxifen alone (10 mg bid × 5 yrs), (b) RT alone (50 Gy), and (c) RT + tamoxifen. After 8-yr follow-up, the IBTR was 16.5% with tamoxifen alone vs. 9.3% with RT alone vs. 2.8% with RT + tamoxifen. There was no difference in OS. No benefit was seen in ER– tumors. CBTR was 0.9%, 4.2%, and 3.0% in the 3 arms, respectively.

Are there pt subgroups with a low risk of LR who can be treated with BCS and systemic therapy alone without RT?

Possibly. 2 recent trials have been conducted to answer the question whether age is a determining factor. The data suggests that the risk is very low only for **pts >70 yo** and possibly in those with **very small tumors (<1 cm),** so a discussion can be made about withholding RT if the pt is being treated with tamoxifen. There is no data whether the same applies for AIs.

Princess Margaret Hospital/Canadian trial (*Fyles AW et al., NEJM 2004*): 769 women ≥50 yo (median age 68 yrs) with T1 or T2 (≤5 cm) –nodes (in women age ≥65 yrs, either clinical or pathologic evaluation was sufficient and sentinel lymph node [SLN] Bx was not routinely done) underwent lumpectomy to –margins and were randomized to (a) tamoxifen alone (20 mg/day × 5 yrs) vs. (b) tamoxifen + RT (40 Gy in 16 fx with a boost of 12.5 Gy in 5 fx). After 8-yrs follow-up, RT reduced LR from 17.6% to 3.5%. But with tumors <1 cm, the risk of relapse was 2.6% vs. 0% for the RT group (*p* = 0.02). In those >60 yo with <1 cm tumor, the risk was no different between the 2 arms (1.2% vs. 0%), but this was unplanned analysis with a short follow-up.

Intergroup trial (*Hughes K.*
women ≥70 yo with T1, cli
were randomized to tamoxifei
after lumpectomy to –margins.
assessed clinically *only*, and axili
discouraged. RT was 45 Gy to tl
boost of 14 Gy. The initial 5-yr L   ...ᵤ vs.
1%, respectively. At 8-yr follow-up ...ᴸF rate in the
tamoxifen alone arm was 7% vs. 1% in RT.

What are some alternative fractionation regimens for whole breast irradiation as part of BCT? What 2 RT regimens can be employed for use in BCT?

Traditionally in the U.S., alternative fractionation regimens include **conventional fractionation at 1.8–2 Gy/fx to 45–50 Gy whole breast → a boost to 60–66 Gy.** However, several recent published trials suggest the same outcomes using a hypofractionated approach.

Canadian regimen (*Whelan TJ et al., JNCI 2002; Whelan TJ et al., NEJM 2010*): RCT using 42.5 Gy in 16 fx (2.65 Gy/fx) vs. 50 Gy in 25 fx (2 Gy/fx) with no boost; 1,234 T1-2N0 pts, all with –SMs. **Women with >25-cm breast width were excluded** (to reduce heterogeneity of dose to the breast). At median follow-up of 69 mos, there was no difference in LC, OS, or cosmesis. Updated 10-yr follow-up: there was no difference in DFS or cosmesis. LR risk was 6.7% in the standard regimen vs. 6.2% in the hypofractionated regimen. Good to excellent cosmesis was equivalent (71.3% standard vs. 69.8% hypofractionated).

British regimen (*START B trials, Lancet 2008*): 2,215 women with pT1-3N0-1 s/p surgery randomized to 50 Gy in 25 fx vs. 40 Gy in 15 fx (2.67 Gy/fx) with no boost given in either arm. After 6-yr follow-up, there was no difference in IBTR (3% vs. 2%). Late adverse events were not greater in the 40-Gy arm (if not a bit better).

How should chemo be sequenced with radiotherapy after BCS?

JCRT sequencing trial ("Upfront-Outback" trial) (*Bellon et al., JCO 2005*): per the initial report (*Recht et al., NEJM 1996*), the 5-yr crude rate of distant recurrence was better in the chemo 1ˢᵗ arm (20% vs. 32%). However, in the 11-yr follow-up update, there was no difference in DFS, LR, DM, or OS. For those with a –margin, the crude LR rate was 6% in the chemo 1ˢᵗ arm vs. 13% in the RT 1ˢᵗ arm. However, the study was not powered to show any differences.

Thus, either sequence is acceptable. However, convention is to give chemo 1ˢᵗ.

**...e max length
... that RT can be
...ayed after BCS before
impacting clinical
outcomes?**

Generally, RT can start whenever the pt is finished healing, which can range from 2-4 weeks, but **possibly no more than 20 wks**. There is recent data to suggest that if there is a delay >20 wks in pts who rcv chemo, the DFS and breast cancer mortality rates increase (British Columbia study: *Olivotto IA et al., JCO 2009*).

**Can accelerated partial
breast irradiation (PBI)
be considered an option
for BCT?**

As of 2010, this is not an option. This is a clinical question being tested in the **NSABP B39/RTOG 0413 trial,** which randomizes women to whole breast RT vs. PBI by 3 methods (interstitial, mammosite, and EBRT).

ASTRO has published guidelines on who may be considered for PBI off trial (*Smith BD et al., IJROBP 2009*). Generally, pts considered "suitable" are >60 yo, ER+, IDC ≤2 cm (no DCIS or ILC), N0 (nor pN[i+]), unicentric, ≥2-mm margin, no LVSI, no EIC, and BRCA1/BRCA2–. Several retrospective studies have demonstrated excellent LC in pts with short follow-up (*Smith BD et al., IJROBP 2009*).

**What are the doses
recommended for PBI if
done off protocol?**

For <u>EBRT</u>, **38.5 Gy in 10 fx** using 3D-CRT. For <u>brachytherapy</u> (interstitial or intracavitary forms), the dose is **34 Gy in 10 fx.**

The target includes the tumor bed and a 1-cm margin for brachytherapy and a 1–1.5 cm for EBRT to account for uncertainties in setup due to respiration.

**Are there subsets of
women who undergo
mastectomy for early-
stage breast cancers
(T1-2N0) who may
benefit from PMRT?**

Yes. PMRT is generally recommended (NCCN, ASCO) in women with T3-4N+ (>4 nodes) Dz according to PMRT RCTs (Chapter 45). PMRT may not be necessary if the margins are clear (≥1 cm). However, consider PMRT for those with SMs **<1 mm.**

In pts treated with mastectomy for early-stage cancer, Vancouver retrospective data suggest that PMRT may also benefit women with certain risk features (**LVSI, grade 3, no chemo, or T2 tumors**). In the presence of 2–3 factors (LVSI + grade 3 or grade 3 + T2 + no chemo), the LRR risk is ~21%–23% without RT. (*Truong PT et al., IJROBP 2005*)

In a separate report from Harvard (*Jagsi R et al., IJROBP 2005*), similar factors predicted for LRR after mastectomy without PMRT (close margin, ≥T2, premenopausal pt, and LVI). 10-yr LRR (80% in the CW) according to risk factors was 0, 1.2%; 1, 10%; 2, 18%; 3, 41%.

How should a Dx of breast cancer be managed in a pregnant woman?	**Depends on the stage of pregnancy.** Generally, adj chemo can be used, though not during the 1st trimester of pregnancy. RT or hormones should be added postpartum. Chemo used during pregnancy utilizes combinations of Adr, cyclophosphamide, and 5-FU.

1st trimester: consider termination. If the pt refuses, consider mastectomy + axillary staging. If chemo is needed, add it during the 2nd trimester. Adj RT and hormones, if needed, should be added postpartum

2nd–3rd trimester: BCT or mastectomy can be considered. Neoadj chemo can be considered. Surgical management and chemo in pregnant women is the same as that used in nonpregnant women, but adj hormones and RT cannot be added until the postpartum period.

(Adopted from *NCCN 2010*)

▌Toxicity

What is the typical recommended follow-up schedule for pts treated for invasive breast cancer?	Invasive breast cancer recommended follow-up after Tx: 1. Interval H&P q4–6mos × 5 yrs, then annually 2. Mammogram annually for contralat breast, q6–12mos for ipsi breast (if conserved) 3. Annual gynecologic exam for women with intact uterus on tamoxifen 4. Bone health assessment (bone mineral density scan) at baseline and periodically during course of use of AIs
For pts who have large breasts with large medial to lat separation (>22–24 cm), what techniques will improve dose homogeneity?	**Photon energy >10 MV to keep max inhomogeneity <10% and field segmentation techniques** (IMRT). Avoid medial wedges to reduce scatter to contralat breast in pts <45 yo.
Which randomized trial demonstrated the superiority of 3D-IMRT compared to 2D tx approaches for minimizing cosmetic changes to the breast?	Royal Marsden (*Donovan E et al., Radiother Oncol 2007*) randomized 306 women to 2D-RT or 3D-IMRT. RT was 50 Gy → boost to 11.1 Gy with electrons. There was a significant cosmetic difference in the breast of 2D-RT (58%) vs. 3D-IMRT (40%) pts. Fewer pts in the IMRT group developed palpable induration. There were no differences in the QOL between the groups. A randomized trial (*Pignol JP et al., JCO 2008*) comparing breast IMRT to standard techniques showed IMRT to be superior with respect to moist desquamation (31% vs. 48%) and improved dose distribution.

Is LABC more common among certain ethnic groups?

Yes. A higher proportion of **black women** have LABC.

What are the histologic subtypes of LABC?

The histologic subtypes are the **same for LABC as for earlier-stage Dz.** Infiltrating ductal carcinoma is still the most common, but favorable histologies, such as tubular, medullary, and mucinous, are less frequently represented.

Are there genetic/ molecular factors associated with LABC?

No. There are no molecular markers that define LABC. However, tumors with HER2/Neu positivity, BRCA1 mutation, and triple-negative (estrogen receptor [ER]–, progesterone receptor [PR]–, HER2–) are associated with aggressive phenotypes. A genomic profile of basal and HER2 subtypes is associated with a poor prognosis as well. The use of Herceptin in HER2+ positive tumors has improved their outcome, though.

▪ Workup/Staging

What is the workup for locally advanced invasive breast cancer?

Invasive breast cancer workup: H&P, CBC, liver profile, ER/PR/HER2 status; diagnostic mammogram and US as necessary; bone scan, CXR (CT chest optional), and CT abdomen; US or MRI abdomen as needed

In a pt with T1-T2 breast cancer and a clinically– axilla, what is the rate of pathologic axillary involvement?

In T2-T3 pts with a clinically– axilla, there is pathologic axillary involvement in ~**30%.**

In a breast cancer pt with a clinically+ axilla, what is the chance that the axilla is negative upon resection?

In pts with a clinically+ axilla, there is a ~**25%** chance for a negative axilla upon resection.

What are the 5 regional LN stations in breast cancer?

Regional LN stations in breast cancer:
  Station I: nodes inf/lat to pectoralis minor
  Station II: nodes deep to pectoralis minor
  Station III: nodes sup/medial to pectoralis minor
  Station IV: supraclavicular nodes
  Station V: internal mammary (IM) nodes

"Infraclavicular" nodes typically refers to the level III axillary nodes by radiation oncology.

How is IBC diagnosed?	IBC is a **clinical Dx,** with characteristics of rapid onset (<3 mos), generalized induration, often **without** an associated mass (classic type), peau d'orange appearance, and a diffuse skin erythema affecting more than two thirds of the breast. Enlargement, flattening and retraction of the nipple with warmth, and tenderness are common. IBC is characterized pathologically by cancer cells in dermal lymphatics (not necessary for Dx). Random Bx of breast parenchyma may yield cancer cells.

■ Treatment/Prognosis

What are the most important factors that predict for LRR?	**Increasing number of LNs with Dz and breast tumor size** are the most important factors that predict for LRR.
What are the basic principles of treating LABC?	Inoperable LABC: neoadj chemo is used to shrink the tumor and potentially convert it to be operable. Neoadj or adj chemo should be included. Operable LABC: Neoadj or adj chemo are used. Modified radical mastectomy (including level I–II axillary LNs) is the definitive locoregional Tx. PMRT is indicated in most circumstances. Hormonal therapy and Herceptin are incorporated as appropriate per receptor status of Dz.
What is a Halsted radical mastectomy?	Halsted radical mastectomy includes **resection of all breast parenchyma, a large portion of breast skin, and major and minor pectoral muscles en bloc with axillary LNs.**
What is spared with a modified radical mastectomy?	Modified radical mastectomy spares the **pectoralis muscle.**
What is spared with a total or simple mastectomy?	In a total or simple mastectomy, only the breast tissue is removed with overlying skin. **Axillary LNs are not dissected.**
What is considered an "adequate" axillary LND for purposes of staging and clearance?	**Oncologic resection of levels I–II** is considered standard and adequate. The LNs and axillary fat pad need to be removed en bloc. If suspicious nodes are present in level III, then level III dissection should be performed.
What is standard systemic chemo?	Standard chemo at present includes an **anthracycline- and taxane-based regimen** (e.g., Adriamycin/cyclophosphamide [AC] and Taxol).
What is meant by "dose-dense" chemo?	Dose-dense chemo is **administered q2wks** as opposed to q3wks.

Has dose-dense chemo been demonstrated to be superior in a prospective randomized trial?

Yes. Intergroup trial C9741 randomized 2,005 node+ pts to AC × 4 > Taxol × 4 given q3wks vs. q2wks. 4-yr DFS improved from 75% to 82% with the q2wk schedule. The risk ratio for OS was 0.69 in favor of the q2wk schedule. Median follow-up was 36 mos. Severe neutropenia was also less frequent with the dose-dense schedule.

What is the rationale for the use of neoadj chemo for LABC?

Neoadj chemo may convert pts with unresectable LABC to resectability. It may also be used to shrink large breast tumor requiring mastectomy in resectable pts to be managed with breast conservation surgery (BCS). Neoadj trials have the advantage of providing pathologic assessment of chemo response at the time of surgery. If the tumor is not responsive to 1 chemo regimen and progresses clinically, a different chemo regimen can be used.

What major study determined whether neoadj chemo improves survival compared to adj chemo in LABC?

NSABP B18 was designed to assess whether preop AC resulted in improved DFS and OS compared to postop AC. Secondary aims were to assess response to preop AC and correlate with survival and LR outcomes. Rates of BCS were also assessed. All women were deemed operable at enrollment, and the majority had T2 or smaller primary and clinically node– Dz. At the most recent follow-up (16 yrs) (*Rastogi et al., JCO 2008*), there has been no significant difference in OS or DFS between the women treated with neoadj vs. adj chemo. There is a trend, however, for women <50 yo for improved DFS and OS when treated preoperatively ($p = 0.09$ and 0.06). There was a 27% conversion rate from mastectomy to BCS.

What procedures should be done prior to starting neoadj chemo for LABC?

Core Bx and wire localization for the Bx bed (in case the pt has a CR to chemo). Perform sentinal lymph node (SLN) Bx if cN0; if cN+, consider FNA Bx.

Does adding Taxol to standard AC chemo improve the outcomes of pts with breast cancer?

Yes. Adding Taxol improves response rates, DFS, and OS.

NSABP 27 randomized operable pts to preop AC, preop AC + Taxol, or preop AC + postop Taxol. Here, the addition of Taxol did not improve survival outcomes but did improve pCR in the preop group (26% vs. 13%). (*Rastogi et al., JCO 2008*)

The **CALGB 9344** study randomized 3,121 operable pts with LN+ Dz and found that adding Taxol q3wks × 4 to AC × 4 improved DFS and OS. (*Henderson IC et al., JCO 2003*)

In a retrospective study of 1,500 pts on **CALGB 9344**, the benefit of Taxol appeared to be in HER2+ tumors and not HER2–/ER+ tumors. (*Hayes DF et al., NEJM 2007*)

ECOG E1199 randomized 4,950 stage II–IIIA breast cancer pts to AC q3wks × 4 → Taxol q3wks × 4, AC q3wks × 4 → Taxol × 12 weekly, AC q3wks × 4 → Taxotere q3wks × 4, and AC q3wks × 4 → Taxotere × 12 weekly. The weekly Taxol arm had improved DFS (HR 1.27) and OS (HR 1.32). The effect was significant in all pts, including those with ER+/HER2– tumors. (*Sparano JA et al., NEJM 2008*)

In NSABP 18 and 27, did pCR at the time of surgery correlate with good OS and DFS outcomes?

Yes. In both **NSABP 18** and **NSABP 27,** pCR at the time of surgery correlated with improved OS and DFS compared to non-pCR pts.

What other seminal neoadj chemo trials addressed neoadj vs. adj chemo and its role regarding BCS?

EORTC 10902 randomized 698 pts with early breast cancer to preop vs. postop chemo (5-FU/epirubicin/cyclophosphamide × 4). Endpoints were BCS, DFS, OS, and tumor response. At 10-yr follow-up, there was no difference in OS or LRR. Neoadj chemo was associated with an improved rate of BCS. (*Van der Hage JA et al., J Clin Oncol 2001*)

In EORTC 10902, was there a difference in the # of BCS between arms? Was there a difference in outcomes between planned breast-conserved pts and breast-converted pts?

BCS increased from 22% to 35% in the preop chemo arm. While the initial follow-up of **EORTC 10902** indicated that converted breast-conserved pts did worse in terms of OS compared to planned pts—an indication that prechemo staging remains relevant. However, the most recent 10-yr follow-up data indicate that there is no difference in survival outcomes between these 2 groups. (*Van der Hage JA et al., J Clin Oncol 2001*)

Postmastectomy radiation therapy (PMRT) was the standard of care for many decades. Why did it fall out of favor?

There have been more than 25 prospective randomized trials evaluating PMRT over more than 50 yrs. Historically, PMRT was typically offered since pts presented at later stages and no chemo was given. **Historical series, while uniformly demonstrating improved LC, did not demonstrate survival benefit.**

Meta-analysis by *Stjernsward* (6 trials) demonstrated a 1%–10% decrease in OS with PRMT. (*Lancet 1974*)

Meta-analysis by *Cuzick et al.* (9 trials) demonstrated no OS survival benefit with PMRT at 10 yrs. (*Cancer Treat Rep 1987*)

An update by *Cuzik* demonstrated that PMRT increased cardiac mortality and slightly decreased breast cancer mortality. (*J Clin Oncol 1994*)

Therefore, with the addition of chemo (i.e., cyclophosphamide/methotrexate/5-FU [CMF]), PMRT went out of favor at the publication of the meta-analysis studies.

What are some criticisms of older PMRT data and meta-analysis?

Criticisms of older PMRT data include the **significant heterogeneity of surgical and RT techniques, old RT techniques with associated cardiac and pulmonary toxicity, and lack of systemic therapy,** implying that clinically undetectable systemic Dz was not well controlled.

What 3 randomized prospective trials are considered to represent the "modern" PMRT experience?

The **Premenopausal Danish Trial (DBCG 82b)** (*Overgaard et al., NEJM 1997*), the **Postmenopausal Danish Trial (DBCG 82c)** (*Overgaard et al., Lancet 1999*), and the **British Columbia PMRT Trial** (*Ragaz et al., JNCI 2005*) represent the "modern" PMRT experience.

What were the design and study outcomes of Premenopausal Danish Trial DBCG 82b?

In **Premenopausal Danish Trial 82b,** 1,708 women were randomized to mastectomy and adj CMF + chemo (8 cycles) or – RT (9 cycles). Inclusion criteria were +axillary LN, tumor >5 cm, or involvement of skin or pectoral fascia. 10-yr OS was 54% (+PMRT) and 45% (–PMRT, $p < 0.001$). Crude cumulative LRR was 32% –PMRT and 9% +PMRT. The survival benefit was seen for all pts (N0-N3).

What are some criticisms of Premenopausal Danish Trial DBCG 82b?

Criticisms of **Premenopausal Danish Trial 82b** include the inadequate surgical Tx of axilla resulting in a median of 7 nodes removed (which is low), an excess of LF occurring in the axilla (44% in the CMF arm was concerning), and the use of outdated CMF chemo.

What were the design and trial outcomes of Postmenopausal Danish Trial 82c?

In **Postmenopausal Danish Trial 82c,** 1,375 postmenopausal women <70 yo were randomized to postmastectomy tamoxifen × 1 yr vs. tamoxifen + PMRT. Inclusion criteria, surgical characteristics, and RT were as for Premenopausal Danish Trial 82b. PMRT significantly improved LR (–PMRT 35% vs. +PMRT 8%), DFS (–PMRT 24% vs. +PMRT 36%), and OS (–PMRT 34% vs. +PMRT 45%) at 10-yrs follow-up (all significant).

What are some criticisms of Postmenopausal Danish Trial 82c?

In **Postmenopausal Danish Trial 82c**, as in Premenopausal Danish Trial 82b, inadequate surgical Tx of the axilla resulted in a median of only 7 axillary LNs removed at surgery. A suboptimal duration of tamoxifen was also employed (1 yr vs. the typical 5 yrs).

What was the surgery in the Danish 82b and 82c trials?

Pts were surgically managed with total mastectomy + axillary LN sampling (aimed at removing at least 5 LNs, full dissection was not required). A median of 7 nodes were removed. 15% had only 0–3 LNs removed, and 75% had <9 LNs removed. This is significantly less than most centers in the U.S., where >10 LNs represent adequate dissection.

How was the RT given in the Danish 82b and 82c trials?

For 82b, PMRT was given after cycle 1 of CMF and 3–5 wks postoperatively. For 82c, PMRT was given 2–4 wks postoperatively. The RT dose was 48–50 Gy given in 22–25 fx to the CW with ant photon fields to cover supraclavicular, infraclavicular, and axillary nodes and an ant electron field to cover the IM nodes and CW. Posterior axillary boost (PAB) was used for pts with a large AP diameter.

What was the design of the British Columbia Trial?

In the British Columbia Trial, 318 premenopausal, high-risk pts with positive axillary LNs were randomized to CMF chemo × 6–12 mos vs. CMF + RT. Surgery involved total mastectomy + axillary LND (median removal of 11 LNs). RT used Co-60 to 37.5 Gy in 16 fx. A 5-field technique was employed, including an en face photon field to cover bilat IM nodes.

What are the relevant outcomes of the British Columbia Trial?

In the British Columbia Trial, at 20-yr follow-up, adj RT improved LRR before DM (13% vs. 39%), DFS (48% vs. 31%), and OS (47% vs. 37%) (all significant). The benefit was extended to those with 1–3 LN+ Dz as well as those with >4 LN+ Dz.

What are some criticisms of the British Columbia Trial?

In the British Columbia Trial, LRF was high compared to many current series, CMF chemo was employed, and the RT fields included en face photons for IM nodal coverage (though no excessive cardiac deaths were observed).

What was demonstrated by the most recent EBCTCG RT meta-analysis?

In the most recent EBCTCG meta-analysis (*EBCTCG collaborators, Lancet 2005*), 78 randomized trials including 42,000 women were included. After BCS, adj RT reduced 5-yr LR from 26% to 7% and increased 15-yr breast cancer mortality from 30.5% to 35.9%. After mastectomy with axillary clearance in node+ pts, PMRT reduced 5-yr LR from 23% to 5% and improved 15-yr breast cancer mortality from 54.7% to 60.1% (both significant); 5.4% in the entire cohort. In pts with node– Dz who had mastectomy with axillary clearance, PMRT reduced 5-yr LR from 6% to 2% ($p = 0.0002$) but caused a 3.6% increase in the 15-yr breast cancer mortality rate. 5-yr tamoxifen use reduced the LR rate by about one half in pts with ER+ Dz. In all pts, chemo reduced the LR rate by one third. RT was associated with excess contralat breast cancer, lung cancer, and cardiac mortality. Many "older" trials were included in this analysis.

What was demonstrated by the Whelan meta-analysis for PMRT?

The Whelan meta-analysis (*Whelan TJ et al., JCO 2000*) included 18 relatively recent trials (1967–1999) with 6,367 pts who had mastectomy and chemo. Adj RT was found to be associated with reduced LR (OR 0.25), all recurrence (OR 0.69), and reduced mortality (OR 0.83). The survival benefit was not significant when the Danish trials were excluded.

What was demonstrated by the Gebski meta-analysis for PMRT?

The Gebski meta-analysis (*Gebski V et al., JNCI 2006*) analyzed 36 unconfounded PMRT trials and stratified these trials according to the appropriate RT dose given (biologic effective dose 40–60 Gy in 2 Gy/fx) and the RT target tissue coverage. Among the 17 series that fit these criteria and had 5-yr follow-up data, adj RT was associated with an absolute 2.9% increase in OS at 5 yrs. Among the 13 series that had 10-yr data, a 10-yr OS benefit of 6.4% was observed.

Have there been any prospective randomized trials evaluating PMRT in pts treated with neoadj chemo?

No. There have been no prospective randomized trials evaluating PMRT in pts treated with neoadj chemo.

What was demonstrated in the retrospective series from MDACC regarding PMRT in pts treated with neoadj chemo?

Huang E. et al. analyzed the outcomes of 542 pts who had been enrolled in prospective clinical trials and treated with neoadj chemo, mastectomy, and RT. These pts were compared to 134 pts enrolled in the same trials who rcv no adj RT. Clinical stage, margin status, and hormone receptor status did not favor the adj RT group. CSS was improved with adj RT in pts with clinical stage IIIB or supraclavicular LN+ Dz, clinical T4 tumors, and pathologically ≥4 +nodes. LRR was improved even for those pts with clinical stage III or supraclavicular LN+ Dz who achieved a pCR on neoadj chemo. (*JCO 2004*)

What are the present ASCO guidelines for PMRT?

PMRT is **recommended for pts with ≥4 +LNs and suggested for T3 tumor with axillary LN Dz or operable stage III Dz.**

What is the rationale for not recommending PMRT to pts with <4 positive axillary LNs?

In numerous studies, Dz involvement of 1–3 LNs has been associated with an increased risk of LR compared to those with no LN Dz. Since RT can result in toxicity-related mortality, **there is concern that PMRT in this population will lead to worse OS.**

What are some arguments for providing PMRT to pts with 1–3 positive axillary LNs?

An argument for treating pts with 1–3 LN Dz with PMRT is that all 3 modern randomized trials (**Danish 82b, Danish 82c, and British Columbia**) showed significant OS benefit with PMRT. This was true in subgroup analysis of this population and even when analysis was restricted to pts who had at least 8 axillary LNs removed in Danish trials. (*Overgaard et al., Radiother Oncol 2007*)

In EBCTCG meta-analysis, pts with 1–3 LN Dz had absolute 5-yr LR benefit of 11.6% with PMRT but did not have OS benefit. This was likely b/c their initial LR risk without PMRT was not that high, so PMRT did not generate larger LR benefit. In the same analysis, pts with absolute 5-yr LR benefit of 10%–20% had OS benefit with PMRT. Therefore, PMRT should be considered for pts with 1–3 LN Dz and other high-risk clinicopathologic factors (such as LVSI, ECE >2 mm, +margin, <35–40 yo) that would further increase their LR risk.

What is the argument that the LF rates (and therefore the benefit of PMRT) in pts with N1 Dz (1–3 LN+) seen in the Danish and British Columbia PMRT trials do not necessarily represent the typical experience in this subset of pts in U.S.?

In the ECOG postmastectomy chemo trials (without adj RT) (*Fowble B et al., JCO 1988*), where the median nodes removed were 12, the 3-yr isolated LRF rate in the 1–3 node pts was 7% but goes up to 15% for 4+ LNs. The cumulative 10-yr LRR +/− DM for pts with 1–3 LN Dz in retrospective review of pts in prospective trials conducted by the NSABP, the ECOG, and MDACC was 4%–13% (*Taghian AG et al., JCO 2004; Recht A et al., JCO 1999; Katz A et al., JCO 2000*).

For pts who undergo mastectomy with 1–3 +nodes, what other clinicopathologic factors should be considered when recommending PMRT?

Retrospective studies from the IBCSG, NSABP, and MDACC have suggested that factors such as **+LVI, high grade, younger age, ECE ≥2 mm, ≤10 LN examined, ≥20% LN+, larger tumor size (T2 or ≥4 cm), and close margins** produce 10-yr LRR >15%. So consider PMRT for these pts.

Under what circumstances should regional LN be covered for PMRT (comprehensive PMRT)?

Comprehensive PMRT (CW + LN) is recommended for most pts who have high LRR risk that warrant PMRT since the benefit of RT of regional LN outweighs in most cases the added toxicity. We consider **CW RT alone** for pts with upfront mastectomy and T3N0 or those with T1-T2N0 who are being treated for +margin only. The results from **EORTC 22922/10925** and SUPREMO trials will give us better indication for PMRT use in pts with 1–3 LN involvement.

Should the IM chain be included in all PMRT fields?

This is **controversial.** Some radiation oncologists believe that since it was covered in the 3 randomized PMRT trials, and a nonrandomized Israeli study (*Stemmer SM et al., J Clin Oncol 2003*) demonstrated that IM nodal irradiation may improve DFS (73% vs. 52%) and trended to improved OS (78% vs. 64%, *p* = 0.08), that it should be the gold standard approach. However, others would argue not to include IM nodes routinely since 3 randomized trials examining the role of IM nodal dissection did not improve OS for these pts (*Veronesi U et al., Eur J Cancer 1999*; *Meir P et al., Cancer 1989*; *Lacour J et al., Cancer 1976*) and that isolated recurrence in the IM is low after whole breast RT without IM node RT, possibly some of the Dz is already included in the tangent field.

A randomized trial (**EORTC 22922/10925**) testing the effects of IM nodal irradiation on LRC and survival has completed accrual with results pending.

Should pts with T3N0 breast cancer who have had a mastectomy without neoadj chemo be treated with PMRT?

This is **controversial.** Traditionally, pts with T3N0 without other risk factors have been treated with CW-only PMRT. However, 2 recent retrospective studies have demonstrated that the LF rates are low for T3N0 pts after mastectomy alone with adj chemo, questioning the role of PMRT. This is an evolving area of research, so pts with pT3N0 without other risk factors should be considered for CW-alone PMRT with appropriate discussion of risk and benefits of RT.

Taghian AG et al., JCO 2006: review of an NSABP postmastectomy chemo trial, with 313 pts with ≥5-cm tumors (N0). The 10-yr isolated LRF was 7.1%, and LRF +/− DM was 10%. 24 or 28 LRR was at the CW. However, the median size of the tumor was 5.5 cm, so the data may not be applicable for very large or infiltrative tumors.

Floyd SR et al., IJROBP 2006: review of a multi-institutional database for ≥5-cm tumors (N0). Out of 70 pts, the 5-yr LRF was 7.6%. LVI was a significant prognostic factor for LF.

How is IBC managed?

IBC is managed using **combined-modality therapy** with neoadj chemo, modified radical mastectomy, and comprehensive PMRT +/− additional chemo (if not completed preoperatively) and hormones (if ER+) and/or Herceptin × 1 yr (if HER2+). Many retrospective studies show 5-yr DFS of 25%–30% and 5-yr OS of ~40%.

What are 2 acceptable PMRT schedules for IBC?	<u>Conventional</u>: 50 Gy comprehensive RT → 66 Gy to CW boost <u>MDACC</u>: hyperfractionated RT: 1.5 Gy bid to 51 Gy to CW and axilla →15 Gy boost in 10 fx bid to 66 Gy The LRC from bid RT is promising, with 5- and 10-yr LRC of 84% and 77%, respectively (*Liao Z et al., IJROBP 2000*).
What are the options for a pt with poor response and unresectable Dz after induction chemo for IBC?	Alternative chemo; if there is still no response, can consider upfront RT (conventional RT or hyperfractionated RT) → consideration for surgery.
For pts who want breast reconstruction after mastectomy, when should the breast reconstruction be done relative to the rest of the adj Tx?	**Breast reconstruction should be done 6–12 mos after RT** since cosmetic outcome is worse if reconstruction is done before RT. A 2-stage delayed implant is recommended. For saline implants, skin-sparing mastectomy with placement of tissue expanders should be done prior to RT. The tissue expander is deflated during RT and re-expanded afterward.

▊ Toxicity

What are the acute and late toxicities of whole breast RT?	<u>Acute</u>: RT dermatitis, fatigue, hyperpigmentation, pneumonitis <u>Late</u>: soft tissue fibrosis, breast size change, telangiectasias, lymphedema, pulmonary fibrosis, precocious cardiovascular Dz, 2nd malignancy
With whole breast RT, what is the rate of acute skin breakdown, and where does it typically occur?	~**20%–30%** of pts experience skin breakdown. The most common sites are the **inframammary fold and axillary sulcus.**
What % of women have a less than good or excellent cosmetic result after whole breast RT and lumpectomy?	After whole breast RT and lumpectomy, ~**20%–30%** have a less than good or excellent cosmetic result.
What is the rate of lymphedema 5 yrs after whole breast RT +/− axillary LND? How does the RT technique affect risk?	Lymphedema occurs in ~**15%–40% of pts after RT + axillary LND.** It occurs in **10%–15% after RT and SLN Bx.** The rate of lymphedema with SLN Bx alone is <2%. Retrospective studies suggest that the use of a supraclavicular field to treat the regional nodes **increases the risk of lymphedema compared to tangents alone, on the order of 15%–20%. Adding PAB to modified radical mastectomy + axillary and supraclavicular RT increases the rate to 40%–45%.**

What is the RR of cardiovascular death after RT?

Studies from the pre-3D planning era suggest that RT for breast cancer is associated with an increase in annual events of cardiovascular death (**relative ratio of 1.25, EBCTCG**) compared to no RT.

What is the risk of 2nd malignancies after whole breast RT?

From EBCTCG, the relative ratio of annual events compared to no RT is ~**1.6–2.**

PART VII Gastrointestinal

46
Esophageal Cancer
Steven H. Lin and Zhongxing Liao

Background

What are the boundaries of the esophagus that divide it into cervical, upper thoracic, mid-thoracic, and lower thoracic regions?

The esophagus spans from the cricopharyngeus at the cricoid to the gastroesophageal (GE) junction. Relative to the incisors, the cervical esophagus spans from 15–18 cm, the upper thoracic from 18–24 cm, the mid thoracic from 24–32 cm, and the lower thoracic from 32–40 cm.

What is the incidence and mortality of esophageal cancer in the U.S.?

In 2009, **16,470 cases** were diagnosed, with **14,530 estimated deaths.** Median age is 69 yrs. (*ACS 2009*)

What is the racial and gender predilection of developing esophageal cancer?

The **racial predilection depends on histology.** Squamous cell carcinoma (SCC) is 3 times more common in blacks, whereas adenocarcinoma is more common in whites. **Males are more commonly affected than females** (nearly 3:1).

What are the risk factors of developing esophageal cancer?

Esophageal SCC risk factors: smoking/alcohol tylosis, Plummer-Vinson syndrome, caustic injury to the esophagus, Hx of H&N cancer, and achalasia. HPV infection has been associated in ~20% cases in high-incidence areas (China, Africa, Japan) but none in low-incidence areas (Europe, U.S.).
Esophageal adenocarcinoma risk factors: obesity/GERD, Barrett esophagus, lack of fruits/vegetables, low socioeconomic status

What are some protective factors for developing esophageal cancers?

Protective factors for developing esophageal cancer include **fruits/vegetables and *Helicobacter pylori* infection** (possible atrophic gastritis).

How do pts with esophageal cancer typically present?

Dysphagia and weight loss (>90%), odynophagia, pain, cough, dyspnea, and hoarseness

What is the pattern of spread of tumors of the esophagus?

Tumors of the esophagus spread **locoregionally through the extensive submucosal lymphatic plexus or distantly through hematogenous routes.**

What histologies predominate based on the tumor location within the esophagus?

The proximal three fourths of the esophagus (cervical to mid thoracic) are mostly **SCCs** (~40%), whereas **adenocarcinoma** generally is found in the distal esophagus (~60%).

What are some other more uncommon histologies seen for tumors of the esophagus?

Adenocytic, mucoepidermoid, small cell, and sarcomatous (leiomyosarcoma) carcinomas (all typically 1% of cases). Extremely rare types are lymphoma, Kaposi sarcoma, and melanoma.

What are the patterns of failure (locoregional vs. distant) relative to the histology and tumor location of esophageal cancers?

The patterns of recurrence from surgical series suggest that there is **predominant LRF in cancers of the upper and middle esophagus** (mostly squamous cell), whereas **distant recurrence is more common in lesions in distal third of the esophagus** (mostly adenocarcinomas). (*Mariette C et al., Cancer 2003; Katayama A et al., J Am Coll Surg 2003*)

What are the common sites of DM seen for esophageal cancers?

Lung, liver, and bone are the most common sites of distant Dz.

What % of pts with esophageal cancers present with localized Dz vs. distant Dz?

The extent of Dz at presentation depends on the location and size of the tumor. Dz at the middle and lower third of the esophagus tends to present with **localized Dz (25%–50%),** whereas upper thoracic Dz tends to be **less localized Dz (10%–25%).** Tumors >5 cm also tend to have greater **metastatic rate (~75%)** than tumors <5 cm.

What is the most important factor that determines nodal mets and DM?

DOI is the most important factor dictating nodal and distant spread. (*Mariette C et al., Cancer 2003*)

What is the extent of submucosal spread of Dz seen for esophageal cancers, and does it differ by histology?

Gao XS et al. reported the following for SCC: proximal and distal spread 10.5 +/− 13.5 mm and 10.6 +/− 8.5 mm, respectively, with 94% of pts having all tumor contained within a 30-mm margin. For adenocarcinoma, spread of Dz to 10.3 +/− 7.2 mm proximally and 18.3 +/− 16.3 mm distally, with a margin of 50 mm required to encompass all tumor in 94% of cases. (*IJROBP 2007*)

▍Workup/Staging

What components of the Hx are important in assessing a pt with dysphagia?

Appropriate parts of the Hx in assessing dysphagia Sx include **onset, duration, solids vs. liquids, other Sx of retrosternal pain, bone pain, cough, hoarseness, Hx of smoking/alcohol, GERD, and Hx of prior H&N cancer.**

What should be included in the workup of pts with suspected esophageal cancers?

Suspected esophageal cancer workup: H&P, labs (LFTs, alk phos, Cr), esophagogastroduodenoscopy with Bx. If cancer, then EUS + FNA for nodal sampling for T&N staging, CXR, bronchoscopy (for upper/mid thoracic lesions to r/o tracheoesophageal fistula), and PET/CT. Laparoscopic staging is done in some institutions, with reports of upstaging and sparing the morbidity of more aggressive Tx in 10%–15% of cases.

To what anatomic extent is esophageal cancer being defined?

Esophageal cancer is defined as **15 cm from the incisors to the GE junction and the proximal 5 cm of the stomach.** Stomach tumors arising ≤5 cm from the GE junction or above is considered esophageal cancer.

What is new about the AJCC 7th edition (2009) of the TNM staging for esophageal cancer?

The new system **distinguishes the number of nodal mets, subclassifies T4 Dz, expands the Tis definition, and removes the M1a-b designation.**

Tis: high-grade dysplasia and CIS
T1a: involves lamina propria or muscularis mucosae
T1b: involves submucosa
T2: invades muscularis propria
T3: invades adventitia (*Note:* No serosal layer.)
T4a: pleural, pericardial, or diaphragm involvement
T4b: other organs (aorta, vertebral body, trachea)

Nx: regional nodes cannot be assessed
N0: no regional node mets
N1: 1–2 regional LN mets, including nodes previously labeled as M1a*
N2: 3–6 regional LN mets, including nodes previously labeled as M1a*
N3: ≥7 regional LN mets, including nodes previously labeled as M1a*
  *M1a (differ by site): upper thoracic includes cervical LN mets; mid thoracic is not applicable; lower thoracic/GE junction includes celiac LN mets. (*Note:* M1a designation is no longer recognized in the 7th edition.)

M1: DM (retroperitoneal, para-aortic LN, lung, liver, bone, etc.)

What are the AJCC 7th edition (2009) stage groupings for esophageal cancer, and what new feature has been added?

Tumor grade (1-3) has been added to the TNM stage groupings, and separate stage groupings are given for SCC and adenocarcinoma.

Stage 0: TisN0M0, G1
Stage IA: T1N0M0, G1-2
Stage IB: T1N0M0, G3; T2N0M0, G1-2
Stage IIA: T2N0M0, G3
Stage IIB: T3N0 or T1-2N1, any G
Stage IIIA: T1-2N2M0, any G; T3N1M0, any G; T4aN0M0, any G
Stage IIIB: T3N2M0, any G
Stage IIIC: T4aN1-2M0, any G; T4b or N3, any G
Stage IV: TXNXM1

Why does SCC have a separate stage grouping from adenocarcinoma in the new staging system?

Tumor location is accounted for in the stage grouping for SCC, with lower regions having a better prognosis compared with upper and middle regions. The only changes compared to adenocarcinoma is in IA, IB, IIA, and IIB stage groupings:

Stage IA: T1N0M0G1, any location
Stage IB: T1N0M0G2-3 any location; T2-3N0M0G1, lower location
Stage IIA: T2-3N0M0G1, upper/middle location; T2-3N0M0G2-3, lower location
Stage IIB: T2-3N0M0G2-3, upper location/middle location; T1-2N1M0 any G, any location

▌Treatment/Prognosis

How are pts with Barrett esophagus and high-grade dysplasia managed?

This is **controversial,** with Tx ranging from esophagectomy to local ablative procedures to active surveillance with acid-suppressive therapies.

What are the pros and cons of doing esophagectomy for pts with high-grade dysplasia?

Pros: prevents progression to invasive carcinoma, removal of unsuspected frank invasive Dz (up to 40% of resected specimens).
Cons: a large morbid procedure for a substantial # of pts with high-grade dysplasia alone, which by itself often does not develop into invasive cancer in the pt's lifetime. Local therapies or surveillance would allow identification of pts with early invasive lesions that are readily curable.

What are the guidelines used for surveillance of high-grade dysplasia of the esophagus?

Serial upper endoscopy at 3- to 6-mo intervals with multiple 4-quadrant Bx at 1- to 2-cm intervals.
In a prospective clinical study (*Schnell TG et al., Gastroenterology 2001*), ~16% pts were subsequently identified with invasive cancer with a follow-up of 7.3 yrs. In this study, 11 of 12 pts were found to have early-stage adenocarcinoma, which was managed curatively.

Does the extent of high-grade dysplasia predict for the presence of occult adenocarcinoma?

No. Although ~40%–45% of esophagectomy specimens contain invasive cancers from pts referred for high-grade dysplasia, the extent of high-grade dysplasia in the esophagus does not predict for occult cancer. (*Dar MS et al., Gut 2003*)

What are some local ablative procedures for the management of early-stage esophageal cancers?

Photodynamic therapy, laser ablation, and argon plasma coagulation are some ablative procedures that should be done on study since experience with these is limited.

What is endoscopic mucosal resection (EMR), and what are the criteria for the use of EMR for dysplasia or early-stage (Tis-T1) adenocarcinoma of the esophagus?

EMR involves **submucosal injection of fluid to lift and separate the lesion from the underlying muscular layer,** and resection is carried out by suction to trap the lesion in a cylinder. *Ell C et al. (Gastrointest Endosc 2007)* reported in 100 pts a 5-yr survival of 98%, with no deaths from esophageal cancers. Recurrent/metachronous Dz was subsequently detected in 11%, and all were managed with successful repeat EMR. In an earlier report (*Ell C et al., Gastrointest Endosc 2000*), the remission rate was 59% for a less favorable group using less strict criteria.

The criteria to use EMR were **lesions with no ulceration, T1N0, no vascular/lymphatic invasion, <2 cm, and well to moderately differentiated.**

What are the most important features that predict for poor outcomes in pts with T1 esophageal cancers treated with surgical resection alone?

T1b Dz, LVI, and tumor length predict poor outcomes in these pts. (*Cen P et al., Cancer 2008; Bolton WD et al., J Thorac Cardiovasc Surg 2009*)

How are localized esophageal cancers (>T1N0) managed?

Local esophageal cancer management: **neoadj chemo alone or CRT → esophagectomy → +/− chemo**

What are the types of surgical procedures employed for the management of esophageal cancers?

Minimally invasive esophagectomy using laparoscopy, thoracoscopy, or a combination. Traditional surgical approaches include **radical esophagectomy, transhiatal, or transthoracic esophagectomies.**

How do transhiatal and transthoracic esophagectomy procedures compare in terms of dissection extent and location of the Dz?

In general: A transhiatal approach may be less morbid but will have less exposure to allow wider tumor clearance or more thorough LND compared to a transthoracic approach. Anastomatic leak for the transhiatal approach is easier to manage than the transthoracic approach (cervical vs. intrathoracic leaks).

Transhiatal esophagectomy: Pros—good for distal tumors with possible en bloc resection, laparotomy and a cervical approach (no thoracotomy) with cervical anastomosis, less morbid with less pain, and avoids fatal intrathoracic anastomotic leak. Cons—poor visualization of upper/mid thoracic tumors, LND limited to blunt dissection, more anastomotic leaks, and more recurrent laryngeal nerve palsy.

Transthoracic esophagectomy: Ivor-Lewis (right thoracotomy) is the most common and preferred route and best for exposure for all levels of the esophagus, whereas left thoracotomy provides access to only the distal esophagus. Ivor-Lewis (right thoracotomy and laparotomy) provides direct visualization and exposure with a better radial margin and a more thorough LND. Cons include intrathoracic leak that can lead to fatal mediastinitis.

Does the # of nodes removed from esophagectomy predict for better outcome?

Yes. Data suggest that the # of nodes removed is an independent predictor of survival. In 1 large study, the optimal number was 23 (*Peyre CG et al., Ann Surg 2008*).

Is there evidence to prove that either transhiatal or transthoracic esophagectomy would be superior for Dz control and outcome?

No. There is no data to date showing that 1 approach is superior than the other. Two large meta-analyses comparing transhiatal with transthoracic esophagectomy have shown equivalence (*Rindani R et al., Aust N Z J Surg 1999; Hulscher JB et al., Ann Thorac Surg 2001*). In general, transthoracic approaches carry greater operative mortality and pulmonary complications, but transhiatal approaches have greater anastomatic leaks and stricture rates as well as recurrent laryngeal nerve injury. 5-yr OS rates are similar between the 2 approaches (20%–25%).

What is the 5-yr OS for pts managed with surgery alone for localized esophageal cancers?

5-yr OS is **20%–25%** for pts managed with surgery alone for localized Dz. This is higher for earlier-stage Dz (T1N0 ~77%) but lower for stage III Dz (~10%–15%).

What is the rationale for adding preop therapies to the Tx of esophageal cancer?

The rationale for preop therapies is the **high rate of both local and distant failure with surgery alone.** LF rates range from 19%–57% and distant Dz ranges from 34%–50% in pts with complete resection. Response rate to neoadj therapy is prognostic, and the LC rate with adding surgery to preop CRT is better than definitive CRT.

Is there evidence to support the use of preop chemo (no RT) for Tx of resectable esophageal cancers?

This is **controversial.** Several phase II studies have demonstrated benefit, and 4 randomized studies have reported conflicting results on the benefit of preop chemo.

US Intergroup trial (*Kelsen DP et al., NEJM 1998*): 467 pts randomized to 3 × 5-FU/cisplatin preop and 2 × 5-FU/cisplatin postop or immediate surgical resection alone. There were no differences in resectability or survival (4-yr OS 26% vs. 23%, respectively; MS 16 mos vs. 15 mos, respectively). Pathologic CR was 2.5%. Pts with complete resection had a 5-yr DFS of 32% vs. 5% with R1-R2 resection.

MRC randomized trial of preop chemo (*MRC, Lancet 2002*): 802 pts randomized to (a) 2 × cisplatin/5-FU preop or (b) immediate surgery. There was a significant benefit of neoadj chemo. MS was 13.3 mos vs. 16.8 mos, respectively, and 2-yr OS was 34% vs. 43%, respectively. The complete resection rate was also improved by chemo (54% vs. 60%, respectively).

MRC Adjuvant Gastric Cancer Infusional Chemo (MAGIC) trial (*Cunningham D et al., Lancet 2008*): pts randomized with gastric, GE junction, and distal esophageal adenocarcinoma (26%) to (a) preop epirubicin/cisplatin/5-FU (ECF) × 3 and postop ECF × 3 or (b) surgery alone showed a survival benefit for chemo. 5-yr OS was 36% vs. 23%, respectively ($p = 0.009$).

German Esophageal Cancer Study Group trial (*Stahl M et al., JCO 2009*): randomized phase III in pts with T3-4NXM0 adenocarcinoma of the GE junction or gastric cardia. The study closed early due to poor accrual (126 out of 354 intended). Randomization: (a) induction chemo → surgery or (b) induction chemo → preop CRT → surgery. Chemo was cisplatin/5-FU/leukovorin. RT was 30 Gy in 15 fx. pCR was better in the preop CRT group (15.6% vs. 2%) and in tumor-free LNs (64% vs. 38%). 3-yr OS trended better in the CRT group (47% vs. 28%, $p = 0.07$). Postop mortality was higher in the CRT group (10% vs. 3.8%, $p = 0.26$).

What is the randomized trial evidence to support preop CRT over surgery alone?

This is **somewhat controversial.** Studies have demonstrated that concomitant CRT does improve outcome over sequential therapies. Randomized trials and a meta-analysis have demonstrated benefit with preop CRT.

Walsh TN et al., NEJM 1996: adenocarcinoma only, 5-FU + cisplatin concurrent with RT to 40 Gy/15 fx vs. surgery alone. CRT improved 3-yr survival of 32% vs. 6%, MS 16 mos vs. 11 mos, pCR was 22%, node+ Dz in 22% preop vs. 82% surgery alone. *Criticism:* Small study ($n = 32$) due to early closure; there was poor outcome in surgery alone compared with historical outcomes.

Urba SG et al., JCO 2007: adenocarcinoma in 75%, 100 pts randomized to cisplatin/vinblastine/5-FU + RT to 45 Gy bid vs. surgery alone. 3-yr OS was 30% vs. 16%, respectively ($p = 0.18$). DM was the same in both arms (60%).

Bosset JF et al., NEJM 1997 (EORTC): SCC only, stages I–II. Cisplatin was given 0–2 days prior to RT, and RT was a split course of 18.5 Gy (3.7 Gy × 5) given on days 1 and 22. There was higher postop mortality in the trimodality approach (12% vs. 4%). There was no improvement in DFS or OS.

Burmeister B et al., Lancet 2007 (TTROG): adenocarcinoma and SCC, 256 pts randomized to cisplatin + 5-FU with RT to 35 Gy/15 fx. Less intensive chemo (5-FU 800 mg/m^2 vs. 1,000 mg/m^2 in other studies) was used. There was no difference in OS, but there was a trend to improved survival in SCC.

CALGB 9781 (*Tepper J et al., JCO 2008*): 56 pts randomized (closed due to poor accrual) to cisplatin + 5-FU with RT to 50.4 Gy. pCR rate was 40%. 5-yr OS was 39% vs. 16% ($p = 0.005$). MS was 48 mos vs. 22 mos.

Meta-analysis (*Gebski V et al., Lancet Oncol 2007*): 10 trials, 1,209 pts, comparing preop CRT vs. surgery alone. Concurrent CRT had a HR of 0.87 (13% reduction in mortality at 2 yrs). There was no difference in histologies. There was no benefit seen for sequential chemo → RT.

What are the advantages of preop CRT for Tx of esophageal cancers?

A lower RT dose and the ability to downstage pts with locally advanced Dz may improve outcomes. Data from phase II–III preop CRT has demonstrated that pCR or min residual Dz has an excellent prognosis with 5-yr OS of 60%–70%.

What are the typical pCR rates after CRT for esophageal cancer?

pCR rates range from **22%–40%** in the randomized trials using cisplatin + 5-FU (on avg, 25%–30%).

Is there a role for preop radiotherapy for esophageal cancers?

No. Studies demonstrate no benefit of preop RT alone.

What is the role of postop radiation vs. preop CRT?

Postop RT alone has failed to demonstrate a benefit in several randomized trials. Incomplete resection should receive definitive CRT or palliative chemo or RT alone. Completely resected stage II–III adenocarcinoma of the GE junction should receive postop CRT based on the Intergroup gastric trial (*MacDonald JS et al., NEJM 2001*).

What is the data demonstrating efficacy of definitive CRT vs. RT alone?

RTOG 85-01 (*Herskovic A et al., NEJM 1992; Cooper JS et al., JAMA 1999*): 123 pts randomized to 64 Gy RT alone vs. 50 Gy RT + cis/5-FU × 2 during RT and 2 cycles after RT. There was SCC in 88% pts. 5-yr OS was 27% vs. 0% for RT alone. 10-yr OS was 20% for CRT. There was no difference between adenocarcinoma and SCC.

RT technique used in this trial: initial RT field was the whole esophagus to 50 Gy (RT alone) or 30 Gy (CRT) → CD to 14 Gy (RT) or 20 Gy (CRT) to tumor + 5-cm sup/inf margin.

Is there a benefit of escalating the RT dose during CRT for esophageal cancer?

This is **controversial,** since **INT 0123** (*Minsky BD et al., JCO 2002*) is a phase III study that randomized pts to 50.4 Gy vs. 64.8 Gy with cisplatin + 5-FU × 2 → adj cisplatin/5-FU × 2. There was no difference in LC (44% vs. 48%). Excessive deaths in 64.8 Gy arm (11 vs. 2) were seen even before the 50.4 Gy dose (7 of 11 deaths). However, separate analysis excluding the early deaths still did not find a benefit to a higher dose.

Is there evidence to suggest that adding surgery to definitive CRT will improve the outcome?

This is **controversial.** Two randomized trials examining CRT + surgery vs. CRT alone demonstrated LC benefit of adding surgery but not OS. This is possibly due to increased postop mortality.

French data (*Bedenne L et al., JCO 2007*): 444 pts enrolled, treated first with CRT (45 Gy or split course 15 Gy × 2); the 230 responding pts (88% SCC) were randomized to surgery or no surgery. LC was better with surgery (66% vs. 57%). There was no difference in survival (34% vs. 40%). The mortality rate was higher in the surgery group (9.3% vs. 0.8%).

German data (*Stahl M et al., JCO 2005*): 172 pts with SCC randomized to induction chemo + 40 Gy/chemo + surgery vs. induction chemo + 65 Gy/chemo alone. PFS was better with surgery (64% vs. 41%). Survival was the same between arms, with a trend to better survival for surgery.

Conclusion from these studies: For good performance status pts with surgery performed at a high-volume center, preop CRT should be considered standard. There is, however, increased interest to identify pts who would be candidates for definitive CRT (i.e., those with a cCR and has less likelihood to recur locally) for organ preservation.

Could salvage therapies (surgery or RT) be performed after definitive CRT or surgery for esophageal cancer management?

Yes. Salvage surgery can be performed for select pts who recur after definitive CRT but with increased operative morbidity/mortality (*Tachimori Y et al., J Thorac Cardiovasc Surg 2009*). Salvage RT can be performed for isolated LR after surgery alone, but the dose should be limited to 45 Gy with concurrent chemo because of gastric pull-through.

Can RT be performed in pts with trancheo-esophageal fistula?

Yes. Although historically it is contraindicated because of fear that RT may worsen the fistula, available studies demonstrate that RT does not worsen the fistula and may even cause healing and closure in 1 series (*Muto M et al., Cancer 1999*).

How are cancers of the cervical esophagus managed in general?

Because of the difficult and morbid surgery (total laryngopharyngoesophagectomy), cancers of the cervical esophagus are managed **like a H&N primary with a nonsurgical approach and definitive CRT.** Case series from MD Anderson using IMRT + 5-FU/cisplatin (*Wang SL et al., WJG 2006*) and *Burmeister et al.* (*AOHNS 2000*) show that a high dose toward 70 Gy (60–66 Gy as done for H&N cancers) offer good LC and response (LC 88% and 5-yr OS 55% from the *Burmeister et al.* series). However, late toxicity, such as esophageal stricture, is a problem.

Can definitive RT be used for early-stage (Tis, IA) esophageal cancers?	**Yes.** With doses 60–72 Gy or 55–60 Gy + a brachytherapy boost, the LC and DFS is ~80%. Tumors >5 cm should rcv CRT because of poorer LC (~50%–60% per *Hishikawa Y et al., Radiother Oncol 1991*).
What are the radiotherapy doses and techniques for the management of esophageal cancer?	Preop CRT: 44–50.4 Gy Definitive CRT: 50.4 Gy Definitive RT: 60–64 Gy Field size (to block edge): 5 cm above and below GTV, 1.5–2.5 cm laterally. If escalated above 50 Gy, CD to 2 cm above and below GTV. Treat with 3D-CRT or IMRT techniques.

■ Toxicity

What are the esophageal stricture rates receiving RT alone?	Based on Emami data (*Emami B et al., IJROBP 1991*), a 5% stricture rate occurs when one third of the esophagus gets 60 Gy, two thirds get 58 Gy, and 55 Gy for entire esophagus.
What is the dose limitation to the heart?	Dose limitations to the heart are as follows: **whole heart to 30 Gy, two thirds to 45 Gy, and one third to 55 Gy.** Try to keep V40 <50% to minimize potential late toxicities.
What are the dose limits for the kidneys, liver, and spinal cord?	Kidneys: keep combined kidneys V18 <30%, or limit one third of 1 kidney to a full dose Liver: V30 <50% Spinal cord: no point dose >45 Gy
What types of toxicities are experienced during radiotherapy, and what measures should be taken to help minimize these toxicities?	Acute: esophagitis, skin irritation, fatigue, weight loss Late: dysphagia, stricture, pneumonitis, laryngeal edema, cardiac injury, renal insufficiency, liver injury Relief is obtained with **topical anesthesia, narcotics, H2 blockers, feeding tube, and limiting the dose to critical structures.**
Per NCCN 2010, what is the appropriate follow-up schedule for pts after completion of Tx for esophageal cancer?	Esophageal cancer follow-up following Tx: H&P every 4 mos for 1 yr, every 6 mos for 2 yrs, then annually; at each visit, basic labs such as CBC/chemistry panel +/− endoscopy as clinically indicated; and dilatation for stenosis and nutritional counseling as needed.
Pts with Tis or T1a esophageal cancer who undergo EMR or ablative procedures should have what type of follow-up schedule/procedures?	Tis/T1a esophageal cancer pts with EMR or ablative procedures follow-up: H&P + endoscopy every 3 mos for 1 yr, then annually (*NCCN 2010*).

47

Gastric Cancer

Steven H. Lin and Salma Jabbour

▮ Background

What is the incidence of gastric cancer in the U.S. and worldwide?

<u>U.S</u>: 21,130 cases/yr (in 2009), with 10,620 deaths (7th leading)

<u>Worldwide</u>: ~875,000 new cases/yr; 2nd-leading cause of death (behind lung cancer)

Where are the high-incidence areas in the world?

The highest incidences are found in **East Asia (Japan and China) > South America > Eastern Europe.**

What are some acquired and genetic risk factors for developing gastric cancer?

<u>Acquired factors</u>: *Helicobacter pylori* infection, high intake of smoked and salted foods, nitrates, diet low in fruits/vegetables, smoking, RT exposure, obesity, Barrett esophagus/GERD, prior subtotal gastrectomy

<u>Genetic factors</u>: E-cadherin (CDH-1 gene) mutation, type A blood group, pernicious anemia, HNPCC, Li-Fraumeni syndrome

How does tumor location relate to the underlying etiology of gastric adenocarcinoma?

Body and antral lesions are associated with *H. pylori* infection and chronic atrophic gastritis, whereas proximal gastric lesions (gastroesophageal [GE] junction, gastric cardia) are associated with obesity, GERD, and smoking.

Which has poorer prognosis: proximal or distal gastric cancer?

Stage for stage, **proximal** gastric cancer has a poorer prognosis.

What are the 2 histologic types of gastric adenocarcinoma? How do these 2 types differ in terms of etiology of the gastric cancer?

Intestinal and diffuse are the 2 histologic types of adenocarcinomas. <u>Intestinal type</u> are differentiated cancers with a tendency to form glands, occur in the distal stomach, and arise from precursor lesions seen mostly in endemic areas and in older people, more commonly men, suggesting an environmental etiology. <u>Diffuse type</u> are less differentiated (signet ring cells, mucin producing), have extensive submucosal/distant spread, and tend to be proximal. They do not arise from precancerous lesions, are more common in low-incidence areas, and are more common in women and younger people, suggesting a genetic etiology.

What is the the Borrmann classification of gastric cancer?	The Borrmann classification is **based on the gross morphologic appearance.** It is divided into 5 types: Type I: polypoid/fungating Type II: ulcerating Type III: ulcerating/infiltrative Type IV: diffusely infiltrating (linitis plastica) Type V: cannot be classified (most aggressive)
What are the lymphatic drainages of the stomach? Please also include the Japanese Research Society (JRS) classification of nodal designation.	1st echelon: N1—perigastric nodes (lesser and greater curvature) and periesophageal nodes (proximal gastric) 2nd echelon: N2—celiac axis, common hepatic, splenic More distant: N3—hepatoduodenal, peripancreatic, mesenteric root; N4—portocaval, PA nodes, middle colic **JRS N1–N4 are not the same as AJCC staging.**
What are the patterns of spread for gastric cancer?	Local extension to adjacent organs, lymphatic mets, peritoneal spread, or hematogenous (liver, lung, bone). Liver/lung mets are generally for proximal/GE junction tumors.
What are the anatomic boundaries and organs for the stomach?	Superior: diaphragm, left hepatic lobe Inferior: transverse colon, mesocolon, greater omentum Anterior: abdominal wall Posterior and lateral: spleen, pancreas, left adrenal, left kidney, splenic flexure of colon
What is the most important prognostic factor for gastric cancer?	**TNM stage** is the most important factor, with the histologic grade and Borrmann types not being independently prognostic apart from tumor stage. However, in general, Borrmann type I and II are more favorable compared to type IV.
Is all nodal involvement equally prognostic for gastric cancer?	**No.** The # and location of nodes are important. Min LN involvement adjacent to the primary lesion is more favorable.

■ Workup/Staging

How do pts with gastric cancer generally present?	Anorexia, abdominal discomfort, weight loss, fatigue, n/v, melena, and weakness from anemia
What aspects of the physical exam are relevant for evaluating a pt for a possible gastric malignancy?	General physical with focus on abdominal mass (local extension), liver mets, ovarian mets (Krukenberg tumor), distant LN mets (Virchow: left SCV; Irish: left axillary; Sister Mary Joseph: umbilical), ascites, Blumer shelf (rectal peritoneal involvement)

What is important in the workup for gastric cancer?

Gastric cancer workup: H&P (onset, duration, Hx of risk factors), CBC, CMP, esophagogastroduodenoscopy + Bx, EUS +/− FNA of regional LN mets, CT C/A/P, and diagnostic laparoscopy to r/o peritoneal seeding

How many layers are seen on EUS when imaging the GI tract?

5 layers are seen on EUS: layers 1, 3, and 5 are hyperechoic (bright), and layers 2 and 4 are hypoechoic (dark). Layer 1 is superficial mucosa, layer 2 is deep mucosa, layer 3 is submucosa, layer 4 is muscularis propria, and layer 5 is subserosa fat and serosa.

What is the rate of upstaging to stage IV using diagnostic laparoscopy?

35%–40% of pts are found to have mets using diagnostic laparoscopy.

Why is PET imaging not routinely used in staging gastric cancer?

In 1 study, only approximately two thirds of primary tumors are FDG avid (*Shah et al., Proc ASCO 2007*), with GLUT-1 transporter rarely present on the common subtypes of gastric cancer (signet ring and mucinous). Therefore, there are too many false negatives.

What is the AJCC 7th edition (2009) T-staging classification for gastric cancer?

Tis: confined to mucosa without invasion to lamina propria
T1a: invades lamina propria or muscularis mucosae
T1b: invades submucosa
T2: invades muscularis propria
T3*: penetrates subserosa without invasion of visceral peritoneum (serosa)
T4a*: invades serosa
T4b: invades adjacent structures
*Tumor is classified as T3 if it penetrates through the muscularis propria with extension into the gastrocolic or gastrohepatic ligaments, or into the greater or lesser omentum without perforation of the visceral peritoneum covering these structures. Tumor is classified as T4 if it penetrates the visceral peritoneum covering the gastric ligaments or the omentum.

What is the AJCC 7th edition (2009) N-staging classification for gastric cancer?

N1: 1–2 LNs
N2: 3–6 LNs
N3: ≥7 LNs
N3a: 7–15 LNs
N3b: >15 LNs

What are the AJCC 7th edition (2009) stage groupings for gastric cancer?

Stage IA: T1N0 (adds to 1)
Stage IB: T1N1, T2a-bN0 (adds to 2)
Stage IIA: T1N2, T2N1, or T3N0 (adds to 3)
Stage IIB: T2N2, T3N1, T4aN0 (adds to 4)
Stage IIIA: T4aN1, T3N2, T2N3 (adds to 5)
Stage IIIB: T4bN0, T4bN1, T4aN2, T3N3 (adds to 6 mostly)
Stage IIIC: T4bN2, T4aN3, T4bN3 (adds to 7 mostly)
Stage IV: TXNXM1

What is the 5-yr OS for the various stages of gastric cancer?

T1N0, 90%; T2N0, 52%; T3N0, 47%; T4N0, 15%; TXN1, 10%; TXN2, 10%; TXN3, 10%; TXN4, 3% (Japanese data: modified from *Noguichi Y et al., Cancer 1989*). These results may not reflect outcomes in the U.S. There is a chance that the biology of gastric cancer is different in Japanese cohorts and that gastric cancer screening is used in Japan to discover early stages of Dz. Surgery is probably easier in the Japanese population because of lower BMIs. Better outcomes may also reflect more extensive LND performed as standard practice.

▌ Treatment/Prognosis

What surgical margin is necessary for resection of gastric cancer?

≥5 cm proximal and distal margin (except for select cases removed endoscopically)

In what tumor location is subtotal vs. total gastrectomy indicated? Is there a benefit of advocating total gastrectomy for most gastric tumors?

Subtotal gastrectomy for distal tumors (antrum/body); total gastrectomy for proximal tumors (cardia, greater curvature)

No. According to the following 2 trials, there is no benefit of advocating total gastrectomy:

Gouzi et al. randomized distal tumors to total gastrectomy vs. subtotal gastrectomy. There were no differences in morbidity/mortality (1.3% vs. 3.2%) or survival outcomes (5-yr OS 48%). (*Ann Surg 1989*)

Italian data from a 2nd randomized trial (*Bozzetti F et al., Ann Surg 1999*) showed no difference in 5-yr survival between subtotal gastrectomy (65%) and total gastrectomy (62%).

Should splenectomy be performed for proximal gastric tumors to get splenic LN clearance?

Avoid splenectomy if possible, since there is no value of splenectomy in a randomized trial (*Csendes A et al., Surgery 2002*). Splenectomy and pancreatectomy had an adverse impact on survival in the Dutch and MRC D1 vs. D2 RCTs (see below).

How are GE junction cancers classified, and how is the classification important therapeutically?

GE junction cancers are classified by the **Siewert classification** as 3 entities:

Type I: adenocarcinoma of distal esophagus, arising from Barrett, that infiltrate GE junction

Type II: adenocarcinoma of cardia portion, arising from cardia and short segment of intestinal metaplasia at GE junction

Type III: adenocarcinoma of subcardial stomach, which may infiltrate GE junction or distal esophagus from below

Type I has lymphatic drainage reminiscent of esophageal primaries (mediatinal and celiac), whereas types II–III drain to celiac, splenic, and para-aortic (P-A) nodes. Esophagectomy is typically recommended for type I tumors, whereas gastrectomy is recommended for type II–III tumors.

What are the types of nodal dissections for gastric cancer?

D0: no nodal dissection

D1: perigastric nodes removed

D2: D1 + periarterial nodes (left gastric, hepatic, celiac, splenic)

D3: D2 + hepatoduodenal, peripancreatic, mesenteric root, portocaval, P-A nodes, middle colic

Is extended lymphadenectomy necessary for surgical cure of gastric cancer?

No. Although results from numerous randomized trials have *not* shown an OS advantage of extended lymphadenectomy, CSS and LRR may be improved with extended dissection in the most recent update of the Dutch trial.

Dutch trial (*Bonenkamp JJ et al., NEJM 1999*): 711 pts randomized to D1 vs. D2 dissection. There was greater mortality in the D2 group (10% vs. 4%, p = SS), and 5-yr OS was 45% vs. 47% (NSS). In the most recent 15-yr update (*Songun I et al., Lancet Oncol 2010*), the 15-yr OS is 21% in the D1 group and 29% in the D2 groups (p = 0.34). However, the gastric cancer–related death rate is significantly higher in the D1 group (48%) vs. the D2 group (37%), while deaths from other Dz were similar in the 2 groups. LR was lower in the D2 group (12% vs. 22%) as well as the regional recurrence (13% vs. 19%) (all SS).

MRC trial (*Cushieri A et al., Br J Cancer 1999*): 400 pts randomized to D1 vs. D2. There was greater mortality in the D2 group (13% vs. 6.5%), and 5-yr OS was the same (35% vs. 33%).

In both trials, splenectomy and pancreatectomy had an adverse impact on survival.

Japanese trial JCOG9501 (D2 vs. D2 + P-A node dissection [PAND]) (*Sasako M et al., NEJM 2008*) demonstrated that although extended LND does not increase morbidity or mortality, there is also no difference in 5-yr OS (69.2% for D2 vs. 70.3% for D2 + PAND) or for LRR.

An **Italian trial** (D1 vs. D2) (*Degiuli M et al., Br J Surg 2010*) has shown no increased morbidity or mortality with extended lymphadenectomy, but clinical outcomes have not yet been reported.

What is the min # of LNs that should be pathologically assessed in a gastrectomy specimen?

In the U.S., at least **15 LNs** should be assessed by the pathologist, since pt survival improves if >15 LNs are examined.

What are the selection criteria for endoscopic mucosal resection (EMR) or limited surgical resection (without nodal evaluation) of gastric cancer?

Favorable early-stage gastric cancer: **Tis-T1 (but not involving submucosa), small (≤3 cm), nonulcerated, well differentiated, N0.** In general, these types of tumors have <5% LN met rate.

When is surgery alone adequate for gastric cancer?

T1N0 or T2N0 (but not beyond the muscularis propria). 5-yr OS for favorable early-stage gastric cancer is 80%–90%. For all others, adj Tx is needed (**Ib** [except T2aN0] **to IIIC** [nonmetastatic]).

What is the relapse pattern after "curative" resection of gastric cancer?

Distant Dz (50%) and LRR. LRR is common in the gastric bed, nearby LNs, anastomotic site, gastric remnant, and duodenal stump. In the classic paper of the University of Minnesota reoperative analysis (*Gunderson L et al., IJROBP 1982*), local-only recurrence was seen in 29%, LR and/or regional LN mets in 54%, and LF as any component of failure in 88% of pts.

What is the evidence that demonstrated the benefit of adj CRT after surgical resection for gastric cancer?

INT-0116 (*Macdonald JS et al., NEJM 2001*): 556 pts, stage IB–IV (nonmetastatic) adenocarcinoma of stomach and GE junction (~20%), randomized after en bloc resection to –margin to (a) observation or (b) CRT (1 cycle bolus 5-FU/leukovorin [LV]) before RT, 2 cycles during 45 Gy RT, and 2 cycles after RT. Median follow-up was 5 yrs. CRT was beneficial in all parameters except for DM 3-yr RFS 48% vs. 31%; 3-yr OS 50% vs. 41%; median OS 36 mos vs. 27 mos; and LR 19% vs. 29%. DM 18% surgery vs. 33% CRT (NSS). Toxic deaths of 1% were seen.

What % of PCA pts have regional node+ Dz at Dx?

~**25%** of PCA pts have regional node+ Dz at Dx.

For PCA, what are the 3 most common sites of DM?

Common sites of DM for PCA include the **liver, peritoneal surface, and lungs.**

Is there a role for screening in PCA?

No. There is no current role for PCA screening. There are studies evaluating the role of screening 1st-degree relatives of PCA with EUS, but this is still experimental.

What % of pancreatic tumors are from the exocrine pancreas?

~**95%** of PCA are from the exocrine pancreas.

What are the 4 most common pathologic subtypes of exocrine pancreatic tumors?

Most common subtypes of exocrine pancreatic tumors:
1. Ductal adenocarcinoma (80%)
2. Mucinous cystadenocarcinoma
3. Acinar cell carcinoma
4. Adenosquamous carcinoma

What is the most common oncogene in PCA?

The **K-ras** oncogene is present in ~85% of PCA.

What are the 2 most common presenting Sx of PCA?

Common presenting Sx of PCA are **pancreatic/biliary duct obstruction, jaundice, and abdominal pain.**

What Dz is commonly diagnosed 1–2 yrs prior to a PCA Dx?

60%–80% of PCA pts are diagnosed with diabetes 1–2 yrs prior to Dx. However, only a small proportion of diabetic pts develop PCA.

Periampullary cancers refer to tumors arising from what 3 structures?

Periampullary tumors are those arising from the **ampulla of Vater, distal common bile duct (CBD), and adjacent duodenum.**

■ Workup/Staging

What is the DDx of a pancreatic mass?

The DDx of a pancreatic mass includes exocrine cancer, islet cell/neuroendocrine cancer, cystic adenomas, papillary cystic neoplasms (e.g., intraductal papillary mucinous tumor), lymphoma, acinar cell carcinoma, and metastatic cancer.

Name 4 appropriate procedures for obtaining tissue from a suspicious pancreatic mass.

Procedures to obtain tissue from a suspicious pancreatic mass:
1. EUS-guided FNA
2. CT-guided FNA
3. Endoscopic retrograde cholangiopancreatography (ERCP)
4. Pancreatic resection (i.e., histologic Dx is not required before surgery)

What is the major advantage of EUS-guided FNA over CT-guided FNA of a pancreatic mass?

EUS-guided FNA is associated with **lower risk of peritoneal seeding** (2% vs. 16%).

What is the workup for suspected PCA?

Suspected PCA workup: H&P, CBC, CMP, CA 19-9, triphasic thin-sliced CT abdomen (pancreas protocol), chest imaging, +/− ERCP/EUS FNA for Dx and/or stent placement

In what circumstance will a PCA pt not excrete any CA 19-9?

If a pt is red cell Lewis antigen A–B negative, then the pt cannot excrete CA 19-9. The Lewis antigen negative phenotype is present in 5%–10% of the population.

What is the significance of a post-resection CA 19-9 >90 U/mL?

In **RTOG 9704,** 53 pts (14%) had CA 19-9 >90 U/mL, and only 2 of these pts survived up to 3 yrs.

What is the NCCN 2010 classification scheme for PCA?

PCA are classified in 4 categories (and per AJCC staging):
1. Resectable (T1-3N0 or N+) (stages I–II)
2. Borderline resectable (T4NX) (stage III)
3. Locally advanced (T4NX) (stage III)
4. Metastatic (TXNXM1) (stage IV)

What is the AJCC 7th edition (2009) T and N staging for PCA?

T1: limited to pancreas and ≤2 cm
T2: limited to pancreas and >2 cm
T3: extends beyond pancreas but without celiac axis or superior mesenteric artery (SMA) involvement
T4: celiac axis or SMA involvement
N1: regional node involvement

What are the AJCC 7th edition (2009) stage groupings for PCA?

Stage 0: Tis
Stage IA: T1N0M0
Stage IB: T2N0M0
Stage IIA: T3N0M0
Stage IIB: T1-3N1M0
Stage III: T4NXM0
Stage IV: TXNXM1

Per the NCCN, what 3 criteria are necessary for a primary pancreatic tumor to be resectable?

NCCN resectability for PCA is defined as follows:
1. Patent superior mesenteric vein (SMV)/portal vein confluence
2. Clear fat plane around celiac artery and SMA
3. No nodal mets or other mets beyond field of resection

Per the NCCN, what pancreatic head/body lesions are considered "borderline resectable"?

NCCN definition of borderline resectability for PCA:
1. Severe unilat SMV/portal confluence impingement
2. Tumor abutment on SMA
3. Gastroduodenal artery encasement up to hepatic artery
4. Tumors with limited involvement of IVC
5. Short segment SMV occlusion with patent vein both proximally and distally
6. Colon or mesocolon invasion

What pancreatic tail lesions are considered "borderline resectable"?

Invasion into the adrenal gland, colon, mesocolon, or kidney are considered borderline resectable for PCA tail lesions.

What location of PCA is associated with higher rates of resectability: head, body, or tail?

PCA **head** tumors are more resectable b/c they cause Sx early (and therefore present with earlier-stage Dz).

What % of pts with resectable PCA tumors by CT imaging will be resectable at the time of surgery?

~**80%** of PCA pts deemed resectable by CT are resectable at the time of surgery.

What is the stage of a PCA pt with positive cytology at time of laparoscopy?

Positive cytology is **stage IV** (M1).

Does the AJCC 7th edition (2009) TNM staging for periampullary adenocarcinoma differ from PCA?

Yes. There is a separate AJCC TNM staging for ampulla of Vater carcinoma, distal CBD carcinoma, and duodenal carcinoma.

■ Treatment/Prognosis

What surgical procedure is required to resect a pancreatic head lesion?

Surgery utilized for pancreatic head resection includes **pylorus-preserving pancreaticoduodenectomy** (PPPD) or **classic pancreaticoduodenectomy** (Whipple procedure).

What anastomoses are performed in the classic pancreaticoduodenectomy (Whipple)?

There are 3 anastomoses performed for the Whipple procedure:
1. Pancreaticojejunostomy
2. Choledochojejunostomy (hepaticojejunostomy)
3. Gastrojejunostomy

What are the 4 most favorable prognostic factors after resection?

Most favorable prognostic factors after resection of PCA:
1. −Margins (R0)
2. Low grade (G1)
3. Small tumor size (<3 cm)
4. N0 status

Is there a benefit to R1 or R2 resection over definitive CRT for PCA?

No. Retrospective evidence suggests that survival is similar between PCA pts who had R1 or R2 resection and definitive CRT. Therefore, planned resections should be done in pts where R0 resections are likely. Debulking surgery does not improve outcome over definitive CRT.

Should pts with resectable PCA undergo extended retroperitoneal lymphadenectomy?

No. Resectable PCA pts should not undergo an extended retroperitoneal lymphadenectomy. There is no survival benefit to extended lymphadenectomy by an RCT (5-yr 25% vs. 31%, NSS). (*Riall TS et al., J Gastrointest Surg 2005*)

Can definitive CRT replace surgical resection for resectable PCA?

No. Surgery alone is superior to CRT alone for pts with resectable PCA per the Japanese PCA Study Group in an RCT of surgery alone vs. definitive CRT (50.4 Gy with continuous infusion [CI] 5-FU). The trial was stopped early due to the benefit of surgery: MS was 12 mos vs. 9 mos, and 5-yr OS was 10% vs. 0%. (*Doi R et al., Surg Today 2008*)

What are adj Tx options for a PCA pt s/p resection?

Adj Tx options after a pancreaticoduodenectomy:
1. Adj gemcitabine (**CONKO-001**)
2. Adj gemcitabine alone → 5-FU/RT→ gemcitabine alone (**RTOG 9704**)
3. Adj 5-FU/RT (**GITSG 91-73**); consider maintenance gemcitabine afterward
4. Adj 5-FU → 5-FU/RT → 5-FU (**RTOG 9704**)
5. Observation alone

What is the standard total dose and fractionation for PCA after surgical resection?

Standard adj RT volumes and doses for adj PCA are as follows: tumor bed and at-risk regional nodes plus a 1–2-cm margin for motion and set-up error to 45 Gy. CD to tumor bed and a margin to 50.4–54 Gy in 1.8 Gy/fx.

What American study 1st reported a benefit of adj CRT vs. no additional Tx for resected PCA? Describe the arms of this study and the major results.

The Gastrointestinal Tumor Study Group (GITSG 91–73) trial 1st reported benefit to adj CRT for PCA in 1985.
Standard arm: postop observation
Experimental arm: Adj CRT using split-course RT to 40 Gy (2-wk break after 20 Gy) with intermittent bolus 5-FU → 2 full yrs of adj 5-FU alone
Improved MS (20 mos vs. 11 mos) and 2-yr OS (42% vs. 15%) in the adj CRT arm (*Kalser MH et al., Arch Surg 1985*)

Did the EORTC 40891 study on PCA support or contest the benefit of adj CRT?

Support. The **EORTC 40891** trial included T1-T2, N0-N1 PCA or T1-T3, N0-N1 periampullary adenocarcinoma. The same randomization was used as that in GITSG 1985, except the Tx arm did *not* rcv maintenance adj 5-FU for 2 yrs. Median PFS was 17 mos (CRT) vs. 16 mos (observation), NSS; MS was 24 mos (CRT) vs. 19 mos (observation), NSS. For the subset of PCA pts, 5-yr OS was 20% (CRT) vs. 10% (observation), $p = 0.09$ (*Klinkenbijl JH et al., Ann Surg 1999*). The authors concluded that routine adj CRT was not warranted, though statistical reanalysis of this study found a significant survival benefit with adj therapy (*Garofalo MC et al. Ann Surg 2006*).

Did the ESPAC-1 study on PCA support or contest the benefit of adj CRT?

Contest. ESPAC-1 included pts with grossly resected adenocarcinoma of the pancreas. The study used a 2×2 factorial design; surgery $+/-$ CRT and $+/-$ adj chemo. Adj CRT was similar to GITSG. Adj chemo was 6 mos of 5-FU. MS was 15 mos (CRT) vs. 16 mos (no CRT), NSS; OS was 20 mos (chemo) vs. 14 mos (no chemo), $p = 0.0005$.

Criticisms: Physicians could have pts randomize into 2×2 or directly into 1 of the 2 randomizations. "Background Tx" was allowed (i.e., observation pts may have rcv chemo and/or RT). There was no central RT quality assurance. (*Neoptolemos JP et al., Lancet 2001*)

Note: Analysis of 2×2 subset suggests that CRT had a deleterious effect; 5-yr OS was 10% (CRT) vs. 20% (no CRT), $p = 0.05$.

How does the presence of a +margin after resection for PCA influence the decision for adj CRT?

UK Clinical Trials Unit meta-analysis of 5 RCTs, including individual data from 4 RCTs, found that the benefit of adj CRT was greater in R1 pts compared to R0 pts, though the difference was not SS. Also, the benefit of adj chemo alone decreased in R1 pts compared to R0 pts, suggesting that CRT may have more important role in R1 pts. (*Butturini G et al., Arch Surg 2008*)

What study supports the role for adj gemcitabine for resected PCA over best supportive care? What subset of pts were excluded from this trial?

CONKO-001 included T1-T4, N0-N1 pts in a RCT of observation vs. adj gemcitabine. Outcomes favored adj gemcitabine: MS was 23 mos vs. 20 mos (SS), and 5-yr OS was 21% vs. 9% (SS) (*Neuhaus P et al., ASCO Abstract 2008*). *Note:* Pts with CA 19-9 >90 were excluded from this trial.

What study compared adj 5-FU to gemcitabine following surgical resection?

ESPAC-3 showed a MS of 23 mos (95% confidence interval: 21.1, 25.0 mos) for pts treated with 5-FU and 23.6 mos (95% confidence interval: 21.4, 26.4 mos) for pts treated with gemcitabine. There was no significant difference between the groups. (*ASCO abstract 2009*)

Did the study RTOG 9704 on PCA support or contest a benefit of gemcitabine-based adj CRT?

This is **controversial**. **RTOG 9704** randomized R0 and R1 PCA pts to CI 5-FU (250 mg/m^2/d) CRT (50.4 Gy) and pre- and post-CRT with either additional 5-FU or gemcitabine. Among all eligible pts, there were no differences. In a preplanned subset analysis of pts with pancreatic head tumors, trends favored gemcitabine: MS was 20.5 mos vs. 16.7 mos, and 3-yr OS was 31% vs. 22%, but results were NSS ($p = 0.09$). The 3-yr LR was significantly better for the gemcitabine arm (23% vs. 28%). (*Regine W et al., JAMA 2008*)

What is the Picozzi regimen for pts with PCA?

The Picozzi regimen is **adj CRT with α-interferon, 5-FU, cisplatin, and RT** (45–54 Gy). 42% of pts were admitted during CRT; however, outcomes were very promising: 5-yr OS was 55%, and MS was not reached (*Picozzi VJ et al., Am J Surg 2003*). Subsequent study results are pending.

What is the Tx paradigm for borderline resectable PCA?

Borderline resectable PCA Tx paradigm: Consider staging laparoscopy, stent placement if jaundice, and neoadj CRT → resection.

What neoadj CRT regimen should be used for borderline resectable PCA?

There is **no standard neoadj Tx for PCA.** Use similar paradigms as for locally advanced cases: (a) 5-FU/RT, (b) gemcitabine/RT, or (c) induction gemcitabine/Taxotere/Xeloda (GTX) → 5-FU/RT, with RT to 45–50.4 Gy in 1.8–2Gy/fx or 30 Gy in 3Gy/fx per the MDACC paradigm (*Breslin TM et al., Ann Surg Oncol 2001*).

What is the Tx paradigm for locally advanced PCA?

Locally advanced unresectable PCA Tx paradigm: Biliary stent (if jaundice) can be done 1st → (a) definitive CRT, (b) induction chemo → restage → CRT, (c) gemcitabine + RT, or (d) gemcitabine-based chemo.

What definitive CRT regimen should be used for locally advanced PCA?

Standard regimen for definitive CRT: 5-FU (CI 250 mg/m^2/d) + RT, with RT to 50–60 Gy in 1.8–2 Gy/fx or 30 Gy in 3 Gy/fx.

Is there a gender predilection for HCC?	**Yes.** Males are 3 times more likely to develop HCC.
Worldwide, where does HCC rank as a cause of cancer death?	Worldwide, HCC is the **4th leading cause of cancer death** (3rd for men), but rates vary dramatically by region.
HCC incidence peaks in what decade of life?	HCC incidence peaks in the **6th decade** of life.
What is the most common clinical presentation of HCC?	The most common clinical presentation of HCC is **rising AFP in the setting of worsening pre-existing liver Dz.**
Who should be screened for HCC and how?	**Pts with cirrhosis, hepatitis B carrier state, or nonalcoholic steatohepatitis** should be screened for HCC. Screen with **AFP and liver US** every 6–12 mos.
Do most pts with HCC present with localized or metastatic Dz?	90% of HCC pts present with **localized Dz.**
In HCC, what are the most common sites of metastatic spread?	HCC most commonly metastasizes to **intra-abdominal LNs and lungs.** Less common sites of mets include bone, brain, and adrenal glands.

▪ Workup/Staging

What is the workup of suspected HCC?	Suspected HCC workup: H&P, AFP, CBC, CMP with LDH, LFTs, PT/INR, hepatitis panel (HBV/HCV studies), triphasic CT abdomen or MRI liver, chest imaging, and percutaneous Bx if necessary
For a pt with suspected HCC, when is a Bx unnecessary to establish the Dx?	In HCC, a Bx is not necessary to establish Dx if: 1. A liver lesion is >2 cm, has classic appearance by 1 imaging modality (CT, US, MRI, angiography), and is associated with AFP > 200 ng/mL 2. A liver lesion is 1–2 cm and has classic appearance by 2 imaging modalities *Note:* If a liver lesion is <1 cm, then the pt should be followed with serial imaging.
In what HCC variant is the AFP level often normal?	AFP levels are normal in the majority of pts with **fibro-lamellar carcinoma** (FLC, a variant of HCC. It is found commonly in females and has a good prognosis. Note that some authors argue that FLC is not truly a variant of HCC since it usually occurs in the absence of cirrhosis.

What are the characteristic triphasic CT and MRI findings of an HCC liver lesion?

On dynamic CT: early phase, tumor is seen as hyperintense b/c of increased vascularity. In the later phase, the tumor is hypodense.

On MRI T1-weighted images: low signal intensity and intermediate signal intensity on T2; HCC appears hypervascular, has increased T2 signal, and shows venous invasion

What is the AJCC 7th edition (2009) TNM staging for HCC?

Note: Bold text highlights 7th edition changes.

T1: solitary tumor without vascular invasion

T2: solitary tumor with vascular invasion or multiple tumors ≤5 cm

T3a: multiple tumors >5 cm

T3b: single tumor or multiple tumors of any size involving major branch of portal or hepatic veins

T4: tumor with direct invasion of adjacent organs other than gallbladder or with perforation of visceral peritoneum

N1: regional LN mets (hilar, hepatoduodenal ligament, **inf phrenic LN** [no longer classified as M1], and caval LNs)

M1: DMs

What are the AJCC 7th edition (2009) stage groupings for HCC?

Note: Bold text highlights 7th edition changes.

Stage I: T1N0

Stage II: T2N0

Stage IIIA: T3aN0

Stage IIIB: T3bN0

Stage IIIC: T4N0

Stage IVA: TXN1M0

Stage IVB: TXNXM1

Name 3 systems (other than AJCC) used to stage HCC internationally.

Staging systems for HCC commonly used outside the U.S.:

1. BCLC (Barcelona Clinic Liver Cancer)
2. CLIP (Cancer of the Liver Italian Program)
3. JIS score (Japanese Integrated Staging)

Applicability of each of these staging systems appears to depend on the Tx method.

What does a Child-Pugh score predict in pts with chronic liver Dz?

The Child-Pugh score was originally used to estimate operative mortality risk but is currently used to **assess OS prognosis** for pts with liver failure. Based on cumulative scores, pts are divided into class A, B, or C, with C being the poorest risk.

What are the 5 components of the Child-Pugh score in chronic liver Dz?

Components of the Child-Pugh score include **total bilirubin, serum albumin, INR, degree of ascites, and degree of hepatic encephalopathy.**

What does the acronym MELD represent, and what does the MELD score predict in chronic liver Dz?	MELD stands for **M**odel for **E**nd-**S**tage **L**iver **D**isease, initially developed to predict the 3-mo mortality after a transjugular intrahepatic portosystemic shunt (TIPS) procedure. Now it is **used to assess severity of chronic liver Dz and the 3-mo OS without a liver transplant.** The MELD score is highly correlated with the Child-Pugh score.
What are the 3 components of the MELD score in chronic liver Dz?	Components of the MELD score include **total bilirubin, INR, and Cr.**

■ Treatment/Prognosis

What 3 features of the HCC pt and the pt's tumors define the appropriate Tx paradigm?	The 3 features that define the Tx options for a pt with HCC are whether the pt (a) has metastatic Dz, (b) has resectable localized tumor, and (c) is medically fit for major surgery.
What are the only 2 curative Tx options for HCC?	The only 2 established curative Tx options for HCC are **partial hepatectomy to –margins and liver transplantation.** Potentially curative RT Tx with hypofractionated photons and proton therapy are being explored.
Partial hepatectomy is an option in which HCC pts?	Partial hepatectomy is a potentially curative option in HCC pts who are medically fit for surgery, have a solitary mass without major vascular involvement, are Childs-Pugh class A with mild or moderate portal hypertension, and have adequate future liver remnant (if no cirrhosis, require >20% of liver; if Childs A cirrhosis, require >30% of liver). Attempt at curative resection in HCC pts with multifocal tumors and major vascular invasion is controversial.
What % of HCC pts will have an LR after partial hepatectomy after 5 yrs?	~75% of pts with HCC will have an LR (new primary or local spread). (*Mathurin P et al., Aliment Pharmacal Ther 2003*)
In pts with localized resectable HCC, what adj Tx improves LC and survival after partial hepatectomy?	A study from China found that in pts with HCC s/p partial hepatectomy, **adj intra-arterial lipiodol I-131** improved LC and possibly OS (*Lau WY et al., Ann Surg 2008*). Confirmatory studies are under way.
What criteria are used to determine if liver transplant is an option for a pt with HCC?	The **United Network for Organ Sharing (UNOS) criteria** are used to determine if liver transplantation is appropriate in a pt with HCC. Per the UNOS criteria, transplantation is an option for medically fit pts with a **single tumor ≤5 cm** or **2–3 tumors ≤3 cm.**

What are the Tx options for an HCC pt with localized Dz who is medically unfit for major surgery?

Tx options for an HCC pt with localized Dz but who is unfit for major surgery:
1. Sorafenib for Child-Pugh A or B pt
2. Tumor ablation procedure (radio frequency, cryoablation, microwave, percutaneous alcohol injection)
3. Tumor embolization procedure (chemoembolization [aka trans-arterial chemoembolization (TACE)], bland embolization, radioembolization)
4. EBRT, including stereotactic body radiation therapy (SBRT) and proton therapy techniques

In the U.S., what isotope is most commonly used for radioembolization for HCC pts?

In the U.S., the most commonly used isotope for radioembolization in HCC pts is **yttrium-90,** a pure β-emitter.

What are the 2 forms of microspheres used for radioembolization in HCC pts, and what is the difference between them?

Microspheres used for radioembolization in HCC pts:
1. TheraSphere (glass microspheres)
2. SIR-Spheres (resin microspheres)

Estimate the response rate of HCC to yttrium-90–labeled microspheres.

The response rate of HCC to yttrium-90–labeled microspheres **varies from 50%–80%** depending on the definition of response used.

What are the EB Tx options with either medically inoperable or technically unresectable HCC?

A number of methods of externally irradiating pts with HCC have been explored:
1. Whole liver RT for palliation (21 Gy in 7 fx)
2. High-dose RT (>50 Gy) with standard fractionation
3. Hyperfractionated RT with chemosensitization
4. Hypofractionated stereotactic RT
5. Proton therapy

Currently, there is no standard EB technique for unresectable or medically inoperable HCC pts.

What are the Tx options for an HCC pt with metastatic Dz?

The only standard active Tx option for metastatic HCC is **sorafenib.** HCC typically does not respond to traditional cytotoxic chemo.

What is the MS in metastatic or inoperable HCC pts treated with sorafenib alone?

The MS of metastatic or inoperable HCC pts treated with sorafenib alone is **10.7 mos.** (*Llovet JM et al., NEJM 2008*)

What are the dose and results of SBRT for HCC?

In a phase I study for HCC and cholangiocarcinoma, 41 pts rcv 6 fx SBRT, with the dose delivered depending on the volume of liver irradiated based on the normal tissue complication probability model (24–54 Gy, median 36 Gy). No radiation-induced liver disease (RILD) or grade 4–5 toxicities were seen. Grade 3 liver enzymes were present in 12% of pts. (*Tse RV et al., JCO 2008*)

Another single institutional experience utilized 12.5 Gy × 3 (<4 cm and no cirrhosis) or 5 Gy × 5 or 10 Gy × 3 (≥4 cm with cirrhosis) with LC rates of 94% and 82% in 1 and 2 yrs, respectively. (*Mendez Romero A et al., Acta Oncol 2006*)

What is the role for proton beam in the management of unresectable HCC?

A Japanese prospective study enrolled 51 pts with tumors >2 cm from the porta hepatis and GI tract were treated with 66 cobalt Gray equivalents in 10 fx. LC was 94.5% at 3 yrs and 87.8% at 5 yrs. There were minor grade 1 acute adverse events, and only 3 pts were rated higher than grade 2. (*Fukumitsu N et al., IJROBP 2009*)

▪ Toxicity

What are the components of the clinical syndrome of RILD?

Signs and Sx of RILD include fatigue, RUQ pain, ascites, anicteric hepatomegaly, and elevated liver enzymes (especially alk phos that occurs 2 wks to 3 mos of the end of RT.

What is the histologic hallmark of RILD?

The pathologic hallmark of RILD is **veno-occlusive Dz with venous congestion of the central portion of the liver lobule.** Hepatocyte atrophy and fibrosis eventually develop.

What is the Emami RILD TD 5/5 for whole liver RT in 2 Gy/fx?

The Emami RILD TD 5/5 for whole liver RT in 2 Gy/fx is **30 Gy.**

What is the Emami RILD TD 50/5 for whole liver RT in 2 Gy/fx?

The Emami RILD TD 50/5 for whole liver RT in 2 Gy/fx is **42 Gy.**

What is the RILD TD 5/5 for whole liver RT in 6 fx?

The RILD TD 5/5 for whole liver RT in 6 fx is ~21 Gy.

What is the RILD TD 5/5 for RT to more than one third of the liver in 1.8 Gy/fx?

The RILD TD 5/5 for RT to more than one third of the liver in 1.8 Gy/fx is ~**68.4 Gy.**

50

Biliary Cancer

Robert C. Susil and Salma Jabbour

Background

What common condition is linked with increased risk for gallbladder cancer?

Cholelithiasis increases the risk for gallbladder cancer (presumably via chronic inflammation).

What 2 medical conditions are most associated with increased incidence of cholangiocarcinoma?

Pts with **primary sclerosing cholangitis or ulcerative colitis** have an increased incidence of cholangiocarcinoma.

What is the most common histology for gallbladder cancer?

Most gallbladder cancers are **adenocarcinomas.**

What pathologic subtype of gallbladder cancer and cholangiocarcinoma is associated with an improved prognosis?

Papillary adenocarcinoma is associated with an improved prognosis compared with other gallbladder adenocarcinomas and cholangiocarcinomas.

What % of gallbladder cancer presents with DM? What 2 sites are most common?

40%–50% of gallbladder cancer presents with DM. **Liver and peritoneal involvement** is most common.

What % of gallbladder cancer presents with LN mets? What 4 nodal regions are most commonly involved?

45% of gallbladder cancer presents with nodal mets. The **cystic, hilar, pericholedochal, and celiac nodes** are most commonly involved. Note that the cystic nodes drain to the pericholedocal nodes, which drain to the retropancreaticoduodenal nodes.

What subtype of adenocarcinoma is the most common form of cholangiocarcinoma?

Mucin-producing adenocarcinoma is the most common form of cholangiocarcinoma.

What is the most common route of spread for gallbladder cancer and cholangiocarcinoma?

Gallbladder cancer and cholangiocarcinoma most commonly spread by **direct extension** (to the liver for gallbladder cancer and along the biliary tree for cholangiocarcinoma).

What are the 3 subsites for cholangiocarcinoma?

Cholangiocarcinoma is divided into **intrahepatic, extrahepatic, and hilar** (i.e., Klatskin tumors) subsites.

321

What is the AJCC 7ᵗʰ edition (2009) T staging for distal bile duct cholangiocarcinoma?

Tis: CIS
T1: tumor confined to bile duct histologically
T2: tumor invades beyond bile duct wall
T3: tumor invades liver, gallbladder, pancreas, and/ or unilat branches of the portal vein (right or left) or hepatic vein (right or left)
T4: tumor invades celiac axis or superior mesenteric artery (SMA)

What is the AJCC 7ᵗʰ edition (2009) T staging for gallbladder cancer?

The gallbladder and cystic duct are included in this current classification:
Tis: CIS
T1: tumor invades lamina propria (T1a) or muscle layer (T1b)
T2: tumor invades perimuscular connective tissue but not into liver or beyond serosa
T3: tumor perforates serosa and/or directly invades liver and/or invades 1 adjacent organ/structure (stomach, duodenum, colon, pancreas, omentum, or extrahepatic bile ducts)
T4: tumor invades main portal vein, hepatic artery, or multiple extrahepatic organs/structures

What is the AJCC 7ᵗʰ edition (2009) N classification for biliary cancers (gallbladder and perihilar)?

Hilar LNs are distinguished separately from other regional LN mets:
N1 (mets to hilar nodes): nodes of cystic duct, CBD, hepatic artery, and/or portal vein
N2: (mets to regional nodes): periaortic, pericaval, SMA, and/or celiac LNs.

What are the AJCC 7ᵗʰ edition (2009) groupings for biliary cancers (gallbladder and perihilar)?

Stage 0: TisN0
Stage I: T1N0M0
Stage II: T2N0M0
Stage IIIA: T3N0M0
Stage IIIB: T1-3N1M0
Stage IVA: T4N0-1M0
Stage IVB: TXN2M0 or TXNXM1

What AJCC stage grouping do distal bile duct cancers have in common?

Pancreatic cancer, including N staging (N0 or N1), since it is managed with similar approaches.

■ Treatment/Prognosis

What % of gallbladder cancer pts have potentially resectable Dz at presentation?

Only **10%–30%** of gallbladder cancer pts have potentially resectable Dz at presentation.

Which gallbladder cancer pts do not require a 2ⁿᵈ surgery after adenocarcinoma is discovered following cholecystectomy for presumed benign Dz?

Following cholecystectomy for presumed benign Dz, **pts with ≤T1a** (not beyond the lamina propria) gallbladder cancer do not require a 2ⁿᵈ surgery.

What 2ⁿᵈ surgery should be performed after ≥T1b gallbladder adenocarcinoma is discovered on cholecystectomy for presumed benign Dz?

Following cholecystectomy for presumed benign Dz, pts with ≥T1b gallbladder cancer require **radical re-resection of the gallbladder bed (2-cm margins), regional nodal dissection, and resection of the port sites.**

What is the preferred surgical management for stage T3-T4 gallbladder adenocarcinoma?

Recommended surgical management for stage T3-T4 gallbladder adenocarcinoma includes **radical cholecystectomy and regional nodal dissection** (porta hepatis, gastrohepatic ligament, and retroduodenal nodes).

What is the preferred surgical management for resectable hilar cholangiocarcinoma? Distal cholangiocarcinoma?

Recommended surgical management for resectable hilar cholangiocarcinoma includes major bile duct resection, Roux-en-Y hepaticojejunostomy, and regional lymphadenectomy. Distal cholangiocarcinomas should be managed with pancreaticoduodenectomy and regional lymphadenectomy.

What is the recommended adj Tx for localized (but >T1a) gallbladder cancer?

Single-institution series suggest that **adj 5-FU–based CRT** may benefit resected gallbladder cancer pts. (*Kresl JJ et al., IJROBP 2002; Yu JB et al., JCO 2008; Gold DJ et al., IJROBP 2009*)

What is the recommended definitive Tx for localized, unresectable gallbladder cancer?

Although outcomes are generally very poor, **definitive 5-FU–based CRT** is an appropriate Tx for unresectable, localized gallbladder cancer. Chemo with 5-FU or gemcitabine is also an appropriate option.

What is the recommended adj Tx for localized, resectable cholangiocarcinoma? Localized, unresectable cholangiocarcinoma?

Single-institution series suggest that **5-FU–based CRT** is an appropriate adj Tx for localized resectable cholangiocarcinoma (*Hughes MA et al., IJROBP 2007; Nelson JW et al., IJROBP 2009; Shinohara T et al., IJROBP 2008*). This is also appropriate for unresectable cholangiocarcinoma (*Pitt HA et al., Ann Surg 1995*).

What are the appropriate targets and doses for adj gallbladder cancer or cholangiocarcinoma RT?

For resected gallbladder cancer or cholangiocarcinoma, **the resection bed and regional nodes** (porta hepatic, gastrohepatic ligament, retroduodenal, and celiac) should be included in the RT Tx volume. Doses from 45–50 Gy for subclinical Dz and 60–65 Gy for microscopic Dz are appropriate.

What 2 familial syndromes, other than FAP and HNPCC, have been associated with a higher risk for developing colon cancer?

Cowden syndrome and **Gardner syndrome** predispose pts to developing colon cancer (in addition to other cancers).

Is smoking a risk factor for colorectal cancer?

Yes. Smoking is a risk factor for colorectal cancer. (*Stürmer T et al., J Natl Cancer Inst 2000*)

Which supplements and which drug have shown promise as chemopreventative agents in colorectal cancer?

Calcium, vitamin D, and folic acid supplementation have shown some benefit in preventing colorectal cancer, while **aspirin** administration has been associated with a lower risk of developing colorectal polyps.

Initial mutation of what tumor suppressor gene leads to a greater chance for developing colorectal cancer? With what familial condition is this mutation associated?

Initial mutation in the **APC** tumor suppressor gene leads to a higher chance for developing colorectal cancer; this mutation is also associated with **FAP.**

Mutation of what oncogene leads to a greater chance for developing colorectal cancer?

Initial mutation in the **K-ras** oncogene leads to a higher chance for developing colorectal cancer.

Most familial HNPCC cases have been associated with mutations in what genes? What do these genes regulate?

Most familial cases identified as HNPCC have been associated with mutations in the **hMLH1 or hMSH2** genes, which **regulate mismatch repair.**

Pts with what chronic inflammatory condition are at an ~20-fold increased risk for developing colorectal cancer?

Pts with **ulcerative colitis** are at an ~20-fold increased risk for developing colorectal cancer.

■ Workup/Staging

What is the most common presenting Sx in rectal cancer?

Hematochezia is the most common presenting Sx in rectal cancer.

What must the physical exam include for pts with suspected rectal cancer?

The physical must include DRE (pelvic exam for women) for presumed rectal cancer pts.

How is the Dx of rectal cancer typically established?

Endoscopic Bx is a typical way of establishing the Dx. A full colonoscopy should be performed to r/o more proximal lesions.

What studies are performed in the workup of rectal cancer pts, and what is the purpose of each modality?

For staging purposes, EUS must be performed in rectal cancer pts. **To r/o metastatic Dz, CT C/A/P is** performed.

What labs are collected as part of the staging workup for colorectal cancers?

Labs for the workup of colorectal cancer: **CBC, Chem 7, LFTs, CEA**

Is a PET scan routinely indicated for pts with rectal cancer?

No. A PET scan is not routinely indicated in pts with localized rectal cancer.

What is the AJCC 7th edition (2009) T staging for colorectal cancer?

The T staging for rectal cancer is based on the DOI:
Tis: CIS or invasion into lamina propria
T1: invades submucosa
T2: invades muscularis propria
T3: invades through muscularis and into pericolorectal tissues
T4a: penetrates surface of visceral peritoneum
T4b: invades or adheres to adjacent organs

What is the AJCC 7th edition (2009) N staging for colorectal cancer?

In the 2002 edition of AJCC, N1 designated involvement of 1–3 regional LNs, whereas N2 designated involvement of ≥4 LNs.

In the **AJCC 7th edition,** N1 and N2 are further broken down:
N1a: mets to 1 regional LN
N1b: mets to 2–3 regional LNs
N1c: tumor deposits in subserosa, mesentery, or nonperitonealized pericolic or perirectal tissues *without* regional LN mets
N2a: mets to 4–6 LNs
N2b: mets to ≥7 LNs

What is the AJCC 7th edition (2009) breakdown of M staging for colorectal cancer?

M1a: DMs to a single organ or site (e.g., liver, lung, ovary, nonregional LNs)
M1b: mets >1 organ/site or deposits in peritoneum

What are the AJCC 7th edition (2009) TNM stage groupings for colorectal cancer?

Stage I: T1-2N0
Stage IIA: T3N0
Stage IIB: T4aN0
Stage IIC: T4bN0
Stage IIIA: T1-2N1 or N1c; T1N2a
Stage IIIB: T3-4aN1 or N1c; T2-3N2a; T1-2N2b
Stage IIIC: T4aN2a; T3-4aN2b; T4bN1-2
Stage IVA: TXNXM1a
Stage IVB: TXNXM1b

What surgical approach for rectal cancer is preferred for sphincter preservation?

LAR spares the sphincter and is therefore a preferred surgical option (if feasible) for rectal cancer pts; in contrast, APR requires a colostomy.

What is the pattern of failure for rectal cancer historically after surgery alone?

For rectal cancer, the pattern of failure after surgery is primarily **locoregional.**

What is the approximate LR rate for T3-T4 or N1 rectal cancer after surgery alone?

The historic LR rate for T3-T4 or N1 rectal cancer is ~**25%.** This is improved with better surgery (i.e., total mesorectal excision [TME], LR 11% [Dutch TME study]).

What is the significance of a positive circumferential margin at the time of surgery for rectal cancer?

A positive circumferential margin predicts for inferior LC, DM, and OS rates after surgery for rectal cancer based on meta-analysis. (*Nagtegaal ID et al., JCO 2008*)

What kind of surgical technique is currently standard in the surgical management of rectal cancer? Why is this important?

TME is a standard surgical technique in the operative management of rectal cancer, as it **helps reduce the rate of positive radial margins and improves LC.**

What are the indications for adj CRT after definitive resection for rectal cancer?

After a definitive resection for rectal cancer, CRT is indicated **if the pathology is node+ or ≥T2.**

What are some options for rectal cancer pts with solitary or oligometastatic Dz to the liver that is resectable?

Surgical resection of the metastatic site is the only modality with proven survival benefit. How these cases should be managed needs to be determined on a case-by-case basis in a multidisciplinary setting. Some options for metastatic (resectable) rectal cancer include:

1. Induction chemo → restaging → resection of the mets → CRT to primary → LAR if possible +/− additional chemo
2. If the pt is symptomatic, consider preop CRT or short-course RT (5 Gy × 5) as done in Europe → surgery of both primary and metastatic site → adj chemo (FOLFOX/Avastin)

What % of rectal cancer pts are technically resectable at presentation?

80% of rectal cancer pts are technically resectable at presentation.

What is the chemo of choice for rectal cancer with RT? How is it given?

5-FU (**225 mg/m^2**) is given concurrently with RT via **continuous infusion** (CI), as the **NCCTG 86-47-51/ Intergroup trial** (*O'Connell MJ et al., NEJM 1994*) showed improved 4-yr OS when compared to bolus administration in the adj CRT setting (70% vs. 60%).

What is the data addressing adj RT alone in rectal cancer, and what does it show?

There are many RCTs (e.g., **MRC 3, NSABP R-01**) that investigated adj RT alone, showing **improvement in LC only** but **no** improvement in OS, DFS, or MFS); this was confirmed by a CCCG meta-analysis (*CCCG, Lancet 2001*).

What major studies established a role for adj CRT in rectal cancer?

GITSG 7175 (*GITSG collaborators, NEJM 1985; Thomas PR et al., Radiother Oncol 1988*) randomized pts after surgery to observation, chemo alone, RT alone, or CRT and found that adj CRT in rectal cancer significantly improved OS (45% vs. 27% at 10 yrs) and LF rates (10% vs. 25%) when compared to surgery alone.

Intergroup/NCCTG 79-47-51 (*Krook JE et al., NEJM 1991*) randomized stage II–III rectal cancer pts to RT alone or CRT (5-FU × 2 > 5-FU + RT > 5-FU × 2) after surgery (50% APR). 5-yr LR, DM, and OS were better for CRT (LR: 14% vs. 25%; DM: 29% vs. 46%; OS: 55% vs. 45%). There was worse acute grade 3–4 diarrhea (20% vs. 5%) but no late complications for the CRT arm.

What are some major criticisms of the rectal cancer trial GITSG 7175?

GITSG 7175 is criticized b/c it was underpowered, 5-FU was given by bolus with semustine (which causes leukemias), randomization was unequal, and there was no intention-to-treat analysis.

Which studies demonstrated that semustine is not a necessary component of CRT in rectal cancer?

GITSG 7180 and **NCCTG 86-47-51** demonstrated that semustine is not a necessary component of CRT in rectal cancer.

Which study compared preop RT to postop RT (without chemo) in rectal cancer?

The **Swedish Uppsala trial** (*Frykholm GJ et al., Dis Colon Rectum 1993*) compared adj to neoadj RT in rectal cancer and found no OS benefit but improved LR rates (13% vs. 22%) and lower SBO rates (5% vs. 11%) with preop RT.

Which study compared surgery alone to preop RT in rectal cancer? What did it find, and what were its limitations?

The **Swedish Rectal Cancer trial** (*NEJM 1997*) compared neoadj RT (25 Gy in 5 fx) to surgery alone in rectal cancer and found a significant **improvement in OS** (38% vs. 30%) and LR (9% vs. 26%) at 13 yrs with neoadj RT. The trial is often criticized b/c TME was not used and there was a high recurrence rate for the surgery alone arm (26%).

Can the use of TME obviate the need for neoadj RT for rectal cancer?

No. TME does not offset the benefit of neoadj RT based on the Dutch TME study (*Peeters KC et al., Ann Surg 2007*). The study compared TME alone to neoadj RT and TME and found no OS benefit, but there was an improved LR rate (6% vs. 11%) with the addition of neoadj RT.

What was the RT dose/ fractionation scheme in the Dutch and Swedish rectal cancer studies? How long after the completion of RT do pts go to surgery?

Both the Dutch and Swedish rectal cancer studies used neoadj RT in **25 Gy in 5 fx** (5 Gy × 5). Pts typically underwent surgical resection **within 1 wk** of RT completion.

What were the arms in the MRC CR07/NCIC C016 rectal cancer study, and what were its main findings?

The **MRC CR07/NCIC C016** rectal cancer study (*Sebag-Montefiore D et al., Lancet 2009*) randomized pts to preop RT (25 Gy in 5 fx) vs. selective postop CRT (45 Gy in 25 fx) and found better outcomes with preop RT in terms of LR (4% vs. 11%, SS) and DFS (77% vs. 71%, SS). OS was similar at 4-yr follow-up. A short neoadj RT course is an acceptable option.

Which major European rectal cancer study compared neoadj CRT to adj CRT, and what were its findings?

The **German Rectal Cancer trial** (*Sauer R et al., NEJM 2004*) compared preop to postop CRT in T3-T4 or node+ rectal cancer (RT was to 50.4 Gy for the neoadj arm and 55.8 Gy for the postop arm with 5-FU chemo (CI 5-FU days 1–5 at 1,000 mg/day, wks 1 and 5). All pts rcv 4 additional cycles of bolus 5-FU (500 mg/m^2/day, days 1–5, q4wks) at 4 wks after completion of initial therapy. The study found a similar 5-yr OS and DFS between the 2 arms but better LR rates (6% vs. 13%), fewer acute (27% vs. 40%) and late toxicities (14% vs. 24%), and better sphincter-preservation rates (39% vs. 19%) in the preop CRT arm. Most of the acute and late toxicities were especially due to acute/chronic diarrhea and anastomatic stricture.

What is the pathologic CR rate for preop CRT for rectal cancer?

According to the German Rectal Cancer trial, the **pCR rate is 8%.**

What % of pts receiving neoadj CRT will be overtreated b/c of having stage I Dz instead of the presumed more advanced Dz?

~**18%** of pts will be overtreated with neoadj CRT b/c of an apparent stage I Dz. This is based on the results of the postop arm of the German Rectal Cancer trial, where 18% of the pts did not rcv postop CRT b/c of T1-T2 N0 Dz found at resection. All of these pts were thought to have T3-T4 or node+ Dz based on EUS.

What was a major criticism of the German Rectal Cancer trial (*Sauer R et al., NEJM 2004*)?

A major criticism of the German Rectal Cancer trial (*Sauer R et al., NEJM 2004*) was that **only 54% of adj pts rcv a full RT dose** (vs. 92% in the neoadj arm).

Did pts in the German Rectal Cancer trial have TME as part of their surgery?

Yes. All pts in the German Rectal Cancer trial (*Sauer R et al., NEJM 2004*) had TME at the time of surgery.

What was the sphincter-preservation rate in the neoadj CRT arm in the German Rectal Cancer trial (*Sauer R et al., NEJM 2004*)?

The sphincter-preservation rate in the neoadj CRT arm in the German Rectal Cancer trial (*Sauer R et al., NEJM 2004*) was **39% at 5 yrs** (compared to 19% in the postop CRT arm).

How long after neoadj CRT should surgery be performed for rectal cancer? Why is this done?

Surgery should be performed ~**6–8 wks** after neoadj CRT for rectal cancer to allow for adequate **down-staging.**

How long after surgery should adj CRT be initiated for rectal cancer?

Adj CRT for rectal cancer should begin **4–6 wks** after surgery.

What did all pts in the German Rectal Cancer trial (*Sauer R et al., NEJM 2004*) rcv after either surgery (neoadj CRT arm) or CRT (adj arm)?

All pts in the German Rectal Cancer trial (*Sauer R et al., NEJM 2004*) rcv 4–5 cycles of **bolus 5-FU** (500 mg/m²/day, days 1–5, q4wks) 4 wks after either surgery (neoadj CRT arm) or CRT (adj arm).

Which 2 major randomized studies compared neoadj RT to neoadj CRT in rectal cancer, and what did they find? How was CRT delivered in both studies? What was a major limitation of these trials?

The **French FFCD 9203** (*Gerard JP et al., JCO 2006*) and **EORTC 22921** (*Bosset JF et al., NEJM 2006*) compared neoadj RT to neoadj CRT in rectal cancer. The French study found no OS difference but did find improved LR with neoadj CRT at 5 yrs (8% vs. 16%, SS). The EORTC study also found no OS difference and improved LR with neoadj CRT at 5 yrs (9% vs. 17%). Grade 3–4 acute toxicity was higher in the CRT vs. RT arms. Both trials used neoadj CRT with 45 Gy (1.8) and 5-FU (350 mg/m²/day, wks 1 and 5 of RT). A small % of pts actually rcv adj CT (EORTC: 43%).

How should rectal cancer pts be simulated in preparation for RT?

Rectal cancer pts should undergo CT simulation **in the prone position, on a belly board, and with a full bladder** (with optional placement of anal/vaginal markers and/or rectal contrast).

What structures should be encompassed within the RT field for rectal cancer?

For rectal cancer, the **tumor bed** (+2–5-cm margin) and **presacral/internal iliac nodes** should be included in the RT fields.

What additional nodal chain needs to be covered in the RT fields with T4 rectal cancer?

The **external iliac nodes** need to be encompassed for T4 rectal lesions (invasion of bladder, vagina, uterus, but may not be necessary for bony sacrum invasion).

What RT fields are generally employed for rectal cancer?

Whole pelvis fields (3 fields) with a PA field and 2 opposed lat fields are typically employed for rectal cancer.

What are the RT doses for rectal cancer?

RT doses for rectal cancer:
Neoadj/postop: initial whole pelvis (3 field) to 45 Gy in 1.8 Gy/fx; CD to tumor bed +2–3 cm (opposed lats only, or 3D-CRT) to **50.4 Gy (preop)** (or **55.8 Gy (postop)** if the small bowel is out of the way)
Definitive/unresectable: initial to 45 Gy, CD1 to 50.4 Gy; consider CD2 with conformal RT to **54–59.4 Gy** (if dose to the small bowel is limited)

Describe the anatomic boundaries of the RT fields for rectal cancer.

Anatomic boundaries for the RT fields in rectal cancer:
Posterior-Anterior: sup at L5-S1, inf at bottom of ischial tuberosity or 3 cm below tumor volume, lat at 1.5 cm from pelvic inlet
Laterals: 1 cm post behind entire bony sacrum, ant behind pubic symphisis for T3 (in front if T4), sup-inf same as PA; blocks applied to spare small bowel

Which border is not altered for the CD fields in the Tx of rectal cancer?

The **post border on the lat fields** usually stays the same (behind the bony sacrum) for the CD portion of the RT for rectal cancer given the high rate of LR in this region.

When is IORT indicated for rectal cancer, and what is the dose?

IORT should be considered in rectal cancer for **close/+ margins or as an additional boost**, especially with T4 tumors or with recurrent tumors. The typical dose is **10–15 Gy** to the 90% IDL.

What study showed a benefit with IORT in colorectal cancer?

A retrospective study from Mayo by *Gunderson et al.* evaluated IORT in addition to EBRT and found improved OS and LR rates with addition of IORT (10–20 Gy) when compared to historical controls. (*IJROBP 1997*)

When can RT be considered in colon cancer? When is it given in relation to surgery and to what dose?

RT can be considered **for fixed T4 colon cancer lesions or with a close/+ margin.** RT is typically **given after resection/debulking to a dose of 45–50.4 Gy.**

What major study investigated the role of adj RT in colon cancer? What did it find? What was the limitation of this study?

The **Intergroup 0130** study (*Martenson JA Jr et al., JCO 2004*) compared adj chemo to adj CRT in colon cancer and found no difference in OS or LC with addition of RT. This study was underpowered to show a difference between groups.

Which randomized study investigated the role of elective para-aortic (P-A) RT in rectal cancer? What did it conclude?

The **EORTC trial by** Bosset et al. evaluated the role of elective P-A RT in rectal cancer (25 Gy to LNs and liver) and found no benefit in terms of OS, DFS, or LC. (*Radiother Oncol 2001*)

Which ongoing RCT is comparing neoadj oxaliplatin/Xeloda to 5-FU/oxaliplatin and Xeloda to CI 5-FU with RT in rectal cancer?

NSABP R04 is enrolling pts with localized rectal cancer to neoadj RT with CI 5-FU vs. Xeloda with a 2nd randomization to include or not include oxaliplatin concurrent with 5-FU and RT. All pts are encouraged to rcv adj chemo.

What is the Tx paradigm for small bowel cancer, and what is the role of adj chemo and/or RT?

Small bowel cancer Tx paradigm: resection → 5-FU–based chemo. CRT is considered in cases of close/+ margins, but retrospective studies have found no convincing benefit (e.g., *Kelsey CR et al., IJROBP 2007*).

Why did NSABP R-03 (*Roh MS et al., JCO 2009*) close prematurely, and what were its findings?

NSABP R-03 closed prematurely b/c of poor accrual. It randomized T3-T4 or node+ rectal cancer pts to neoadj CRT vs. postop CRT (5-FU based). There was improved 5-yr DFS (65% vs. 53%, SS) with neoadj CRT but no difference in LR or OS. The pCR rate was 15%.

■ Toxicity

How does the toxicity of CI 5-FU differ from that of bolus administration?

Bolus administration of **5-FU confers greater hematologic toxicity,** whereas **CI confers greater GI toxicity.** (*Smalley SR et al., JCO 2006*)

What was a major late complication of neoadj RT in the Swedish Rectal Cancer trial?

SBO was more likely in the neoadj RT arm in the Swedish Rectal Cancer trial (RR 2.5) (*Birgisson H et al., Br J Surg 2008*), maybe a limitation of a hypofractionated regimen (5 Gy × 5).

What 3 toxicities were worse with neoadj RT in the Swedish Rectal Cancer trial?

Median bowel movement frequency (20 movements/ wk vs. 10 movements/wk, SS), fecal incontinence (62% vs. 27%, SS), and impaired social life (30% vs. 10%, SS) were worse in the neoadj RT arm when compared to surgery alone in the Swedish Rectal Cancer trial.

What should the small bowel RT dose be limited to in rectal cancer?

The small bowel dose should be limited to **45 Gy** in the Tx of rectal cancer.

In anal cancers, what are the most important prognostic factors for LC and survival?	**Tumor size and DOI** predict for LC. The **extent of inguinal or pelvic LN involvement** predicts for survival.

■ Workup/Staging

What are 4 common presenting Sx in anal cancer?	Bleeding, pain/sensation of mass, rectal urgency, and pruritus
What does the workup for anal cancer pts include?	Anal cancer workup: H&P (including gyn exam for women with cervical cancer screening), labs (HIV if risk factors), imaging, Bx of lesion, and FNA of suspicous LN
What imaging studies are typically done for anal cancer pts?	Transanal US (to assess for perirectal nodes/assess invasion), CXR or CT chest, CT abdomen/pelvis, and PET/CT
What features of anal lesions need to be appreciated on physical exam? Why?	The **degree of circumferential involvement and anal sphincter tone** should be appreciated, as these **may dictate Tx.**
What is the approach to suspicious inguinal LNs in anal cancer pts?	**FNA Bx** should be performed for suspicious inguinal LNs.
On what is the T staging for anal cancer based? Define T1-T4.	T staging for anal cancer is based on the **size of the lesion.** **T1:** ≤2 cm **T2:** >2–5 cm **T3:** >5 cm **T4:** invasion of adjacent organs (vagina, urethra, bladder)
Does tumor invasion of sphincter muscle by anal cancer constitute a T4 lesion?	**No.** Direct invasion of the rectal wall, perirectal skin, subcutaneous tissue, or sphincter muscle are *not* classified as T4.
Most pts with anal cancer present with what T stage?	Most anal cancer pts present at stage **T2 or T3.**
What is the N staging of isolated perirectal nodal involvement in anal cancer?	Isolated perirectal nodal involvement is staged as **N1.**
What is the N staging of unilat inguinal or internal iliac LNs in anal cancer?	Unilat inguinal or internal iliac LNs are staged as **N2.**

What N stage is an anal cancer pt with both perirectal and inguinal LNs?	Perirectal and inguinal LNs reflect stage **N3.**
What N stage is an anal cancer pt with bilat inguinal or internal iliac LNs?	Bilat inguinal or internal iliac LNs reflect stage **N3.**
What anal cancer pts have AJCC stage III Dz?	**Node+ or T4 pts** have AJCC stage III Dz.
What is the AJCC 7th edition (2009) stage grouping for anal cancer?	**Stage I:** T1N0 **Stage II:** T2N0 or T3N0 **Stage IIIA:** T1-3N1 or T4N0 **Stage IIIB:** T4N1 or TXN2 or N3 **Stage IV:** TXNXM1
What are the 5-yr OS and LR rates after surgical resection alone for anal cancer?	The 5-yr OS rate after complete surgical resection is ~**70%,** and the LR rate is ~**40%.** (Mayo review of 118 pts: *Boman BM et al., Cancer 1984*)
What % of pts who relapse develop local recurrent Dz as part of the total failure pattern?	~80% develop local recurrent Dz. (*Boman BM et al., Cancer 1984. Note:* This was also a surgical series.)
What are the OS and sphincter preservation rates for all-comers with anal cancer at 5 yrs after definitive CRT?	**OS is ~70%** (**RTOG 9811**) and **sphincter preservation rate is 65%–75%** after CRT alone.

■ Treatment/Prognosis

What are the criteria for local excision alone in anal cancer? What are the LC rates in such carefully selected pts?	Small T1 lesion (<2 cm), well differentiated, −margins, <40% circumferential involvement, no sphincter involvement, compliant pts. For these well selected pts, there is >**90% LC.** (*Boman BM et al., Cancer 1984*)
Can radiotherapy alone be employed for early-stage anal cancer?	**Yes.** However, it can be employed only for **T1N0** lesions. There were excellent LC rates of 100% and CR rates of 96% in 1 series (*Deniaud-Alexandre E et al., IJROBP 2003*).
What was the standard surgical procedure for anal cancer before the advent of CRT? What was the disadvantage of this approach?	**Abdominoperineal resection** (APR) is the standard surgical procedure, but the disadvantage is that it **requires permanent colostomy.**

Can MMC be removed from the standard regimen of 5-FU/MMC for the Tx of anal cancer? What major study addressed this question?

No. MMC cannot be deleted from the standard regimen.

RTOG 87-04 (*Flam M et al., JCO 1996*): 291 pts, MMC/5-FU + RT vs. 5-FU + RT. RT was 45–50.4 Gy. There was no difference in OS (76% vs. 67%, $p = 0.31$), but MMC improved the CR rate (92% vs. 22%) and colostomy rate (9% vs. 22%) at 4 yrs. Grade 4 or 5 heme toxicity was worse (26% vs. 7%).

Can cisplatin be substituted for MMC in the Tx of anal cancer? What 2 major studies addressed this question?

This is **controversial.** 2 randomized studies are conflicting on the possibility of cisplatin substituting for MMC.

RTOG 98-11 (*Ajani JA et al., JAMA 2008*): 644 pts, all stages except T1 or M1; excluded AIDS or prior cancers; randomized to standard therapy vs. 2 cycles of cisplatin/5-FU → cisplatin/5-FU × 2 with RT. RT was 45 Gy to the pelvis, with boost for T2 residual to 10–14 Gy. Only the **5-yr colostomyfree survival rate was better in the standard arm** compared to the cisplatin/5-FU arm, but not in DFS, LR/DM, or OS. 5-yr colostomyfree rate: 10% vs. 19%, $p = 0.02$; 5-yr DFS: 60% vs. 54%, $p = 0.17$; LRF (HR 1.32 with cisplatin, $p = 0.07$), DM (HR 1.38 with cisplatin, $p = 0.14$), 5-yr OS: 75% vs. 70%, $p = 0.1$. Acute grade 3 or 4 severe heme toxicity was worse in the MMC arm (61% vs. 42%, $p < 0.001$) but not in long-term toxicities (11% vs. 10%). *Major criticism:* Neoadj chemo on the experimental arm may have confounded the results.

ACTII (*James R et al., ASCO 2009*): 2 × 2 design, 940 pts (T1-T2 [50%], T3-T4 (43%), 30% N+, 85% anal canal, 15% anal margin) treated with 5-FU (1,000 mg/m^2/day, days 1–4, days 29–32) and RT (50.4 Gy) and randomized to concurrent MMC (12 mg/m^2, day 1) or CDDP (60 mg/m^2, days 1 and 29). 2nd randomization involved adding maintenance therapy (4 wks after CRT) to 2 cycles 5-FU/CDDP or no maintenance. Median follow-up was 3 yrs. *Results:* No difference in CR rate (94% vs. 95%) and # of colostomies (18 vs. 14), and no difference in RFS or OS with maintenance therapy. MMC had more acute grade 3–4 heme toxicities (25% vs. 13%, $p < 0.001$) but no worse sepsis or non-heme toxicities.

When is neoadj chemo an option for anal cancer?

For advanced T3-T4 lesions and/or bulky N2 or N3, especially if an abscess or fistula. Induction cisplatin or cisplatin/5-FU × 2 per **CALGB 9281** → definitive CRT (*Meropol NJ et al., JCO 2008*) can be used. This phase II study demonstrated an 82% CR rate, with a 4-yr OS of 68% and 50% colostomyfree survival in these poor-risk pts.

What is the role of brachytherapy in anal cancer?

Brachytherapy is **generally not done** in the U.S. due to poor LC (<30% for large lesions) and higher complication rates. An older French experience showed favorable results with combined interstitial (Ir-192) and EB RT (*Papillon J & Montbarbon JF, Dis Colon Rectum 1987*).

What is the recurrence rate after definitive CRT for anal cancer, and what are the salvage rates at 5 yrs?

The recurrence rate is **30%,** and the salvage rates at 5 yrs are **40%–60%.**

Describe the RTOG AP/PA technique for anal cancer and the corresponding doses.

The initial AP/PA from L5-S1 is 30.6 Gy (at 1.8 Gy/fx), then reduced AP/PA from the bottom of the sacroiliac joints (and off inguinals after 36 Gy if node–) to 45 Gy, then conformal CD to tumor + 2–2.5-cm margin (and electron boost if node+) to 55–59.4 Gy. The dose to the inguinals is supplemented by bilat electron fields that make up for lack of dose contribution from the PA field to the appropriate doses (to 36 Gy or to the final boost volume for node+ Dz).

How is the anal cancer pt simulated for the AP/PA RTOG technique?

Pt is simulated supine with full bladder and oral contrast and with hips in frog-leg position immobilized with vac-lock cradle, with placement of rectal tube, anal BB, and bolus over inguinal nodes.

How is the AP field different from the PA field for the AP/PA RTOG technique in anal cancer?

The AP field is wider (to the edge of the greater trochanter) than the PA field. As well, the PA field is typically of lower energy (6 MV) than the AP field (18 MV). This technique spares the dose to the femoral head and neck.

Per RTOG 98-11, which anal cancer pts need to receive a boost beyond 45 Gy?

Pts with **T3, T4, or node+ lesions or T2 lesions with residual Dz after 45 Gy** need a boost >45 Gy.

What is the dose per fx for anal cancer per RTOG 98-11?

Per **RTOG 98-11**, the dose per fx for anal cancer is **1.8 Gy/fx to 45 Gy initially, then 2 Gy/fx to 55–59 Gy total for the CD portion**.

What is the min Rx depth for adequate inguinal node coverage in anal cancer?

The min Rx depth is **3 cm.**

How far caudally should inguinal nodes be covered in anal cancer?

Inguinal nodes should be covered to the **inf border of the lesser trochanter.**

What is the MDACC technique for the Tx of anal cancer?

Field setup is similar as in the RTOG technique for the 1st 30.6 Gy. After this dose, the pt is placed prone on a belly board and a 3-field technique is employed, with portal weighted 2 (PA): 1 (right lat): 1 (left lat), energy is 15–18 MV, prescribed to 95% IDL, with the sup border reduced to bottom of the sacroiliac joint. This 3-field plan treats the mini-pelvis to 50.4 Gy. A boost is given to the primary and involved nodes to 55 Gy. The contribution to the inguinals from the 3-field approach is 5–7 Gy. Daily electron boost supplements the needed dose for the involved inguinal area.

What are some of the challenges in HIV+ pts?

Challenges for HIV+ pts include lower LC (by one half) and more side effects (2 times) when compared to HIV– pts. OS is similar, though (*Oehler-Janne C et al., JCO 2005*). Consider substituting MMC for cisplatin/5-FU–based CRT.

What is the role/evidence for IMRT in anal cancer?

Few retrospective studies have shown decreased toxicity and comparable efficacy (French experience: *Menkarios C et al., Radiat Oncol 2007*; University of Chicago experience: *Milano MT et al., IJROBP 2000*). This is being prospectively tested in a phase II evaluation through RTOG 0529 using dose-painting techniques. Early results in 51 pts demonstrate significantly better grade 2–3 GI/GU, and skin toxicities compared to RTOG 98-11, with promising clinical response rates (*Kachnic LA et al., ASCO-GI 2010*)

◼ Toxicity

What RT dose should the bowel be kept under in anal cancer pts?

The bowel should be kept to a dose **<45–50.4 Gy.**

What is the main toxicity of MMC?

MMC has **acute hematologic toxicities** but does not contribute to late toxicities.

Most anal cancer recurrences are within what time frame?

Most anal cancers recur within **2 yrs.**

According to the NCCN, what is the post-Tx follow-up for anal cancer?

Post-Tx anal cancer follow-up: Evaluate in 8–12 wks after Tx with DRE. Bx only if there is suspicious persistent Dz, progressive Dz, or new Sx (e.g., pain, bleeding). If there is complete remission, perform exam q3–6mos for 5 yrs with nodal evaluation, DRE, and anoscopy. Perform pelvic CT annually × 3 yrs (optional if T3-T4 or node+ Dz).

What is the mean time to tumor regression after CRT?

The mean time to tumor regression after CRT is **3 mos (but can be up to 12 mos);** therefore, there is no benefit to routine post-Tx Bx. (*Cummings BJ et al., IJROBP 1991*)

If a pt has Bx-proven persistent Dz 3 mos after completing Tx, should the pt be referred immediately for salvage surgery?

No. According to the NCCN (*2010*), the pt can be re-evaluated again in 4 wks. If there is still no regression, or if there is progression, Bx again and restage if necessary. However, if there is evidence of regression, then continue observation and evaluation in 3 mos.

53

Low-Risk Prostate Cancer

Russell K. Hales and Justin E. Bekelman

Background

What is the annual incidence and mortality of prostate cancer in the U.S.?

~**230,000 Dx** of and ~**27,000 deaths** from prostate cancer annually in the U.S.

1 in how many American men will develop prostate cancer during his lifetime?

~**1 in 6** American men will be diagnosed with prostate cancer during his lifetime.

What are the 4 zones of the prostate?

Zones of the prostate:
1. Peripheral zone
2. Central zone
3. Transitional zone
4. Anterior fibromuscular stroma

Prostate cancers develop most commonly in which zone?

Two thirds of prostate cancers arise in the **peripheral zone.**

Benign prostatic hypertrophy (BPH) develops in which zone?

BPH develops in the **transitional zone.**

What is median lobe hypertrophy?

Median lobe hypertrophy refers to a characteristic transitional zone hypertrophy (BPH) that mushrooms superiorly into the rest of the prostate and bladder. The term does not refer to enlargement of the central zone, which is typically small and compressed in older men.

What is the name for the nerves responsible for penile erections, and where are these nerves located with respect to the prostate?

The **neurovascular bundles** are paired nerves **located along the posterolat edge of the prostate** and are responsible for penile erection.

Name the 3 histologic cell types seen in the normal prostate.

Histologic cell types seen in the normal prostate:
1. Secretory cells (produce PSA and involute with hormonal deprivation)
2. Basal cells (flattened basement membrane where stem cells that repopulate the secretory layers reside)
3. Neuroendocrine cells

Describe the Gleason score and what it represents.

The Gleason score is a grade assigned to prostate cancer specimens that reflects the degree of aggressiveness based on the tumor's resemblance to normal glandular tissue. A primary (or predominant) pattern is recorded followed by a secondary or lesser pattern. The Gleason score is the sum of the primary and secondary pattern values and can be between 2 and 10.

Grade 1: small, well-formed glands, closely packed
Grade 2: well-formed glands, but more tissue between them
Grade 3: darker cells, some of which have left the gland and are invading the surrounding tissue
Grade 4: few recognizable glands with many cells invading the surrounding tissue
Grade 5: no recognizable glands; sheets of cells throughout the surrounding tissue

How often is higher-grade Dz diagnosed in a radical prostatectomy specimen (upstaging) than that seen in Bx specimens?

One third of cases are higher grade in post-prostatectomy specimens than that diagnosed in Bx specimens.

What racial groups are associated with the highest and lowest risks for prostate cancer?

Black men are at highest risk for the development of prostate cancer (and their Dz presents more aggressively [higher Gleason score, more advanced stage]). **Asians are at the lowest risk** for the development of prostate cancer. A 30- to 50-fold difference in the incidence of the Dz is observed between native Asians and black men (*Ross R et al., Cancer 1995*).

Describe 5 clinical factors associated with the Dx of prostate cancer.

Clinical factors associated with the Dx of prostate cancer:
1. Advanced age
2. African American race
3. Past prostate Bx showing prostatic intraepithelial neoplasia (PIN; especially high-grade PIN)
4. Obesity
5. High dietary intake of fats

In a recent European-based study, PSA screening has shown what in terms of prostate cancer Dx and deaths?

In a randomized European study comparing PSA screening to no screening, 182,000 men were enrolled. With a median follow-up of 8 yrs, the cumulative incidence of prostate cancer was 8.2% in the screened group and 4.8% in the control group. The rate ratio for death from prostate cancer in the screening group vs. control group was 0.8 ($p = 0.04$). **1,410 men need to be screened and 48 prostate cancers need to be treated to prevent 1 death from prostate cancer.** (*Schroder FH et al., NEJM 2009*)

Annual DRE and PSA screening in the American population has shown what in terms of prostate cancer Dx and deaths?

In phase III of the U.S. Prostate, Lung, Colorectal, and Ovarian Cancer screening trial (PLCO), ~76,700 men were screened with annual PSA and DRE. After 7 yrs of follow-up, the incidence of prostate cancer was higher in the screened group (116 cases/10,000 person-yrs vs. 95 cases/10,000 person-yrs). The incidence of death was similar between the groups (screened: 2 cases/10,000 person-yrs vs. 1.7 cases/10,000 person-yrs). (*Andriole GL et al., NEJM 2009*)

What are some of the critiques of the PLCO screening trial for prostate cancer?

Critiques of the PLCO screening trial for prostate cancer:
1. 40%–52% of the control group were screened with PSA testing and 41%–46% of the control group were screened with DRE.
2. As of 2009 publication, the study only had a median follow-up of 7 yrs and the complementary European study did not show a divergence in the survival curves until after 7 yrs. (*Andriole GL et al., NEJM 2009*)

What is the most common presentation of prostate cancer?

In the PSA era, most pts present with an **abnl PSA and no associated Sx.**

In men with symptomatic prostate cancer, what local Sx may arise at Dx?

Local Sx that may arise at Dx in men with prostate cancer Sx:
1. Lower tract Sx such as urgency, frequency, nocturia, dysuria
2. Hematuria
3. Sx of rectal involvement, such as hematochezia, constipation, intermittent diarrhea, reduced stool caliber
4. Renal impairment from bladder outlet obstruction

What is the most common site of metastatic spread of prostate cancer?

Bone is the most common site of metastatic spread.

What organ is frequently the site of metastatic Dz in other tumors yet almost never harbors metastatic Dz in prostate cancer?

The **brain** is a frequent site of metastatic Dz in non-prostate carcinoma but almost never is a site of mets in prostate cancer.

Workup/Staging

Name 4 important aspects of a focused Hx to include in a pt with newly diagnosed prostate cancer.

Important aspects of a focused Hx to include in a pt with newly diagnosed prostate cancer:

GI/GU Sx: may be a clinical presentation of the cancer itself but also may inform the most appropriate type of therapy given the baseline GI/GU function

Comorbid illnesses: such information may inform appropriate types of therapies for the pt; specifically and ascertain a Hx of inflammatory bowel Dz, hernia repair, or previous bowel surgeries (is the pt a surgical candidate; hormone suppression candidate?)

Medications: ask about current use of α-blockers or androgen suppression

New-onset bone pain: should result in a thorough evaluation for bone mets

The lab workup for prostate cancer includes what tests?

Prostate cancer lab workup: PSA, CBC, and BMP. Consider free PSA (if cancer Dx uncertain), alk phos (to assess for bone mets), or LFTS (if androgen receptor blockers will be used, as these are associated with hepatotoxicity).

Describe the AJCC 7th edition (2009) clinical TNM staging of prostate cancer.

Note: Per the AJCC, clinical T staging *may* use imaging. However, for research purposes, investigators should specify that the staging was based on DRE only or on DRE and imaging.

cT1: clinically inapparent tumor not palpable or visible by imaging

cT1a: incidental histologic finding in ≤5% of tumor resected

cT1b: incidental histologic finding in >5% of tissue resected

cT1c: tumor identified by needle Bx

cT2: organ-confined Dz

cT2a: tumor involves less than or equal to one half of 1 lobe

cT2b: tumor involves more than one half of 1 lobe (but not both lobes)

cT2c: tumor involves both lobes of prostate

cT3: tumor extends through prostatic capsule

cT3a: ECE

cT3b: seminal vesicle involvement

cT4: adjacent organ involvement (bladder neck, external sphincter, rectum, pelvic wall or levator muscles

N1: regional LN mets

M1: DMs

M1a: nonregional LNs

M1b: bone(s)

M1c: other sites

What % of men with low-grade, early-stage Dz will eventually need definitive management with curative intent b/c of progressive Dz?

In a prospective cohort study at the JHH of men undergoing active surveillance, after median follow-up of 3 yrs, **25% of men underwent definitive management based on Dz progression on Bx or pt preference.** Of these men with progressive Dz on Bx, those who opted for surgical management at the time of follow-up had a proportion with curable Dz that was similar to those men who would be qualified for expectant management upfront but instead chose to undergo upfront surgery (*Carter HB et al., J Urol 2007*). In a prospective, single-arm cohort of 450 men undergoing active surveillance, the 10-yr prostate cancer actuarial survival was 97.2%. Overall, **30%** of men were found to have progressive Dz and were offered definitive therapy (*Klotz L et al., JCO 2009*).

What 3 standard Tx options are available to an otherwise healthy man with no adverse GI/GU Sx and low-risk Dz by D'Amico criteria?

Standard Tx options available to an otherwise healthy man with no adverse GI/GU Sx and low-risk Dz (by D'Amico criteria):
1. Active surveillance (in carefully selected pts)
2. Radical surgery
3. RT (brachytherapy [brachy] or EBRT alone)

Does dose escalation improve outcomes in men with low-risk prostate cancer?

Yes. Dose escalation improves biochemical FFS in men with low-risk prostate cancer. This has been seen in at least 2 randomized trials that included men with low-risk Dz: **PROG 9509** (*Zietman AL et al., JCO 2010*) and the **MDACC RCT** (*Kuban D et al., IJROBP 2008*).

Describe the design and outcomes of PROG 9509, which evaluated dose escalation in prostate cancer.

PROG 9509 included 392 men with low-risk prostate cancer (cT1b-T2b, PSA <15 ng/mL, Gleason <7). All men were treated with 50.4 Gy using photon RT and then were randomized to a proton boost to a total dose of 70.2 GyE vs. 79.2 GyE. **Dose escalation improved 10-yr biochemical failure (32.2% vs. 16.7%).**

Describe the design and outcomes of the MDACC trial that evaluated dose escalation in prostate cancer.

The MDACC dose escalation trial enrolled 301 pts with cT1b-T3 prostate cancer. 21% were low risk, 47% were intermediate risk, and 32% were high risk. Pts were randomized to 70 Gy vs. 78 Gy. **Dose escalation improved 8-yr freedom from failure (78% vs. 59%).** This improvement was seen in the low- and high-risk subsets but not in the intermediate-risk subset. 8-yr CSS was not significantly different (99% vs. 95%), nor was 8-yr OS (78% vs. 79%). (*Kuban D et al., IJROBP 2008*)

What RCTs have compared surgery, EBRT, and brachy for low-risk prostate cancer?	**Currently, no RCTs have compared surgery, EBRT, and/or brachy for low-risk prostate cancer.** Multiple trials comparing definitive modalities for low-risk pts have been attempted, but all have failed due to inadequate accrual. ProtecT is a large UK-based trial designed to address this question and has closed to accrual.
What data support the use of prostatectomy, EBRT, or LDR brachy alone for low-risk prostate cancer?	Numerous retrospective studies suggest similar outcomes for low-risk prostate cancer pts treated with prostatectomy, EBRT, or LDR brachy. *D'Amico et al.* reviewed low-risk pts treated at the University of Pennsylvania or the Joint Center in Boston and found **no difference in 5-yr biochemical FFS (~88%)** in men treated with prostatectomy, EBRT, or brachy alone (*JAMA 1998*). *Kupelian et al.* reviewed low-risk pts from the Cleveland Clinic and Memorial Sloan Kettering and found **similar 5-yr biochemical FFS (~81%–83%)** for men treated with prostatectomy, LDR brachy, and EBRT (to total doses >72 Gy). However, in a subset of men treated with EBRT to <72 Gy, 5-yr biochemical FFS was significantly worse (51%) (*Kupelian P et al., IJROBP 2004*).
Describe the setup of a pt with prostate cancer undergoing CT imaging to plan RT Tx.	A pt undergoing CT imaging to plan RT Tx can be simulated in the prone or supine position. Some institutions use a pelvic MRI or a urethrogram to locate the urogenital diaphragm and, hence, the apex of the prostate. The pt is often instructed to have a full bladder and an empty rectum, though techniques vary at institutions.
Describe 4 techniques to verify prostate position in daily RT Tx.	Techniques to verify prostate position in daily RT Tx: 1. 2D-IGRT + fiducials 2. 3D-IGRT +/− fiducials 3. Implantable radiofrequency transponder 4. BAT US

Toxicity

What are the most common side effects after radical prostatectomy?	The most common significant side effects after radical prostatectomy are **erectile dysfunction, urinary incontinence, and urethral stricture.**
In men with intact erectile function prior to radical prostatectomy, what % retain erectile function after a nerve-sparing procedure?	In men with intact erectile function prior to surgery, at least **50%** will retain erectile function after a nerve-sparing prostatectomy, depending on surgeon volume.

■ Workup/Staging

By the D'Amico criteria, which localized prostate cancer pts are considered to have intermediate-risk Dz?

A pt has intermediate-risk prostate cancer if he has any or all of the following 3 risk factors (but no high-risk factors): **stage T2b, Gleason 7, and pre-Tx PSA 10–20 ng/mL.** (*D'Amico A et al., J Urol 2001*)

By the D'Amico criteria, which localized prostate cancer pts are considered to have high-risk Dz?

A pt has high-risk prostate cancer if he has any or all of the following 3 risk factors: **stage ≥T2c, Gleason ≥8, and pre-Tx PSA >20 ng/mL.** (*D'Amico A et al., J Urol 2001*)

What is the Roach equation that estimates risk of pathologic ECE in prostate cancer pts?

Roach equation for ECE risk:

$$\text{ECE\%} = ([3/2] \times \text{PSA}) + ([\text{Gleason} - 3] \times 10)$$

What is the Roach equation that estimates risk of pathologic seminal vesicle involvement in prostate cancer pts?

Roach equation for seminal vesicle risk:

$$\text{SV\%} = \text{PSA} + ([\text{Gleason} - 6] \times 10)$$

What is the Roach equation that estimates risk of pathologic LN involvement in prostate cancer pts?

Roach equation for LN risk:

$$\text{LN\%} = ([2/3] \times \text{PSA}) + ([\text{Gleason} - 6] \times 10)$$

The Roach equations were developed from prostate cancer pts who had surgery in which yrs?

The Roach equations were developed from prostate cancer pts who had surgery between 1982–1996 (i.e., mainly in the **pre-PSA era**). These tools likely overestimate risks in pts diagnosed in the post-PSA era.

What is the sensitivity and specificity of endorectal coil MRI for determining the presence of prostatic ECE?

The estimates for the sensitivity and specificity of endorectal coil MRI as a predictor of prostatic ECE vary widely, between **13%–95% (sensitivity)** and **49%–97% (specificity).** The experience of the radiologist appears to play an important role in the accuracy of the tool.

What is the sensitivity and specificity of endorectal coil MRI for determining the presence of seminal vesicle invasion by prostate cancer?

The estimated sensitivity of endorectal coil MRI to predict seminal vesicle invasion by prostate cancer varies widely from 23%–80%. The estimates for specificity of seminal vesicle invasion are superior and vary between 81%–99%.

If an endorectal coil MRI is ordered as part of the workup for prostate cancer, how long after Bx should it take place?

There is no consensus on the role of endorectal coil MRI as part of the workup for prostate cancer. However, if an MRI is ordered, wait **6–8 wks after Bx to avoid artifact** caused by post-Bx hemorrhage.

■ Treatment/Prognosis

What are the Tx options for a man with localized intermediate-risk prostate cancer?

Tx options for a man with intermediate-risk prostate cancer:
1. EBRT $+/-$ short-term androgen suppression (AS) (4–6 mos) $+/-$ brachytherapy (brachy) boost
2. Brachy $+/-$ AS
3. Prostatectomy (less ideal for pt with >1 intermediate risk factor).

If he has a life expectancy <10 yrs, also consider active surveillance.

What are the Tx options for a man with localized high-risk prostate cancer?

Tx options for a man with high-risk prostate cancer:
1. EBRT + long-term AS (2–3 yrs) $+/-$ pelvic node RT $+/-$ brachy boost
2. Prostatectomy (less ideal for high-risk pts)

Estimate the 5-yr biochemical failurefree survival (bFS) for D'Amico intermediate- and high-risk prostate cancer pts treated with prostatectomy alone.

After prostatectomy alone, 5-yr bFS is ~**65% for intermediate-risk** and ~**35% for high-risk prostate cancer pts.** (*D'Amico A et al., J Urol 2001*)

Estimate the 10-yr bFS for prostate cancer pts with cT2b and ≥cT2c Dz treated with prostatectomy alone.

After prostatectomy alone, 10-yr bFS is ~**62% for cT2b** and ~**57% for ≥cT2c.** (*Han M et al., Urol Clin N Am 2001*)

Estimate the 10-yr bFS for prostate cancer pts with Gleason 3 + 4 = 7 and 4 + 3 = 7 Dz treated with prostatectomy alone.

After prostatectomy alone, 10-yr bFS is ~**60% with Gleason 3 + 4 = 7 and ~33% with 4 + 3 = 7.** (*Han M et al., Urol Clin N Am 2001*)

Estimate the 10-yr bFS for prostate cancer pts with Gleason 8–10 Dz treated with prostatectomy alone.

After prostatectomy alone, 10-yr bFS is ~**29%** with Gleason 8–10 Dz. (*Han M et al., Urol Clin N Am 2001*)

Estimate the 10-yr bFS for prostate cancer pts with a pretreatment prostate-specific antigen (pPSA) from 10–20 and >20 ng/mL treated with prostatectomy alone.

After prostatectomy alone, 10-yr bFS ~57% with pPSA 10–20 ng/mL and 48% with pPSA >20 ng/mL are **57% and 48%,** respectively. (*Han M et al., Urol Clin N Am 2001*)

Describe the study design and results of RTOG 8610, which studied the benefit of short-course AS in locally advanced prostate cancer.

RTOG 8610 enrolled 456 men with cT2-T4 (bulky) prostate cancer. N1 pts were eligible if below the common iliac. All were treated with EBRT (65–70 Gy) and randomized to 4 mos of AS (beginning 2 mos prior to EBRT) or observation with AS at relapse. **10-yr OS and MS favored the short-course AS arm (43% vs. 34% and 8.7 yrs vs. 7.3 yrs, respectively) though the difference was NSS.** Short-course AS improved 10-yr CSM (23% vs. 36%) and distant failure (35% vs. 47%). (*Roach M et al., JCO 2008*)

Describe the study design and results of RTOG 9408, which studied the benefit of short-course AS in locally confined prostate cancer.

RTOG 9408 enrolled 2,028 pts with T1b-T2b, PSA ≤20, prostate cancer. Pts were randomized to EBRT alone (68.4 Gy) +/− 4-mo AS beginning 2 mos prior to EBRT. **12-yr OS favored the short-course AS arm (51% vs. 56%).** (*McGowan DG et al., abstract IJROBP 2010*).

Describe the study design and results of TROG 96.01, which studied the benefit of short-course AS in locally advanced prostate cancer.

TROG 96.01 enrolled 818 pts with T2b-T4 prostate cancer treated with EBRT (66 Gy in 2 Gy). Pts were randomized to 0, 3, or 6 mos of AS starting 2 mos prior to EBRT. With only a median follow-up of 5.9 yrs, the 3- and 6-mo AS arms had improved LF, biochemical failure, and freedom from salvage Tx compared to the no-AS arm. The 6-mo arm also had improved distant failure and prostate cancer–specific survival (PCSS) compared to the no AS arm. As of yet, there are no OS differences among any of the 3 arms and no consistent cancer control differences between 3- and 6-mo arms. (*Denham JW et al., Lancet Oncol 2005*)

Describe the study design and results of the RCT by *D'Amico et al.*, which studied the benefit of short-course AS in locally advanced prostate cancer.

D'Amico et al. (DFCI trial) enrolled 206 men with cT1b-T2b and 1 of the following: PSA 10–40 ng/mL or Gleason 7–10 or ECE/seminal vesicle invasion by MRI. Pts were randomized to EBRT alone (70 Gy) +/− 6 mos of AS beginning 2 mos prior to EBRT. **The AS arm had improved 8-yr OS (74% vs. 61%).** Unplanned subset analysis suggested that benefit may be limited to men without significant comorbidities. (*JAMA 2008*)

When should AS be started in a prostate cancer pt being treated with EBRT and AS?

In prostate cancer pts being treated with EBRT + AS, **AS is usually started 2 mos prior to the start of EBRT.** Preclinical experiments suggest that neoadj AS may improve prostate cancer RT sensitivity compared to concurrent AS, possibly due to improved tumor oxygenation with neoadj AS. Furthermore, the RCTs that established the role of short-course AS started it neoadjuvantly (**RTOG 8610, D'Amico trial, TROG 96.01**). However, **RTOG 9413,** which compared neoadj/concurrent vs. adj short-course AS showed no bPFS benefit (or detriment) to neoadj AS.

Describe the study design and results of RTOG 9413, which studied the benefit of the sequence of short-course AS and pelvic node RT in locally advanced prostate cancer.

RTOG 9413 had a 2 × 2 factorial design. It randomized 1,323 intermediate- and high-risk pts to 4 mos of AS beginning 2 mos prior to or immediately following EBRT. The 2nd randomization was regarding RT field size: whole pelvis (WP) RT vs. prostate and seminal vesicles only (PSVO). After a median follow-up of 7 yrs, there was **no difference in PFS in the neoadj vs. adj AS arms and no difference in PFS in the WP and PSVO arms.** Interpretation of this trial is limited by the fact that there was an unexpected interaction between the 2 randomizations of this study. (*Lawton C et al., IJROBP 2007*)

What is the appropriate duration of neoadj AS prior to EBRT in prostate cancer pts?

Prostate cancer pts who are treated with neoadj AS usually rcv 2 mos of AS prior to EBRT. However, there is only 1 published RCT on the optimal duration of neoadj AS in localized prostate cancer: *Crook et al. (IJROBP 2009)*. This RCT enrolled 378 men with localized prostate cancer of any risk group, and all were treated with EBRT (66–67 Gy) without concurrent AS. Pts were randomized to 3 mos vs. 8 mos of neoadj AS. 5-yr freedom from failure (FFF) did not differ between the Tx arms. In an unplanned subgroup analysis, 5-yr DFS was improved for high-risk pts (71% vs. 42%) (*Crook J et al., IJROBP 2009*). **RTOG 9910** evaluated 2 mos vs. 7 mos of neoadj therapy, though no results have yet been reported.

What studies support the role of long-term AS in localized high-risk prostate cancer pts treated with EBRT?

An OS benefit of long-term AS in high-risk pts after EBRT was 1st shown in **RTOG 8531.** Multiple subsequent RCTs have also shown improved prostate cancer outcomes: **the Casodex Early Prostate Cancer trial, EORTC 22863, RTOG 9202, and EORTC 22961.**

Describe the study design and results of RTOG 8531, which studied the benefit of the long-term AS in locally advanced prostate cancer.

RTOG 8531 enrolled 945 men with cT3 (nonbulky), pT3 after prostatectomy, or N1 prostate cancer. All were treated with EBRT (definitive dose: 65–70 Gy; postop dose: 60–65 Gy) and randomized to adj AS indefinitely or observation with AS at relapse. **Adj AS improved 10-yr OS (49% vs. 39%), 10-yr CSM (16% vs. 22%), 10-yr LF (23% vs. 38%), and 10-yr distant failure (24% vs. 39%)** (WP). On subset analysis, benefits were limited to the subset with Gleason ≥7 and were especially important in the subset with Gleason ≥8 (*Pilepich MV et al., IJROBP 2005*).

Describe the study design and results of the Casodex Early Prostate Cancer trial, which studied the benefit of the long-term adj Casodex in locally advanced prostate cancer.

The Casodex Early Prostate Cancer trial randomized 8,113 men with prostate cancer to observation or long-term Casodex after local therapy (RT, prostatectomy, observation). The duration of Casodex was either 2 yrs or until progression. In the subgroup of RT pts (1,730 men), after a median follow-up of 7.2 yrs, adj long-term Casodex did not result in OS or PCSS. However, in the subgroup of locally advanced pts (cT3-T4 or N1), there was an OS and PCSS benefit. These findings, however, were the results of an unplanned subset analysis. (*See WA et al., J Cancer Res Clin Oncol 2006*)

Describe the study design and results of EORTC 22863, which studied the benefit of long-term AS in locally advanced prostate cancer.

EORTC 22863 enrolled 412 men with cT3-T4/any grade or cT1-T2/WHO grade 3 prostate cancer. All were treated with EBRT (70 Gy) and randomized to 3 yrs of adj AS (beginning with EBRT) or observation with AS at relapse. Long-term AS improved **5-yr OS (78% vs. 62%), CSS (94% vs. 79%), LF (1.7% vs. 16.4%), and distant failure (9.8% vs. 29.2%).** (*Bolla M et al., Lancet 2002*)

Describe the study design and results of RTOG 9202, which studied the benefit of the long-term AS in locally advanced prostate cancer.

RTOG 9202 enrolled 1,541 men with cT2c-T4, PSA <150. All were treated with 2 mos of neoadj AS and 2 mos of concurrent AS + EBRT (65–70 Gy). Pts were randomized to an additional 2 yrs of adj AS or observation with AS at relapse. Long-term AS was not associated with OS in the entire cohort, though it did show improved 10-yr CSS (89% vs. 84%), local progression (12% vs. 22%), and DM (15% vs. 23%). In an unplanned subgroup analysis, long-term AS improved 10-yr OS in pts with Gleason ≥8 (45% vs. 32%). (*Horwitz EM et al., JCO 2008*)

Describe the study design and results of the EORTC 22961 RCT, which compared short-course and long-term AS with EBRT in localized prostate cancer.

EORTC 22961 enrolled 1,113 men with cT2c-T4/N0 or cT1c-T2b/pN1-N2 prostate cancer and randomized to EBRT (70 Gy) with 6 mos vs. 3 yrs of neoadj, concurrent, and adj AS. **Men receiving 3 yrs of AS had superior OS (5-yr OS 85% vs. 81%) and CSM (5-yr CSM 3.2% vs. 4.7%).** Long-term overall QOL did not significantly differ between the 2 arms. (*Bolla M et al., NEJM 2009*)

What is the appropriate duration of long-term AS in localized high-risk prostate cancer pts treated with EBRT?

RTOG 9202 and EORTC 22961 suggested that long-term (2–3 yrs) AS is superior to short-course AS in high-risk pts. However, the optimum duration of long-term AS has not been well studied.

What is the role of pelvic nodal RT in localized intermediate- and high-risk prostate cancer?

The major RCTs that established the role of RT in locally advanced prostate cancer generally irradiated pelvic nodes. However, the role of pelvic nodal RT in localized prostate cancer has been specifically studied in 3 RCTs: **RTOG 7706, RTOG 9413, and GETUG-01,** and none showed a cancer control benefit to irradiating pelvic nodes. Yet, all of these trials included men who may have been at low risk for harboring nodal Dz. Pelvic nodal RT may still be warranted in men at very high risk of harboring nodal Dz, though who these pts are is controversial.

What is the appropriate EBRT dose for intermediate- and high-risk prostate cancer?

Men with intermediate- and high-risk prostate cancer who do not rcv AS should be treated to total EBRT doses of ≥74 Gy (in 2 Gy/fx). There have been at least 4 EBRT dose escalation studies including intermediate- and high-risk pts: the **MDACC dose escalation trial, PROG 9505, the Dutch dose escalation trial, and the MRC RT01 trial.** All 4 RCTs have shown at least improved biochemical control with dose-escalated EBRT. The role of high-dose EBRT is less clear in the setting of AS. The Dutch dose escalation trial allowed AS, but only a minority of men rcv it (22%; *Peeters ST et al., JCO 2006*). The **MRC RT01** trial mandated neoadj and concurrent AS, and 5-yr outcomes favored dose escalation.

Describe the study design and results of the MDACC RCT that studied the benefit of dose escalation in localized prostate cancer.

The MDACC dose escalation trial enrolled 301 pts with cT1b-T3 prostate cancer. None were treated with AS. 21% were low risk, 47% were intermediate risk, and 32% were high risk. Pts were randomized to 70 Gy vs. 78 Gy. **Dose escalation improved 8-yr FFF (78% vs. 59%).** This improvement was seen in the low- and high-risk subsets but not in the intermediate-risk subset. **8-yr CSS was not significantly different (99% vs. 95%), nor was 8-yr OS (78% vs. 79%).** (*Kuban D et al., IJROBP 2008*)

Describe the study design and results of the PROG 9508 RCT, which studied the benefit of dose escalation in localized prostate cancer.

The **PROG 9509** RCT on dose escalation enrolled 393 pts with T1b-T2b, PSA <15 ng/mL prostate cancer. Pts were randomized to 70.2 Gy or 79.2 Gy. CD RT to the prostate only was given by proton RT prior to 50.4 Gy with photon RT to the prostate and seminal vesicle. **Dose escalation improved 5-yr freedom from biochemical failure (80% vs. 61%) and 5-yr LC (48% vs. 55%).** In an unplanned analysis, a significant improvement in freedom from biochemical failure was seen in both low- and intermediate-risk subsets. (*Zietman AL et al., JAMA 2005*)

Describe the study design and results of the MRC RT01 RCT, which studied the benefit of dose escalation in the setting of neoadj and concurrent AS for localized prostate cancer.

The **MRC RT01** trial enrolled 843 men with cT1b-T3a, PSA <50 prostate cancer. All men were treated with 3–6 mos of neoadj and concurrent AS and randomized to EBRT 64 Gy or 74 Gy. The **dose escalation arm improved 5-yr bPFS (71% vs. 60%).** LC, freedom from salvage AS, and DMFS favored the dose escalation arm, though these endpoints were not statistically different. (*Dearnaley DP et al., Lancet Oncol 2007*)

What is the role of primary AS alone for localized high-risk prostate cancer?

AS alone for localized high-risk prostate cancer may be considered for men who cannot tolerate local management or who have a short life expectancy (<5 yrs). However, **SPCG-7** showed that the addition of EBRT to long-term AS conferred a survival advantage in high-risk men.

Describe the design and results of the Scandinavian RCT (SPCG-7) that studied the long-term AS +/− EBRT in locally advanced prostate cancer.

SPCG-7 enrolled 875 men with cT1b-T2, N0 WHO grade 2–3 or cT3, any grade, N0 prostate cancer. All men were treated with total AS for 3 mos → an antiandrogen alone (flutamide) indefinitely. Pts were randomized to EBRT (70 Gy) starting after 3 mos of AS or no local therapy. With median follow-up of 7.6 yrs, the addition of **EBRT improved 10-yr OS (70% vs. 61%) and 10-yr CSS (88% vs. 76%).** The 10-yr prostate cancer–specific mortality was reduced by half with EBRT (12% vs. 24%). (*Widmark A et al., Lancet 2009*)

What is the role of definitive prostate RT in men with node+ prostate cancer?

There has been no RCT to determine whether men with node+ prostate cancer benefit from local RT. A retrospective review by *Zagars et al.* (*J Urol 2001*) suggested that **EBRT in addition to long-term AS confers an OS benefit to node+ pts.** Subset analyses from **RTOG 8531** suggest that long-term AS + EBRT confers OS benefit compared to EBRT alone in node+ pts. However, long-term biochemical control (PSA <1.5 ng/mL) was still poor (10% at 9 yrs) (*Lawton C et al., JCO 2005*).

▪ Toxicity

What are the most common acute and late side effects of definitive prostate RT?

<u>Acute side effects</u>: fatigue, urinary urgency/frequency, proctitis/diarrhea

<u>Late side effects</u>: erectile dysfunction (inability to maintain an erection for intercourse), cystitis, proctitis (frequency/bleeding)

Estimate the rate of grade 3 or higher late GU or GI RT toxicity with IMRT for prostate cancer.

Numerous retrospective studies suggest that grade 3 or higher late GU or GI RT toxicity is rare (≤1%).

Estimate the rate of erectile dysfunction in previously potent men 2+ yrs after Tx with definitive prostate RT.

Approximately **50%** of men who were previously potent will no longer be able to maintain erections for intercourse 2+ yrs after definitive prostate RT. (*Robinson JW et al., IJROBP 2002*)

Does the use of short-course or long-term AS affect acute or late GU and GI RT toxicity in prostate cancer pts?

No. Multiple studies have evaluated the effect of AS on GU and GI RT toxicity. There appears to be no strong effect.

What are the common short-term and long-term side effects of AS?

Short-term side effects: hot flashes, decreased libido, fatigue

Long-term side effects: gynecomastia, anemia, decreased muscle mass, decreased bone density, obesity, mood changes, dyslipidemia, insulin resistance, possibly diabetes and coronary artery Dz

(*Higano CS, Urology 2003*; *Keating NL et al., J Clin Oncol 2006*)

What are common side effects associated with antiandrogen therapy, and how long is the Tx course?

Common side effects of bicalutamide, which is most commonly prescribed due to its favorable toxicity profile, include **breast tenderness and gynecomastia** (50%) as well as **loss of libido, diarrhea, and hepatotoxicity.** It is generally prescribed for the 1st 2–4 wks with a GnRH analog.

55

Adjuvant and Salvage Treatment for Prostate Cancer

Jing Zeng and Howard M. Sandler

■ Background

What % of newly diagnosed prostate cancers are cT3 Dz or higher?

12%–28% of men with newly diagnosed prostate cancer have cT3 Dz or higher.

In which portion of the prostate is ECE most commonly found?

ECE is most commonly found in the **posterolat portion of the prostate, near the prostatic neurovascular bundle.**

What are the indications for adj RT after prostatectomy, and what studies support its role?

The indications for adj RT after prostatectomy have been refined due to reports from 3 recent RCTs that included men with **pT3N0 prostate cancer or positive surgical margins** and showed improved 5-yr biochemical PFS with adj RT compared to observation: **SWOG 8794, EORTC 22911, and ARO 96-02.** The SWOG 8794 study, which has the longest follow-up, found an OS benefit with adj RT. Subset analyses using centralized pathologic review from the EORTC study suggest that the benefit may be limited to men with +margins after surgery.

Describe the study design and results of the SWOG 8794 RCT that compared adj RT and observation in pts with high-risk features after prostatectomy.

SWOG 8794 enrolled 431 men with pT3N0 prostate cancer or +margin after prostatectomy and randomized to adj RT (60–64 Gy). **Adj RT improved MS (15.2 yrs vs. 13.3 yrs).** Global QOL was initially worse in the adj RT arm but was similar after 2 yrs of follow-up and superior thereafter. (*Thompson IM et al., J Urol 2009*)

Is there any evidence that salvage RT post prostatectomy improves survival compared with observation?

Yes. There are no randomized trials comparing salvage RT post prostatectomy against other Tx strategies. However, there is a suggestive retrospective series from the Johns Hopkins Hospital (*Trock BJ et al., JAMA 2008*) that evaluated 635 pts s/p prostatectomy with biochemical recurrence. Tx included observation, RT alone, or RT + hormone therapy. Adjusted for prognostic factors, **cancer-specific survival was prolonged in pts who rcv salvage RT, regardless of hormone therapy (5-yr CSS 96% vs. 88%).**

Is there randomized data comparing adj vs. salvage RT in men with locally advanced prostate cancer or biochemical recurrence s/p prostatectomy?

No. There are no published randomized trials comparing adj vs. salvage RT in men with locally advanced prostate cancer or biochemical recurrence s/p prostatectomy. The 3 randomized trials on adj therapy (**SWOG 8794, EORTC 22911, and ARO 96-02**) compared adj RT vs. observation, without strict salvage guidelines at the 1st sign of Dz recurrence. **Nonrandomized series on salvage RT appear to produce results somewhat comparable to adj RT.**

What should be the Tx volume in adj and salvage RT post prostatectomy?

The appropriate Tx volume in adj and salvage RT post prostatectomy has not been prospectively determined. Randomized trials in adj RT (**SWOG 8794, EORTC 22911, and ARO 96-02**) used **small-field RT and did not include regional pelvic nodal irradiation. RTOG-0534** is an ongoing trial looking at extent of pelvic RT, but only in men also receiving hormone therapy.

What should be the RT dose in adj and salvage RT post prostatectomy?	There are no randomized studies addressing the issue of dose in adj and salvage RT post prostatectomy. **Retrospective series typically report better outcomes when doses are >65 Gy.** The ASTRO consensus panel recommends >64 Gy. Often, pts with higher levels of pre-RT PSA or with palpable nodules will rcv higher doses of PORT.
Is there randomized data supporting the addition of hormone therapy to salvage RT post prostatectomy?	**No.** There are no published randomized trials addressing the addition of hormone therapy to salvage RT post prostatectomy. **RTOG-9601,** which randomized pts to salvage RT +/− Casodex, has been completed and publication is pending. Based on retrospective series, **it is reasonable to recommend hormone therapy for pts with very unfavorable risk factors, such as high Gleason score or high pre-RT PSA.**
Is there a role for salvage prostatectomy for biochemical recurrence after RT for prostate cancer?	**Yes.** For biochemical recurrence after RT for prostate cancer, salvage prostatectomy can provide long-term Dz control in a significant portion of pts. However, salvage prostatectomy is associated with a higher risk of urinary incontinence and rectal injury, though pts treated with modern IMRT may have better outcomes. Careful pt selection is key. Outcome is better with pts with lower preop PSA. Based on retrospective series, **5-yr PFS is up to 86% for a PSA <4, 55% for a PSA 4–10, and 28% for a PSA >10.**
Is there a role for cryotherapy for biochemical recurrence after RT for prostate cancer?	This is **uncertain.** There are no prospective studies comparing cryotherapy against prostatectomy in the salvage setting post-RT with biochemical recurrence. Relative efficacy and safety are uncertain between the 2 modalities. Since cryotherapy can destroy tissue beyond the prostate, it may be an option for pts with extraprostatic extension of Dz.
Is there a role for brachytherapy (brachy) for biochemical recurrence after EBRT for prostate cancer?	This in **uncertain.** There is not sufficient data to support the widespread use of brachy for biochemical recurrence after EBRT for prostate cancer over the other available modalities, such as prostatectomy and cryotherapy. Small series have shown promise with good Dz control and low levels of toxicity in carefully selected pts, but further study is needed before it is considered a standard approach.

How sensitive and specific is MRI at detecting metastatic Dz?	The role of MRI in this setting has not been thoroughly evaluated. A prospective study of 66 pts with high-risk prostate cancer found the sensitivity/specificity of axial MRI to be 100%/88% compared to bone scan–X-ray sensitivity/specificity of 63%/64% in detecting mets. (*Lecouvet FE et al., J Clin Oncol 2007*)
What is ProstaScint?	ProstaScint is indium-111 capromab pendetide, which is a radiolabeled monoclonal antibody used to target prostate-specific membrane antigen. It is FDA approved for detecting localized Dz recurrence after radical prostatectomy but not metastatic Dz.
Is ProstaScint useful in diagnosing localized and/ or metastatic prostate cancer?	The data are mixed regarding the utility of ProstaScint. Most studies have shown it to have a poor PPV for detecting extraprostatic Dz (*Nagda SN et al., Int J Radiat Oncol Biol Phys 2007; Thomas CT et al., J Clin Oncol 2003*). B/c its interpretation is confounded by reader experience and the timing of imaging, it is not commonly included as part of the workup for localized or metastatic recurrence.
Is there a role for prostate Bx after biochemical failure in pts initially treated with RT?	Based on an ASTRO consensus statement (1999), re-Bx should be considered if the pt is considering additional local therapy and is >2 yrs s/p completion of RT. (*Cox JD et al., J Clin Oncol 1999*)

▊ Treatment/Prognosis

What is 1st-line systemic therapy for metastatic prostate cancer?	AS by orchiectomy or, more commonly, the use of a GnRH analog is considered 1st-line therapy for metastatic prostate cancer.
What is the premise behind androgen deprivation in the Tx of prostate cancer?	Seminal studies by *Huggins et al.* revealed that androgen deprivation through castration and estrogen administration leads to the death of prostate cancer cells. (*Cancer Res 1941*)
Is GnRH agonist therapy superior to orchiectomy for the Tx of metastatic prostate cancer?	Randomized trials and meta-analyses have confirmed equivalent long-term outcomes. Secondary to the irreversibility and psychological morbidity associated with orchiectomy, GnRH agonists are generally considered 1st-line therapy. This therapy has been shown to mainly improve PFS, not OS. (*Kaisary AV et al., Br J Urol 1991; Turkes AO et al., J Steroid Biochem 1987; Vogelzang NJ et al., Urology 1995*)
What are 3 commonly used GnRH agonists?	Most commonly used GnRH agonists: 1. Goserelin (Zoladex) 2. Leuprolide (Lupron) 3. Triptorelin (Trelstar) All 3 are available as depot formulations.

What other modalities of AS are utilized?

GnRH antagonists, antiandrogens (AAs; nonsteroidal competitive androgen receptor antagonists), estrogens, and ketoconazole (antifungal agent, blocks cyt P450 enzymes involved in steroidogenesis)

Should AS be initiated for biochemical recurrence after definitive RT in the absence of clinically evident mets?

The data are mixed, and the answer is therefore **controversial.** There are ongoing RCTs designed to address this issue (ELAAT, OCOG). Until these data are available, in our practice, the authors initiate AS in pts with high-risk features (such as Gleason score >7 and rapid PSA-DT). (*Faria SL et al., Urology 2006; Walsh PC et al., J Urol 2001*)

Should AS be initiated for radiographically evident but asymptomatic mets?

Yes. Studies have shown improved PFS with upfront AS as compared to deferring therapy until signs and Sx of clinical progression. (*MRC Prostate Cancer Group, Br J Urol 1997; Nair B et al., Cochrane Database Syst Rev 2002*)

Is intermittent AS as efficacious as continuous AS?

This is **uncertain.** The premise behind the use of intermittent AS is to help reduce side effects, cost, and progression to hormone-refractory Dz. Phase II studies have validated feasibility and improved QOL, and phase III trials are ongoing with preliminary data suggesting at least similar outcomes. (*Hussain M et al., J Clin Oncol 2006; Salonen AJ et al., J Urol 2008; Shaw GL et al., BJU Int 2007*)

Can AAs be used as monotherapy for AS?

Randomized trial data are **mixed.** A meta-analysis of several trials showed a trend toward OS benefit with medical/surgical castration compared to nonsteroidal AA therapy (*Seidenfeld J et al., Ann Int Med 2000*). As a result, **common practice involves both use of GnRH alone or in combination with a nonsteroidal AA.**

Should GnRH analogs be used alone or in combination with AAs (combination androgen blockade [CAB])?

Possibly. Several randomized trials and meta-analyses have shown a small but significant OS benefit with CAB (*PCTCG, Lancet 2000; Samson DJ et al., Cancer 2002*). GnRH monotherapy may also cause an initial flare of Sx, which can be prevented by preceding therapy with a short course of AAs (*Kuhn JM et al., NEJM 1989*). CAB should be recommended if the side effects can be tolerated.

Typically, how long after initiating AS does it take before a pt's prostate cancer becomes androgen independent?

Androgen independence usually occurs **within 2–3 yrs of starting AS.** (*Eisenberger MA et al., NEJM 1998; Sharifi N et al., BJU Int 2005*)

What is the anticipated 5-yr OS for metastatic prostate cancer treated with CAB?

A meta-analysis by the Prostate Cancer Trialists Collaborative Group reported a **25.4%** 5-yr OS rate for pts with metastatic prostate cancer treated with CAB. (*PCTCG, Lancet 2000*)

How are pts with castrate-resistant prostate cancer commonly treated?

If CAB is being administered, withdrawal of the AA may result in PSA decline. If a GnRH analog is being given, switching to AA may help. Additionally, megestrol acetate may be used. Consider palliative focal or systemic radiotherapy as appropriate in conjunction with a bisphosphonate (refer to Chapter 88).

What is the role of ketoconazole in the Tx of metastatic prostate cancer?

Ketoconazole, a commonly used antifungal, inhibits steroidogenesis and is cytotoxic to prostate cancer cells. It is commonly prescribed for castration-resistant prostate cancer with hydrocortisone to prevent adrenal insufficiency and often results in GI and liver toxicity. Its use is associated with a 20%–50% reduction in PSA with a 3–6 mo duration of response. (*Ryan CJ et al., Curr Oncol Rep 2005*)

What are chemotherapeutic options for pts with metastatic hormone-refractory prostate cancer?

Docetaxel/prednisone is now the standard of care for metastatic, hormone-refractory prostate cancers based on 2 key randomized trials, **TAX 327** and **SWOG 9916.**

The **TAX-327** trial (*Tannock IF et al., NEJM 2004*) randomized 1,006 men to 3 Tx arms: 2 doses of docetaxel (30 mg weekly or 75 mg q3wks) and mitoxantrone in progressive metastatic, hormone-refractory prostate cancer pts who were chemo naive. All 3 groups rcv prednisone and were continued on AS. The mitoxantrone arm had significantly worse OS compared to the q3wk docetaxel arm, but was not significantly worse than the qwk docetaxel arm (MS was 18.9 mos vs. 17.4 mos vs. 16.5 mos, in q3wks, qwk docetaxel, and mitoxantrone arms, respectively). There was greater improvement in PSA, pain, and QOL with docetaxel but increased grade 3–4 toxicity (neutropenia, n/v, diarrhea).

The **SWOG 9916** trial (*Petrylak DP et al., NEJM 2004*) randomized 770 men to estramustine/docetaxel/dexamethasone vs. mitoxantrone/prednisone. The docetaxel arm had significantly improved MS (17.5 mos vs. 15.6 mos) and PSA response (50% vs. 27%). There were more grade 3–4 toxicities (neutropenic fever, n/v, cardiovascular events) in the docetaxel arm.

What is the potential advantage of degarelix in the Tx of prostate cancer?

Degarelix, a newly FDA-approved GnRH antagonist, can produce a faster reduction of testosterone levels and avoid the initial flare. Common side effects, however, include local and systemic inflammatory reactions.

What novel therapies are being considered for metastatic prostate cancer?	Novel therapies considered for metastatic prostate cancer:

1. Gene transfer immunotherapies are designed to express immune-stimulating compounds (e.g., GM-CSF [Gvax] and PROSTVAC). Phase III data is pending.
2. Gene transfer cytoreduction is designed to express lytic viruses (e.g., CV706/E1a) that preferentially target prostate cancer cells.
3. Endothelin receptor antagonists (e.g., ZD4054, atrasentan) are designed to prevent inhibition of apoptosis in prostate cancer cells. RCTs have not shown benefit of atrasentan compared to placebo. **SWOG 0421** is under way.
4. Monoclonal antibody therapies (e.g., cetuximab, trastuzumab) are being explored in phase I–II studies.
5. 17α-hydroxylase/17,20 lyase inhibitors (e.g., abiraterone) are in phase III trials in both chemo-naive castrated pts and in those with prior docetaxel therapy.
6. Selective androgen receptor modulators (e.g., MDV3100) are undergoing phase III evaluation in castrated pts who have failed 1–2 prior chemo regimens.
7. Mature data is awaited on 1st-line docetaxel and prednisone $+/-$ bevacizumab in castrated pts with metastatic Dz.

■ Toxicity

What are the common short-term and long-term side effects of AS?	Short-term effects: hot flashes, ↓ libido, fatigue Long-term effects: gynecomastia, anemia, ↓ muscle mass, ↓ bone density, obesity, mood changes, dyslipidemia, insulin resistance, possibly diabetes and coronary artery Dz (*Higano CS, Urology 2003; Keating NL et al., J Clin Oncol 2006*)
What are common side effects associated with AA therapy, and how long is the Tx course?	Common side effects of bicalutamide, which is most commonly prescribed due to its favorable toxicity profile, include breast tenderness and gynecomastia (50%) as well as loss of libido, diarrhea, and hepatotoxicity. It is generally prescribed for the 1st 2–4 wks with a GnRH analog.

What is pubic arch interference, and how can it be avoided?

Pubic arch interference is when the needle paths are obstructed by the pubic arch. It occurs more frequently in pts with large glands and affects the ant and lat needles. To evaluate for interference, one can use TRUS to compare the largest prostate cross section with the narrowest portion of the pubic arch. Other than hormonal downsizing, the use of an extended lithotomy position (Trendelenburg) may also alleviate some pubic arch interference.

What sources are typically used in permanent seed prostate brachy?

I-125 and Pd-103 are the sources typically used in prostate brachy. Cesium-131 (Cs-131) has also been utilized more recently.

What are the half-lives of the 3 most common sources used in prostate brachy?

Half-lives of the 3 most common sources:
1. I-125 (60 days)
2. Pd-103 (17 days)
3. Cs-131 (10 days)

What doses are typically prescribed when using monotherapy with I-125, Pd-103, and Cs-131?

Doses typically prescribed for brachy monotherapy:
<u>I-125</u>: 145 Gy
<u>Pd-103</u>: 125 Gy
<u>Cs-131</u>: 115 Gy

How far outside of the prostate gland are Rx IDLs able to reach?

Rx IDLs are able to reach **3 mm** outside of the prostate gland.

What can be done to place sources into the tissues surrounding the prostate to provide extracapsular coverage?

In order to reliably place sources into tissues surrounding the prostate, **linked seeds embedded in vicryl sutures** can be placed in the peripheral portions of the prostate.

Prior to the closed transperineal approach, what other method of seed implantation was used?

Prior to the transperineal approach, an **open retropubic laparotomy** method of seed implantation was used.

In prostate LDR brachy, to what do "D90" and "V100" refer and what are the recommended values for these parameters?

In prostate LDR brachy, the **D90 refers to the min dose that covers 90% of the postimplant prostate volume** (given as a % of the prescribed dose). The goal **D90 is >90%** of the Rx dose. The **V100 refers to the volume of the prostate receiving 100% of the Rx dose.** The goal **V100 is >90%.** While D90 and V100 are strongly correlated, D90 is used to describe how hot or cold an implant is with respect to the Rx dose and V100 is used to describe how well the implant covers the desired target.

In prostate brachy, why is the D90 parameter used and not the D100?

D90 is used instead of D100 to evaluate postimplant dosimetry b/c **retrospective studies have identified D90 as a better predictor of long-term biochemical control.** D90 may be a better predictor of outcomes b/c it is less sensitive to small differences in the way a prostate is contoured between users on postimplant CTs. (*Potters L et al., IJROBP 2001*)

In prostate brachy, to what do "RV100" and "Ur150" refer?

RV100 is the volume of the rectum in cubic cm receiving 100% of the Rx dose. Ur150 is the volume of the urethra receiving 150% of the Rx dose.

What are the goal RV100 and Ur150 in prostate brachy planning?

At the JHH, the goal is to limit RV100 to <0.5 cc and Ur150 to <30% of the urethra.

What isotope is typically used in HDR brachy for prostate cancer?

Ir-192 is typically used for HDR brachy to treat prostate cancer.

What is the half-life for Ir-192?

The half-life for Ir-192 is **73.8 days.**

What are the dose/ fractionation schedules that have been used with HDR brachy as monotherapy for low-risk prostate cancer?

HDR dose/fractionation schedules for prostate cancer monotherapy:
1. William Beaumont Hospital schedule: 38 Gy in 4 fx (9.5 Gy/fx) bid (1 implant/day required) (*Martinez AA et al., IJROBP 2009*).
2. California Endocurietherapy Center schedule: 42 Gy in 6 fx (7 Gy/fx) in 2 separate implants 1 wk apart.

Have there been any studies comparing EBRT + brachy boost to EB alone?

Yes. *Hoskin et al.* enrolled 220 pts with T1-T3, local-ized prostate cancer and PSA <50 and randomized to EBRT alone (55 Gy/20 fx [2.75 Gy/fx]) or EBRT + HDR brachy (EBRT 35.75 Gy/13 fx [2.75/fx] and then 8.5 Gy HDR × 2 over 2 days). Mean PSA RFS (using the 1997 ASTRO definition) was 5.1 yrs (combined) vs. 4.3 yrs (EBRT alone). The results of this study are difficult to interpret given the nonstandard fractionation in the control arm. (*Radiother Oncol 2007*)

■ Treatment/Prognosis

Estimate the long-term (8–10 yr) biochemical control in low-risk pts treated with LDR brachy.

Estimates of long-term (8–10 yr) biochemical control vary from **82%–94%.** (*Koukourakis G et al., Adv Urol 2009*)

Is bladder cancer more common in men or women?	In the U.S., bladder cancer is diagnosed **3 times more frequently in men** than women. For squamous histology, the incidence between men and women are equal.
What is the most common histologic subtype of bladder cancer in developed and developing countries?	In developed countries, **90% of bladder cancers are transitional cell carcinomas (TCCs).** In developing countries, **75% of bladder cancers are SCCs.**
What are the different histopathologic types of bladder cancer in order of decreasing frequency?	The most common histology of bladder cancer in the U.S. is TCC/urothelial carcinoma (94%) > SCC (3%) > adenocarcinoma (2%) > small cell tumors (1%).
What % of newly detected bladder tumors are Ta/Tis/T1 lesions?	~**70%** of all newly diagnosed bladder cancers are exophytic papillary tumors, with 70% of these confined to the mucosa (Ta/Tis) and 30% confined to the submucosa (T1). (*Herr HW et al., Cancer: Principles and practice of oncology. 6th ed. 2001*)
What are important prognostic factors in pts with bladder cancer?	Bladder cancer prognostic factors: 1. Tumor grade 2. DOI 3. Stage 4. Histologic subtype
Approximately what % of bladder cancer pts have metastatic Dz at presentation, and what are the common sites of mets?	~**8%** of newly diagnosed bladder cancer pts have metastatic Dz at presentation, usually involving the bone, lungs, or liver.

▊ Workup/Staging

What are the common presenting signs and Sx of bladder cancer?	In pts with bladder cancer, the most common presenting Sx is **hematuria** → urinary frequency and pelvic/flank pain.
What are the initial steps in the workup of a pt suspected to have bladder cancer? What additional workup is needed after a cancer Dx is made?	Pts suspected to have bladder cancer should 1st obtain **urine cytology or undergo cystoscopy.** If a lesion is identified, they should proceed to have a **transurethral resection of bladder tumor (TURBT) and EUA.** If the lesion identified by cystoscopy is solid, of high grade, or suspicious for muscle invasion, then **CT abdomen/pelvis should be performed.** If a cancer Dx is made, **image the upper urinary tract** (intravenous pyelogram, retrograde pyelogram, renal US, or MRI urogram) **and chest** (CXR or CT). Consider bone scan if there is locally advanced Dz. Recommended blood work includes **CBC/CMP.** (*NCCN 2010*)

In the initial TURBT sample of a bladder tumor, what should be present in the pathologic specimen?

The Bx specimen should contain **muscle from the bladder wall** to properly stage the tumor. If there is presence of muscle-invasive Dz, the pathology specimen should also contain **perivesicular fat** to assess the extent of Dz.

What are the indications for re-resection after initial TURBT?

Repeat resection should be performed after initial TURBT when there is **incomplete initial resection, no muscle in tissue sample, a large lesion, any T1 lesion, or insufficient sample to definitively call a T2 lesion.**

What is the AJCC 7th edition (2009) T-stage criteria for bladder cancer?

Ta: noninvasive papillary carcinoma
Tis: CIS ("flat tumor")
T1: tumor invades subepithelial connective tissue
T2a: tumor invades superficial muscularis propria (inner half)
T2b: tumor invades deep muscularis propria (outer half)
T3a: microscopic invasion of perivesical tissue
T3b: macroscopic invasion of perivesical tissue (extravesical mass)
T4a: tumor invades prostatic stroma, uterus, vagina
T4b: tumor invades pelvic wall, abdominal wall

What is the probability of pelvic nodal involvement based on the T stage of a bladder tumor?

Pelvic node involvement by bladder cancer T stage based on the surgical series by *Stein JP et al.*:
Overall: 24% LN+
T0-T1: 5%
T2: 18%
T3a: 26%
T3b: 46%
T4: 42%

(*JCO 2001*)

What is the AJCC 7th edition (2009) N- and M-stage criteria for bladder cancer?

N0: no regional LN mets
N1: single LN in true pelvis (hypogastric, obturator, external iliac, or presacral)
N2: multiple LNs in true pelvis
N3: mets to common iliac LN
M0: no DM
M1: DM

Define the AJCC 7th edition (2009) bladder cancer stage grouping based on TNM status.

Stage 0a: Ta, N0, M0
Stage 0is: Tis, N0, M0
Stage I: T1, N0, M0
Stage II: T2, N0, M0
Stage III: T3 or T4a, N0, M0
Stage IV: T4b or N+ or M1

Is there a role for RT alone in the management of locally advanced bladder cancer?

Rarely. Multiple nonrandomized trials and 1 RCT (*Coppin CM et al., JCO 2006*) suggest superior results with CRT, as well as cystectomy, compared to RT alone in the management of pts with muscle-invasive bladder cancer. RT alone, or in combination with a low-dose radiosensitizer (e.g., cisplatin or 5-FU), may be considered if surgery or full-dose chemo cannot be tolerated.

Is there data to support preop RT → cystectomy over definitive RT alone?

Yes. Several RCTs have compared preop and immediate cystectomy to RT alone for the Tx of bladder cancer, and results favor the surgery arms. Therefore, consider preop RT (or preop CRT) to convert unresectable to resectable tumors.

Danish National Cancer Group: 183 pts, 40 Gy + cystectomy vs. 60 Gy. 5-yr OS was not different, but local/pelvic failure favored the surgery arm (7% vs. 35%). (*Sell A et al., Scand J Urol Neph 1991*)

MDA RCT: 67 pts, 50 Gy + cystectomy vs. 60 Gy. 5-yr OS favored the surgery arm (45% vs. 22%, SS). (*Miller LS, Cancer 1977*)

What % of pts with muscle-invasive bladder cancer treated for bladder preservation achieve a CR after induction cisplatin-based CRT?

~**70%** of pts with muscle-invasive bladder cancer achieve a CR after Tx with induction cisplatin-based CRT. (*Shipley WU et al., Urology 2002*)

What % of pts with muscle-invasive bladder cancer achieve a CR after preop chemo?

~**38%** of pts with muscle-invasive bladder cancer achieve a CR with preop methotrexate/vinblastine/doxorubicin/cisplatin (MVAC). (*Grossman HB et al., NEJM 2003*)

What % of pts with muscle-invasive bladder cancer achieve a CR after preop TURBT alone?

~**15%** of pts with muscle-invasive bladder cancer achieve a CR after preop TURBT alone. (*Grossman HB et al., NEJM 2003*)

What are the 5-yr OS outcomes of pts treated with cystectomy vs. bladder preservation?

CRT-based bladder preservation has not been directly compared to cystectomy alone in an RCT.

5-yr OS estimates for cystectomy alone:
Ta: 95%
T1: 50%–80%
T2: 60%–80%
T3b-T4: 20%–40%
pN+: 15%–30%

5-yr OS estimates for bladder preservation:
T2: 60%
T3b-T4: 45%

(*Shipley WU et al., Urology 2002; Rodel C et al., J Clin Oncol 2002*)

What are the predicted 5-yr OS rates based on stage?

Relative 5-yr OS rates for bladder cancer based on SEER data:

Stage 0: 98%
Stage I: 88%
Stage II: 63%
Stage III: 46%
Stage IV: 15%

What is considered 1st-line chemo (neoadj, adj, or metastatic) in the management of bladder cancer?

Gemcitabine/cisplatin is the 1st-line chemo used in the neoadj, adj, or metastatic setting for pts with bladder cancer. This combination has led to equivalent outcomes but an improved toxicity profile when compared to MVAC in RCTs. (*Roberts JT et al., Ann Oncol 2006*)

What is the Tx strategy for pts with unresectable (cT4, fixed bladder mass, LN+) bladder cancer?

For pts with unresectable bladder cancer, **chemo × 2–3 +/− RT** is administered → restaging with cystoscopy and CT scan. If the tumor becomes resectable, the pt should proceed to cystectomy. If not, consolidation chemo +/− RT is indicated. For those who achieve a CR, consider observation.

How is locally recurrent bladder cancer treated after initial Tx with bladder preservation?

The type of intervention for LF after bladder preservation for bladder cancer is dependent on the extent of Dz. **Recurrent noninvasive Dz may be treated with intravesical BCG. Invasive Dz is treated with radical cystectomy.** In the case of bulky Dz recurrence following >65 Gy EBRT, chemo alone may be considered.

How is metastatic bladder cancer treated?

Combination chemo (**gemcitabine** 1,000 mg/m^2 days 1, 8, and 15 of a 28-day cycle and **cisplatin** 70 mg/m^2 on day 2) should be used for pts with metastatic bladder cancer who have good performance status, no visceral or bone involvement, and normal alk phos and LDH levels. Alternatively, MVAC or taxane-based regimens may be considered. **Pemetrexed may be used in cisplatin-refractory Dz.** Local therapy (surgery or RT) may be considered depending on the extent of response to chemo.

What is the MS for untreated vs. treated metastatic bladder cancer?

MS is **<6 mos for untreated** and **13 mos for treated** metastatic bladder cancer.

How should the histologic variants of urothelial carcinomas (e.g., SCC, adenocarcinoma, sarcomatoid, nested micropapillary subtypes, etc.) be treated?

Chemotherapeutic agents should be selected that target the individual variant histologies of bladder cancer.

What is the best established risk factor for testicular cancer?

A **Hx of cryptorchidism** increases the risk of testicular cancer by ~5 times. The higher the undescended testicle (inguinal canal vs. intra-abdominal), the higher the risk. Orchiopexy prior to puberty lowers this risk. 5%–20% of tumors in pts with a Hx of cryptorchidism develop in the contralat, normally descended testis. The risk is greatest in cases of bilat cryptorchidism.

In a pt with a prior Dx of testicular cancer, what is the cumulative incidence (at 25 yrs) of contralat testicular seminoma?

At 25 yrs following the primary Dx, the cumulative incidence of contralat testicular seminoma is **3.6%.**

What is the most common chromosomal abnormality in testicular GCTs?

A **12p isochromosome** (i.e., a chromosome with 2 copies of the short arm of chromosome 12) is the most common testicular GCT chromosomal abnormality.

Name the layers of tissue surrounding the testes from outer to inner.

Layers of tissue surrounding the testes (outer to inner):
1. Skin
2. Tunica dartos
3. External spermatic fascia
4. Cremaster muscle
5. Internal spermatic fascia
6. Parietal layer of tunica vaginalis
7. Visceral layer of tunica vaginalis
8. Tunica albuginea

Compare and contrast lymphatic drainage of the left vs. right testis.

Lymphatic drainage from testicular tumors goes directly to the para-aortic (P-A) nodes. The left testicular vein drains to the left renal vein, and nodal drainage is primarily to the P-A nodes, directly below the left renal hilum. The right testicular vein drains to the IVC; paracaval and interaortocaval nodes are most commonly involved. Lymphatic drainage from the right testes commonly crosses over to the left, but the reverse is rare.

What is the chance of pelvic/inguinal nodal involvement from testicular cancer? What increases this risk?

Pelvic/inguinal nodes are rarely (<3%) involved by testicular cancer. Risk of involvement increases with:
1. Prior scrotal or inguinal surgery
2. Tumor invasion of the tunica vaginalis or lower one third of epididymis
3. Cryptorchidism

What is the DDx of a testicular mass?

The DDx of a testicular mass includes tumor, torsion, hydrocele, varicocele, spermatocele, and epididymitis.

What is the classic presentation of testicular cancer?

A **painless testicular mass** is the classic presentation of testicular cancer. However, up to 45% of pts will present with pain.

■ Workup/Staging

What imaging modality is preferred for primary evaluation of a testicular mass?

Transscrotal US is preferred for primary evaluation of a testicular mass. Testicular tumors are typically hypoechoic.

What is the preferred primary surgical Tx for a unilat testicular tumor?

Transinguinal orchiectomy is the preferred surgical Tx for unilat testicular tumor.

What are 3 tumor markers that should be drawn before orchiectomy for testicular tumor?

Before orchiectomy for a testicular tumor, levels of **β-HCG, AFP, and LDH** should be drawn.

What are the half-lives of β-HCG and AFP?

The half-life for **β-HCG is 22 hrs.** The half-life for **AFP is 5 days.**

How commonly are β-HCG and AFP elevated in testicular seminoma vs. NSGCT? What are unrelated etiologies for elevated β-HCG and AFP?

β-HCG is elevated in 15% of seminomas. AFP is never elevated in seminoma. 1 or both markers will be elevated in 85% of NSGCTs. The use of marijuana can elevate β-HCG, and reagent cross reaction with LH can cause falsely elevated results. Hepatocellular carcinoma, cirrhosis, hepatitis, and pregnancy can elevate AFP.

What imaging studies, labs, and evaluation should be ordered following transinguinal orchiectomy for seminoma?

Following transinguinal orchiectomy for seminoma, chest imaging (CXR), CT abdomen/pelvis, AFP, β-HCG, and LDH should be ordered. If the CT is positive, bone scan should be added. Pts should also have fertility evaluation and consider sperm banking.

Describe the AJCC 7th edition (2009) TNM and S staging for testicular tumors.

T1: limited to testis and epididymis with no LVSI or tunica vaginalis involvement
T2: LVSI or involvement of tunica vaginalis
T3: involvement of spermatic cord
T4: scrotal invasion
N1: single or multiple regional nodes, all ≤2 cm in greatest dimension
N2: single or multiple regional nodes, any >2–5 cm in greatest dimension
N3: single or multiple regional nodes, any >5 cm in greatest dimension
M1a: nonregional nodal or pulmonary Dz
M1b: nonpulmonary visceral mets
S0: normal LDH, β-HCG, and AFP
S1: LDH <1.5 times normal, β-HCG <5,000 mIU/mL, and AFP <1,000 ng/mL
S2: LDH 1.5–10 times normal, β-HCG 5,000–50,000, or AFP 1,000–10,000
S3: LDH >10 times normal, β-HCG >50,000, or AFP >10,000

Summarize the AJCC 7th edition (2009) stage grouping for testicular tumors.

Stage I: no Dz beyond testis/scrotum (i.e., T1-4N0M0S1-3)

Stage II: regional nodal involvement and S0-S1 tumor markers (IIA = N1, IIB = N2, IIC = N3)

Stage III: S2-S3 tumor markers with N1-S3 Dz, or M1 Dz

What is the stage group distribution for testicular seminoma at presentation?

Most testicular seminoma pts present with stage I Dz (70%–80%), 15%–20% have stage II Dz, and 5% have stage III Dz.

In addition to AJCC staging, what is another common staging system for testicular seminoma?

In addition to AJCC staging, **Royal Marsden staging** is also used for testicular seminoma. This staging is largely similar to the AJCC stage grouping:

Stage I: confined to testis
Stage IIA: node <2 cm
Stage IIB: node 2–5 cm
Stage IIC: node 5–10 cm
Stage IID: node >10 cm
Stage III: nodes above/below diaphragm
Stage IV: extralymphatic mets

▪ Treatment/Prognosis

Following transinguinal orchiectomy, what is the optimal Tx for stage I seminoma, stage IIA–IIB seminoma, and stage IIC or greater seminoma?

Following transinguinal orchiectomy, pts with stage I seminoma may rcv adj RT, surveillance, or chemo. Pts with stage IIA–IIB Dz should rcv adj RT. Pts with stage IIC or greater Dz should be treated with chemo.

When observing stage I seminoma pts, what is the relapse rate? Where do most relapses occur?

When observed following transinguinal orchiectomy for stage I seminoma, **15% of pts will relapse.** 85% of relapses are in the **P-A nodes.**

What 2 pathologic factors are associated with increased risk of relapse following transinguinal orchiectomy for stage I seminoma?

Pooled analysis of pts observed following transinguinal orchiectomy for stage I seminoma from 4 centers show that tumor size >4 cm (RR 2.0), rete testis involvement (RR 1.7), or both (RR 3.4) increased the risk for relapse. (*Warde P et al., J Clin Oncol 2002*)

Following P-A relapse in pts observed following transinguinal orchiectomy for stage I seminoma, what are the appropriate Tx options?

Following P-A relapse in pts observed following transinguinal orchiectomy for stage I seminoma, **retroperitoneal RT** (for nodes <5 cm) **or chemo** are reasonable Tx options.

For pts treated with P-A RT following transinguinal orchiectomy for stage I seminoma, what is the relapse rate? Where do relapses occur?

For pts treated with P-A RT following transinguinal orchiectomy for stage I seminoma, relapse occurs in 0.5%–5% of pts. Most relapses occur within 2 yrs. In-field relapses are extremely rare; most relapses are mediastinal, lung, left supraclavicular, or (if risk factors are present) inguinal.

What data supports the option of adj chemo for stage I seminoma following transinguinal orchiectomy?

MRC-UK randomized 1,447 stage I seminoma pts between adj RT (2 Gy/fx to 20 or 30 Gy) and 1 cycle of carboplatin. There was no difference in 3-yr relapse rates (3.4% for RT vs. 4.6% for carboplatin). (*Oliver R et al., Lancet 2005*)

In a stage I seminoma pt, what factors would favor adj RT over surveillance? What factors favor surveillance?

In a stage I seminoma pt, risk factors such as >4-cm primary or rete testis invasion favor adj RT. Concern over pt adherence with follow-up also favors RT. Hx of inflammatory bowel Dz, horseshoe kidney, or prior RT favor surveillance. Concern over 2nd malignancy also favors surveillance.

Why is P-A RT not part of the definitive management of pts with stage IIC seminoma?

P-A RT is not part of the definitive management of pts with stage IIC seminoma due to **high rates of distant failure** (mediastinal, lung, supraclavicular, or bone). Thus, chemo is needed. In 1 series, 5-yr RFS among IIC pts treated with orchiectomy and RT alone was only 44% (*Chung PW et al., Eur Urol 2004*).

What is the appropriate Tx for pts with stage I–IIB seminoma following relapse after adj P-A RT?

Pts with stage I–IIB seminoma who relapse following adj P-A RT should be treated with **salvage chemo.**

How should seminoma pts with stage IIC or greater be treated?

4 cycles of cisplatin/etoposide (+/− bleomycin) are appropriate for seminoma pts with stage IIC or greater.

What is the appropriate RT field for stage I seminoma pts?

Stage I seminoma pts (if receiving adj RT) should have the P-A nodes treated. **MRC-UK TE 10** randomized 478 pts to P-A RT +/− pelvic RT and found equivalent RFS (96%) (*Fossa SD et al., J Clin Oncol 1999*). 4 pelvic failures occurred in the P-A group (vs. none in the P-A + pelvic group).

For adj stage I seminoma, what are the borders for a P-A field?

Borders for a P-A field (for adj stage I seminoma):
    <u>Superior</u>: T10-11
    <u>Inferior</u>: L5-S1
    <u>Lateral</u>: 2 cm on vertebral bodies. If left-sided
        primary, give 1-cm border on left renal hilum
        and sacroiliac joint.

What is the appropriate field for a stage IIA–IIB seminoma pt?

A stage IIA–IIB seminoma pt should have a "dogleg" or "hockey stick" field treated (including P-A and ipsi pelvic nodes). The sup border is at T10-11, and the inf border is at the obturator foramen. Per **MRC-UK TE 10:**

Superior: T10-11

Inferior: mid obturator foramen

Ipsilateral: renal hilum down as far as disk between 5th lumbar and 1st sacral vertebrae (L5-S1), then diagonally to lat edge of acetabulum, then vertically downward to mid obturator level

Contralateral: inclusion of processus transversus in P-A area down to L5-S1, then diagonally in parallel with ipsi border, then vertically to median border of obturator foramen

What is a reasonable dose and fractionation schedule for stage I seminoma?

For stage I seminoma, doses from 20–25 Gy are commonly prescribed. 125 cGy/fx to 25 Gy is a common schedule (favored at Princess Margaret Hospital). The **MRC-UK TE 18** trial compared 2 Gy/fx to 20 Gy vs. 30 Gy and found equivalent relapse rates at 5 yrs (*Jones WG et al., J Clin Oncol 2005*).

What is a reasonable dose and fractionation schedule for stage IIA–IIB seminoma?

For stage IIA–IIB seminoma, the "dogleg" field may be treated with 125 cGy/fx to 25 Gy. Gross LAD may be boosted with an additional 10 Gy (30 Gy for IIA, 36 Gy for IIB).

What pathologic subtype of seminoma can be uniformly treated with orchiectomy alone?

Spermatocytic seminoma can be treated with orchiectomy alone. This tumor is seen in older pts and, while the precursor cell is unknown, is probably not a true seminoma.

▨ Toxicity

What RT dose can induce temporary azoospermia? Doses greater than what may cause permanent aspermia?

RT doses as low as 20–50 cGy will cause temporary azoospermia. Doses >50 cGy can cause extended or permanent aspermia.

What is the RR of a 2nd non-GCT in pts who rcv adj RT for testicular seminoma?

The RR of a 2nd non-GCT in pts who rcv adj RT for testicular seminoma is **2**. (*Travis LB et al., JNCI 2005*)

What should be done to reduce the testicular RT dose during Tx for testicular seminoma?

During RT for testicular seminoma, a **clamshell should be used** to reduce the dose to the contralat testis.

How does the recommended follow-up differ for stage I pts treated with single-agent carboplatinum vs. a P-A field?

Per NCCN 2010 guidelines, pts treated with single-agent carboplatinum require **the same intensive follow-up as pts being surveilled**—i.e., H&P, LDH, AFP, and β-HCG q3–4mos for yrs 1–3, q6mos for yrs 4–7, then annually. CT abdomen/pelvis should be performed at every visit and CXR at every other visit. **Pts who were treated with P-A RT require less intensive follow-up:** H&P, LDH, AFP, and β-HCG q3–4mos for yr 1 only, q6mos for yr 2, then annually. CT pelvis is required annually only for the 1st 3 yrs (and only for pts who did not get their pelvic nodes treated).

60

Testicular Nonseminomatous Germ Cell Tumor

Kristin Janson Redmond and Thomas J. Guzzo

▌ Background

Approximately how many cases of germ cell tumor (GCT) are diagnosed annually in the U.S.?

~**8,000 cases/yr** in the U.S.

What % of testicular malignancies are GCTs?

~**95%** of testicular malignancies are GCTs.

What is the most common solid tumor in men age 15–34 yrs?

GCT is the most common solid tumor in men age 15–34 yrs.

How has the incidence of GCTs changed in the past 40 yrs?

The incidence of GCTs has **more than doubled** in the past 40 yrs.

Name 5 risk factors for GCTs.

Risk factors for GCTs:
1. Prior personal Hx of GCT
2. Positive family Hx
3. Cryptorchidism
4. Testicular dysgenesis
5. Klinefelter syndrome

Per the International Germ Cell Cancer Collaborative Group, what 3 factors must be met to be classified as *intermediate*-risk NSGCT?

Per the International Germ Cell Cancer Collaborative Group (*JCO 1997*), intermediate-risk NSGCT must meet *both* of the following:
1. Testicular or retroperitoneal primary tumor
2. No nonpulmonary visceral mets

and any of the following intermediate risk factors:
3a. AFP 1,000–10,000 ng/mL
3b. β-HCG 5,000–50,000 mIU/mL
3c. LDH 1.5–10 times the upper limit of normal

Per the International Germ Cell Cancer Collaborative Group, the presence of any of which 5 factors leads to classification of *poor*-risk NSGCT?

Per the International Germ Cell Cancer Collaborative Group (*JCO 1997*), poor-risk NSGCT has *any* of the following:
1. Mediastinal primary tumor
2. Nonpulmonary visceral mets
3. AFP >10,000 ng/mL
4. β-HCG >50,000 mIU/mL
5. LDH >10 times the upper limit of normal

▪ Treatment/Prognosis

Per NCCN 2010, what is the Tx of stage I good- or intermediate-risk NSGCT?

The Tx of stage I good- or intermediate-risk NSGCT is **observation** after orchiectomy if compliant vs. retroperitoneal lymph node dissection (RPLND) vs. bleomycin/etoposide/cisplatin (BEP) chemo × 2 cycles (stage IB only).

What is the risk of relapse after orchiectomy alone for stage I good- or intermediate-risk NSGCT if tumor markers are normal postoperatively?

The risk of relapse after orchiectomy alone for stage I good- or intermediate-risk NSGCT if tumor markers are normal postoperatively is ~**30%.**

Per NCCN 2010, how should pts with stage I NSGCT be monitored in an observation protocol?

Observation in pts with stage I NSGCT should consist of visits, tumor markers, and CXR q1–2mos for yr 1, q2mos yr 2, q3mos yr 3, q4mos yr 4, q6mos yr 5, and q12mos if >6 yrs. CT abdomen/pelvis should be done q2–3mos yr 1, q3–4mos yr 2, q4mos yr 3, q6mos yr 4, and q12mos if >5 yrs.

What did the Medical Research Council Trial TE08 show for pts with stage I NSGCT?

MRC TE 08 randomized 414 pts with stage I NSGCT s/p orchiectomy with normal serum markers (10% high risk with LVI) to CT chest/abdomen at 3 and 12 mos vs. CT scans at 3, 6, 9, 12, and 24 mos. At median follow-up of 3.3 yrs, 2-yr RFS was 79% with 2 scans vs. 84% with 5 scans (NSS). The 1st indication of relapse was markers in 39% and CT abdomen in 39%. The conclusion is that CT scans at 3 and 12 mos after orchiectomy might be reasonable in low-risk pts and that chest CT may be unnecessary. (*Rustin GJ et al., JCO 2007*)

What is the chance of positive nodes on RPLND despite a negative CT scan in pts with stage I NSGCT?

The risk of positive nodes on RPLND despite negative CT scan in pts with stage I NSGCT is **30%.**

What is the relapse rate in pts with stage I NSGCT after orchiectomy → RPLND?

The relapse rate in pts with stage I NSGCT after orchiectomy → RPLND is **5%–10%,** most commonly to the lungs.

Per NCCN 2010, how should pts with NSGCT and persistently positive tumor markers after orchiectomy be treated?

Pts with NSGCT and persistently positive tumor markers after orchiectomy should be treated with either BEP × 3 cycles or cisplatin/etoposide (EP) × 4 cycles.

What did the German Testicular Study Group AUO trial AH 01/94 show for pts with stage I NSGCT?

The **AUO AH 01/94** trial randomized 382 pts with clinical stage I NSGCT to RPLND vs. BEP × 1 cycle. At median follow-up of 4.7 yrs, 2-yr RFS was 92% with surgery and 99% with BEP (HR 7.9, SS). The authors concluded that 1 course of BEP is superior to RPLND in clinical stage I Dz. (*Albers P et al., JCO 2008*)

Per NCCN 2010, how should pts with stage II NSGCT with a +node diagnosed only after RPLND be treated?

Stage II NSGCT with a +node diagnosed only after RPLND should be treated with **2 cycles of BEP chemo.**

Per NCCN 2010, what is the Tx of pts with bulky stage II or III NSGCT?

Pts with bulky stage II or III NSGCT should be treated with **either BEP × 3 cycles or EP × 4 cycles.**

What is the role of RT in the primary Tx of NSGCT?

Although RT may be used for palliation of metastatic Dz, there is no established role for RT in the primary Tx of NSGCT.

Per NCCN 2010, what is the follow-up for pts with NSGCT with CR to chemo and/or RPLND?

Surveillance of pts with NSGCT after CR to chemo and/or RPLND should consist of visits, tumor markers, and CXR q2–3mos yrs 1–2, q4mos yrs 3–4, q6mos yr 5, and q12mos if >6 yrs. CT abdomen/pelvis should be done q6mos yr 1, q6–12mos yr 2, q12mos yrs 3–5, and q12–24mos if >6 yrs.

■ Toxicity

What is the major toxicity associated with RPLND?

The major toxicity associated with RPLND is **retrograde ejaculation resulting in infertility;** however, nerve-sparing techniques can preserve ejaculation in 95% of cases.

What is the pathognomonic complication of bleomycin chemo?

Bleomycin-induced pneumonitis

61

Penile Cancer

Jing Zeng and Alexander Lin

Background

What is the estimated annual incidence of penile cancer Dx in the U.S.? What % of male cancers does this represent? How is this different in developing countries?

There are ~**1,500 new cases/yr** of penile cancer in the U.S., representing <**1% of male cancers.** In developing countries, it can account for 10%–20% of all male cancers.

Name 3 factors associated with the risk of developing penile cancer.

Risk factors for penile cancer:
1. Lack of circumcision
2. Phimosis
3. HPV infection
4. HIV infection

Others factors that may also be associated include smoking, PUVA therapy, and family Hx.

What causes condyloma acuminata?

Condyloma acuminata, more commonly known as genital warts, are associated with **HPV infection.** They are usually benign but can undergo malignant transformation.

What is the difference between erythroplasia of Queyrat (EQ) and Bowen Dz?

Both EQ and Bowen Dz are CIS conditions. **EQ** occurs within the penile mucocutaneous epithelium (**glans and prepuce**), whereas **Bowen Dz** occurs within follicle-bearing epithelium (**penile shaft**).

What are the 2 most common anatomic locations for penile cancer?

The **glans and prepuce** are the 2 most common locations for penile cancer. Less common locations include the coronal sulcus and the shaft. Lesions can appear as a mass, ulceration, or inflammation.

To what LNs do penile cancers primarily drain to 1st?

Inguinal LNs are the initial site of nodal involvement in penile cancers → iliac and pelvic nodes.

What is the anatomic position of the penis?

The anatomic position of the penis is **erect;** the descriptors *dorsal* and *ventral* refer to the anatomic position.

Approximately what % of men with penile cancer and palpable inguinal LAD have pathologically positive nodal mets?

Overall, ~**58%** of palpable inguinal nodes in pts with penile cancer are actually positive for cancer mets on pathology. The rest of the nodes are reactive.

In men with penile cancer and clinically negative nodes, what is the likelihood of occult nodal mets?

In men with penile cancer and clinically negative nodes, the likelihood of occult nodal mets depends on the tumor stage, grade, and presence of LVI. Roughly, it can be **11%–20% for T1 lesions** and up to **60%–75% for T2-T3 lesions.**

What % of men with penile cancer present with DM lesions?

Hematogenous spread of penile cancer is rare until late in the Dz course and is found in only **1%–10%** of men at initial presentation.

What are the most common sites for DM in penile cancer?

Lung, liver, and bone are the most common sites for DM in penile cancer.

What is the most common histology in penile cancer?

Squamous cell carcinoma accounts for 95% of penile malignancies. Other histologic subtypes such as sarcoma, urethral tumors, lymphoma, and basal cell carcinoma are extremely rare.

■ Workup/Staging

What is the workup for penile cancer?

Penile cancer workup: H&P, CBC, chemistry panel, MRI penis/pelvis. **Consider PET/CT and inguinal sentinal LN Bx.**

How should clinically negative LNs in penile cancer be evaluated?

Clinically negative LNs in penile cancer should be evaluated with **CT, MRI, or PET scan,** but the FPR and FNR are both high regardless of the imaging modality. Inguinal sentinel LN Bx is promising (FNR 7%).

Should clinically negative nodes in penile cancer undergo inguinal dissection?

The toxicity of inguinal LND should be weighed against the likelihood of occult nodal mets in penile cancer. **LND may be considered for ≥T2 tumors or for high-grade lesions.** Recent studies suggest that sentinel LN Bx may be a reasonable alternative (*Leijte JA et al., JCO 2009*).

How should clinically positive LNs in penile cancer be evaluated?

Historically, palpable inguinal LNs in penile cancer can be managed by a 6-wk trial of antibiotics. Newer, alternative approaches include FNA or open Bx.

What is the AJCC 7th edition (2009) T staging for penile cancer?	**Tis:** CIS only **Ta:** noninvasive verrucous carcinoma **T1a:** invades subepithelial connective tissue without LVI and is not poorly differentiated (i.e., not grades 3–4) **T1b:** invades subepithelial connective tissue with LVI or is poorly differentiated **T2:** invades corpora spongiosum or cavernosum **T3:** invades urethra **T4:** invades other adjacent structures
What is the AJCC 7th edition (2009) clinical and pathologic N staging for penile cancer?	**cN1:** palpable mobile unilat inguinal LN **cN2:** palpable mobile multiple or bilat inguinal LN **cN3:** palpable fixed inguinal nodal mass or pelvic LAD **pN1:** single inguinal LN **pN2:** multiple or bilat inguinal LN **pN3:** LN ECE or pelvic LN
What is the AJCC 7th edition (2009) stage grouping for penile cancer?	**Stage I:** T1a, N0, M0 **Stage II:** T1b-T3, N0, M0 **Stage IIIa:** T1-3, N1, M0 **Stage IIIb:** T1-3, N2, M0 **Stage IV:** T4 or N3 or M1

■ Treatment/Prognosis

How are noninvasive penile cancers treated?	CIS of the penis can be treated with **topical 5-FU** with good LC and excellent cosmetic outcome. Other methods that are acceptable include **laser surgery, cryotherapy, photodynamic therapy, and local excision.** Fulguration alone has a high recurrence rate and is not an acceptable option.
What are the Tx options for pts with early-stage penile cancer (T1-T2, <4 cm)?	Early-stage penile cancer Tx options include **penectomy (partial or total)** or an organ preservation approach using **EBRT, brachytherapy, or CRT** (cisplatin based).
How are locally advanced (T3-T4) penile cancers managed?	For locally advanced penile cancers, consider **CRT, with surgery reserved for salvage or total penectomy.** Induction chemo → penile-preserving Tx is under investigation.
What surgical margin is typically required for total or partial penectomy for Tx of invasive penile cancer?	For penile cancer resection, a **2-cm proximal margin is needed to ensure a 10–15-mm histologic margin,** which appears to give good LC.

What length of corpus cavernosum is required in order for 50% of men to be able to have sexual intercourse?

~45% of men are able to have adequate sexual intercourse with about **4–6 cm** of corpus cavernosum.

What residual penile length is required for men to be able to urinate in the standing position?

~**2.5–3 cm** of residual penile length is required for men to be able to urinate in the standing position.

Name 3 penile-sparing techniques for treating penile cancer.

Mohs surgery, laser therapy (mostly for smaller T1-T2 tumors), and **RT** are all penile-sparing techniques for treating penile cancer.

What surgical procedure should accompany any RT for penile cancer?

Circumcision should accompany any RT for penile cancer in applicable pts. This allows for better inspection and staging of the lesion as well as helps to alleviate some of the side effects of RT.

In megavoltage EBRT for penile cancer, should bolus be used?

Yes. Bolus should be used in megavoltage EBRT for penile cancer for dose buildup at the surface (usually a wax or plastic cast with the penis suspended above the abdomen or secured against the abdomen if also treating nodes).

In EBRT for penile cancer, what is the CTV and what dose is typically prescribed?

In EBRT for penile cancer, the **CTV is the entire penile length** and typically goes to **45–50 Gy,** with a 10–20 Gy boost to the tumor + a 2-cm margin. Pelvic fields + inguinal nodes are treated to 45 Gy if the pelvic nodes are included in the Tx. Boost to any clinically **gross Dz (65–70 Gy).**

What types of penile cancer lesions are acceptable for brachytherapy?

Penile cancer lesions that can be treated with brachytherapy are typically **<4 cm in diameter** and have **<1 cm of corpora invasion (T1-T2).**

What are 2 ways of delivering brachytherapy in penile cancer, and what is the dose prescribed?

Brachytherapy for penile cancer can be delivered by either (a) using **molds containing sources** such as iridium-192 (less appropriate for pts with short penile length) or (b) using **interstitial implants** by placing catheters 1–1.5 cm apart, perpendicular to the penile axis and afterloading with sources. The **target dose is 55–60 Gy,** with the urethral dose limited to 50 Gy.

How are pts with penile cancers simulated for EBRT?

Simulation for EBRT for penile cancer Tx: supine position and frog-legged, Foley catheter, and penis surrounded with bolus material. If treating pelvic and inguinal nodes, the penis is secured cranially into the pelvic field.

▪ Treatment/Prognosis

What factors affect the Tx strategy of urethral cancer?

Location (ant vs. post), size, DOI, and presence of nodal mets or DMs are the major factors affecting prognosis and Tx strategy.

Does location correlate to the stage/prognosis of urethral cancer?

Yes. Proximal lesions more often present at a higher stage and thus carry a worse prognosis.

What types of surgical resections have been used for male urethral cancer pts?

Multiple forms of conservative resections have been used for very early Dz (Tis-T1), including transurethral resection, laser ablation, and microsurgical resection. Radical resections, which have been the historical standard, include partial and total penectomy and penectomy with cystoprostatectomy.

What are the desired margins for a partial penectomy in urethral cancer?

A **2-cm margin** is desired for a partial penectomy.

What is expected outcome for early-stage (Tis-T1) male pts treated with surgery alone?

Based on the MSKCC experience, among 10 male pts (Tis-T1) treated with various surgical strategies, **DFS at 5 yrs was 83%.** (*Dalbagni G et al., Urology 1999*)

What is the expected outcome for advanced-stage (≥T2) male pts treated with surgery alone?

Based on the MSKCC experience, among 36 male pts (T2-T4) treated with various surgical strategies, **DFS at 5 yrs was 45%** (*Dalbagni G et al., Urology 1999*). Of note, 6 pts were treated with surgical salvage after initial Tx with RT.

What are the outcomes for early-stage (Tis-T1) male pts treated with RT alone?

There is very little data for RT alone in treating male pts with urethral cancer. Only very small series are available. A series of 5 men with early-stage urethral cancer described LC in 4 of those men (*Heysek R et al., J Urol 1985*).

What types of surgical resections have been used for female urethral cancer pts?

Early-stage Dz (Tis-T1) has been treated with local excision, laser excision, transurethral resection, and partial urethrectomy. Radical resection for locally advanced Dz (≥T2) includes ant exenteration, which involves removal of pelvic nodes, the uterus, and appendages, and en bloc resection of pubic symphysis and inf rami.

In locally advanced female urethral cancer (≥pT2), what is the 5-yr OS and LF after ant exenteration alone?

The **5-yr OS is <20%, with a >66% LF rate** in female pts with locally advanced urethral cancer treated with exenteration alone. (*Narayan P, Urol Clin North Am 1992*)

What are outcomes for early-stage (variable definition of early stage includes ant, node— pts without T stage) urethral cancer in female pts treated with RT alone?

A meta-analysis of RT alone in female pts with urethral cancer showed a **5-yr OS of 75% with early-stage Dz and 34% with advanced-stage Dz.** (*Kreig R, Oncology 1999*)

What is the OS for female pts with advanced Dz (variable in definition but in general refers to >T1 Dz, post Dz, or node+ Dz) treated with combined surgery and RT?

Meta-analysis of 34 pts treated in this manner revealed **5-yr OS of 29%** (*Kreig R et al., Oncology 1999*). The single-largest series revealed a 25% OS at 5 yrs among the 20 pts treated (*Grabstald H et al., JAMA 1966*).

What is typical single-modality RT Rx for female urethral cancer?

RT is often given as brachytherapy alone or brachytherapy + EB. Typical Rx include brachytherapy alone to 50–60 Gy and EBRT to 40–45 Gy → brachytherapy to 20–25 Gy. Inguinal nodes should be included.

What are the outcomes for advanced-stage pts treated with CRT?

A number of case reports have shown good results with combined RT and 5-FU/mitomycin-C in both men and women with advanced Dz. A retrospective study of 18 pts from the University of Texas–San Antonio, including male and female pts, demonstrated that among the 8 advanced-stage pts (T3-4N1M1), DFS was 45.2 mos for those treated with CRT compared to 23.3 mos for those treated with surgery alone. Chemo from this study was based on histology and included 5-FU/cisplatin for SCC and carboplatin/Taxol for TCC. There were 8 total high-stage pts in this study. (*Eng T et al., Am J Clin Onc 2003*)

■ Toxicity

What are the expected acute and late RT toxicities associated with Tx of urethral cancer?

Acute toxicities: dermatitis, urinary Sx, diarrhea
Late toxicities: urethral stricture/stenosis, urethrovaginal fistulas, incontinence

▪ Workup/Staging

How is RCC diagnosed?

RCC requires a tissue Dx. Often, nephrectomy is both diagnostic and therapeutic. Percutaneous Bx can also be employed for surgically unfit pts.

What % of biopsied pts have benign Dz?

~**33%** of small renal masses may be characterized as benign according to the specimen obtained.

What imaging is important in the initial workup of RCC?

Imaging workup typically includes contrast-enhanced CT or MRI scan of the abdomen and chest imaging. Consider bone scan and MRI brain if clinically indicated.

Summarize the AJCC 7th edition (2009) T staging for RCC.

T1: limited to kidney and ≤7 cm
T1a: ≤4 cm
T1b: 4–7 cm
T2: limited to kidney and >7 cm
T2a: >7 cm but ≤10 cm
T2b: >10 cm
T3: invades into major veins or perinephric tissues but not into ipsi adrenal gland and not beyond Gerota fascia
T3a: grossly extends into renal vein or its segmental branches, or extends into perirenal and/or renal sinus fat but not beyond Gerota fascia
T3b: extends into vena cava below diaphragm
T3c: extends into vena cava above diaphragm or invades wall of vena cava
T4: invades beyond Gerota fascia, including contiguous extension into ipsi adrenal gland

Summarize the AJCC 7th edition (2009) stage grouping for RCC.

Stage I: T1N0M0
Stage II: T2N0M0
Stage III: T1-2N1M0 or T3N0-1M0
Stage IV: T4 or M1

What other staging systems are widely used for RCC?

The **Robson modification system, Flocks and Kadesky system, and Jewett-Strong classification system** have been used to stage RCC.

Name 3 prognostic factors for RCC.

Prognostic factors for RCC:
1. TNM stage
2. Performance status
3. Furhman grade

▪ Treatment/Prognosis

Describe 4 invasive Tx for locally confined RCC.

Invasive Tx for locally confined RCC:
1. Open nephrectomy
2. Laparoscopic nephrectomy
3. Percutaneous CT-guided cryosurgery
4. Percutaneous radiofrequency ablation
5. Partial nephrectomy

Are there any studies comparing laparoscopic resection with that of open resection in pts with RCC?

Yes. There is retrospective data that compared laparoscopic resection vs. open resection of RCC. There was no difference in DFS. (*Luo JH et al. World J Urol 2009; Marszalek M et al., Eur Urol 2009*)

Are there surgical options for pts with bilat RCC or unilat RCC with a diseased contralat kidney?

Yes. Pts with bilat RCC or a diseased contralat kidney can be treated with nephron-sparing nephrectomy or partial nephrectomy if the renal mass is small.

When is recurrence most likely to occur following surgery for RCC?

Recurrence of RCC is most likely to occur 3–5 yrs after nephrectomy.

Name 4 predictors of RCC recurrence after nephrectomy.

Predictors of RCC recurrence after nephrectomy:
1. Nuclear grade (Fuhrman grade)
2. TNM stage
3. DNA ploidy
4. Genetic RCC syndromes

What are the most common sites of RCC recurrence after nephrectomy?

Most common sites of RCC recurrence after nephrectomy:
1. Lung
2. Bone
3. Regional LNs

What follow-up imaging is recommended for RCC pts after nephrectomy?

RCC pts after nephectomy should be followed with **CXR/CT chest and CT/MRI abdomen.**

For how long should pts with RCC treated with nephrectomy be followed?

Pts with RCC treated with nephrectomy should be followed **for life** (sporadic RCC recurrences have been documented ≥40 yrs later).

Are there any prospective randomized studies examining the role for adj therapy in pts with RCC treated with initial nephrectomy?

Yes. IFN α-2b within 1 mo after surgery vs. Tx only after postsurgical relapse demonstrated no EFS or OS benefit. (*Messing EM et al., JCO 2003*)

What is the 1st-line Tx for pts with metastatic RCC?

1st-line Tx for pts with metastatic RCC:
1. Cytoreductive nephrectomy
2. Metastatectomy for oligomets
3. Sunitinib
4. Temsirolimus
5. Bevacizumab and IFN
6. High-dose recombinant interleukin-2
7. Sorafenib

Cytotoxic chemo for non–clear cell histologies may be considered.

What is the mechanism of action of sorafenib? Of sunitinib?	Sorafenib inhibits multiple kinase pathways, including Raf kinase, PDGF, VEGF receptor 2 and 3, and c-Kit. Sunitinib also inhibits multiple kinase pathways, including PDGF, VEGF, c-KIT, RET, CSF-1R, and flt3.
Is there a role for palliative nephrectomy in pts with RCC?	**Yes.** Palliative nephrectomy is still encouraged to relieve local Sx of pain as well as systemic Sx related to the primary tumor.
What is the data for using cytoreductive surgery in combination with immunotherapy?	Cytoreductive surgery utilized before immunotherapy **may delay time to progression and improve survival of pts with metastatic Dz** (median duration of survival 17 mos vs. 7 mos, SS). (*Mickisch GH et al., Lancet 2001*)
Is there a role for resection of metastatic lesions in pts with RCC?	**Yes.** A retrospective study by *Kavolius et al.* suggests that curative resection of metastatic lesions in pts with RCC improves survival compared to the subtotal resection of pts or those with noncurative salvage attempts (44%, 14%, and 11%, respectively). (*JCO 1998*)
Is there a role for RT to brain mets from RCC?	**Yes.** RCC is widely regarded as a radioresistant tumor. When clinically and technically appropriate, consider SRS for pts with RCC brain mets. (*Jagannathan J et al., Neurosurgery 2010; Te BS et al., Clin Genitourinary Ca 2007*)

▌ Toxicity

What toxicities are associated with sorafenib and sunitinib?	Sorafenib and sunitinib are associated with fatigue, diarrhea, HTN, rash, hand-foot syndrome (sorafenib), and mucositis (sunitinib).

PART IX Gynecology

64

Cervical Cancer
Jing Zeng and Lilie Lin

Background

What is the annual incidence of cervical cancer in the U.S.?	**~11,000 cases/yr** of cervical cancer in the U.S.
What is the mean age of presentation for cervical cancer?	The mean age of presentation for cervical cancer is **47 yrs** in the U.S.
Name 5 lifestyle factors associated with an increased risk of cervical cancer.	Lifestyle factors associated with increased risk of cervical cancer: 1. Early onset of sexual activity 2. Multiple sexual partners 3. Exposure to high-risk partners 4. Hx of STD 5. Smoking 6. High parity 7. Prolonged use of oral contraceptives
HPV is detectable in what % of cervical cancer?	HPV is detectable in **>99%** of cervical cancer.
Roughly what % reduction in mortality has been achieved with PAP screening for cervical cancer?	There has been an **~70% reduction** in cervical cancer mortality with PAP screening.
What does ASCUS stand for (on a PAP result), and how should it be managed?	ASCUS stands for **atypical squamous cells of unknown significance.** About two thirds can resolve spontaneously. Pts can undergo **repeat PAP in 6 mos and then colposcopy if abnl.**
How should LGSIL seen on PAP be managed?	LGSIL resolves spontaneously ~40% of the time; therefore, like with ASCUS, pts can undergo **repeat PAP in 6 mos with colposcopy if abnl.**

How should an HGSIL result from a PAP be managed?

All pts with high-grade SIL should undergo **colposcopy with Bx.** One third of these pts can still resolve spontaneously, but waiting without further investigation is not recommended due to concern for progression.

What % of HGSIL progress to invasive cancers?

~**22%** of HGSIL progress to invasive cancer. This is in contrast to ASCUS (<1%) and LGSIL (~5%).

What % of cervical cancers are caused by HPV 16 and 18?

>**70%** of cervical cancers are caused by HPV 16 and 18.

What HPV subtypes cause most cases of benign warts?

HPV subtypes **6 and 11** cause most cases of benign warts.

In the U.S., what % of cervical cancers are squamous cell carcinomas vs. adenocarcinomas?

With regard to cervical cancers in the U.S., **70% are squamous cell carcinomas,** while ~**25% are adenocarcinomas.**

Name 3 histologic subtypes of adenocarcinoma of the cervix.

Subtypes of adenocarcinoma of the cervix:
1. Mucinous
2. Endometrioid
3. Clear cell
4. Serous

Name 3 common presenting Sx of cervical cancer.

Common presenting Sx of cervical cancer:
1. Abnl vaginal bleeding
2. Postcoital bleeding
3. Abnl vaginal discharge

What specific area of the cervix is the most common point of origin for cervical cancer?

The **transformation zone** is the most common point of origin for cervical cancer. It is a dynamic area between the original and present squamocolumnar junction.

■ Workup/Staging

What should be included in the workup for a pelvic mass?

Pelvic mass workup: H&P, including a careful pelvic exam in the office, basic labs, and EUA with Bx, with cystocopy and proctoscopy for any visible lesions. Studies such as CT, PET, MRI can be obtained for Tx planning purposes (but do not enter FIGO staging of the pt).

What are the areas at risk for local extension of cervical cancer?

Cervical cancer can spread locally to the **corpus, parametria, and vagina.** These should be carefully assessed during a physical exam. Tumor size and parametrial involvement are best assessed by rectovaginal exam.

Name 3 routes of lymphatic drainage from the cervix.

Routes of lymphatic drainage from the cervix:
1. Lat to the external iliac nodes
2. Post into common iliac and lat sacral nodes
3. Post-lat into internal iliac nodes

What imaging studies are allowed in FIGO staging of cervical cancer? What common imaging modalities are not allowed?

CXR and intravenous pyelogram data are allowed in FIGO staging of cervical cancer, as are procedures such as cystoscopy, proctoscopy, and hysteroscopy. **CT, PET, MRI, bone scan, lymphangiography, and laparotomy/laparascopy data are not allowed** to be used for staging but can be used in Tx planning.

What is the utility of PET scans in cervical cancer?

PET is generally fairly sensitive (85%–90%) and specific (95%–100%) for detection of para-aortic (P-A) nodes in pts with locally advanced cervical cancer. There is less agreement about its utility in detecting pelvic nodal mets.

In what group of cervical cancer pts is evaluation of the urinary tract required?

Cervical cancer **pts with more than microscopic Dz** require imaging of the urinary tract. This can be performed with CT, MRI, or intravenous pyelogram.

What is the FIGO (2008) staging for cervical cancer?

Stage IA: microscopic Dz, with ≤5 mm DOI and ≤7 mm horizontal spread. It is further delineated into IA1 (tumors ≤3 mm depth and ≤7 mm wide) and IA2 (tumors >3 mm but ≤5 mm deep and ≤7 mm wide)

Stage IB: clinically visible tumor or >IA2, with IB1 ≤4 cm, and IB2 being bulky tumors >4 cm

Stage IIA: invades beyond uterus but not to pelvic wall, lower 3rd of vagina, or parametrial invasion, with IIA1 lesions ≤4 cm and IIA2 lesions >4 cm

Stage IIB: invades beyond uterus and into parametria but not into pelvic wall or lower 3rd of vagina

Stage IIIA: invades lower 3rd of vagina but no extension into pelvic wall

Stage IIIB: invades pelvic sidewall and/or causes hydronephrosis or nonfunctioning kidney

Stage IVA: invades beyond true pelvis or mucosa of bladder or rectum (must be Bx proven); bullous edema of bladder or rectum does not count

Stage IVB: DMs

How does the AJCC (TNM) staging system for cervical cancer compare with the FIGO system?

In AJCC cervical cancer staging, the **T stage corresponds to the FIGO stage, except for FIGO stage IVB.** AJCC stage 3 includes T3N0-1, and stage 4 includes T4NX or M1 Dz.

What factors are predictive of pelvic nodal involvement in cervical cancer?

Factors that predict for nodal involvement in cervical cancer include **DOI, FIGO stage, and LVSI** (10% without vs. 25% with).

Estimate the risk of pelvic LN involvement based on the following DOIs of a cervical cancer: <3 mm, 3–5 mm, 6–10 mm, and 10–20 mm.

Risk of pelvic nodal involvement by DOI:
  $\leq$3 mm: <1%
  3–5 mm: 1%–8%
  6–10 mm: 15%
  10–20 mm: 25%

Estimate the risk of pelvic LN involvement based on the FIGO stage of cervical cancer.

Pelvic LN+ rates for cervical cancer based on the FIGO stage:
  Stage IA1: 1%
  Stage IA2: 5%
  Stage IB: 15%
  Stage II: 30%
  Stage III: 50%
  Stage IVA: 60%

Estimate the risk of P-A nodal involvement based on the FIGO stage of cervical cancer.

P-A LN+ rates for cervical cancer based on the FIGO stage:
  Stage IA: 0%
  Stage IB: 5%–8%
  Stage IIA: ~10%
  Stage IIB: 20%–30%
  Stage III: 30%
  Stage IVA: 40%

What are the 5-yr OS rates based on the FIGO stage?

5-yr OS based on FIGO stage:
  Stage I: 82%
  Stage II: 64%
  Stage III: 38%
  Stage IV: 14%

(*Benedet et al., J Epi Biostat 1998*)

■ Treatment/Prognosis

What is the most important prognostic factor in cervical cancer?

Tumor stage is the most important prognostic factor in cervical cancer → LN status.

What is removed in a radical trachelectomy as Tx for cervical cancer?

In a radical trachelectomy, **all cervical cancer is removed with the margin**, but the internal os is left behind and stitched closed, with a small meatus for menses to escape. This procedure allows future pregnancy, delivered via a C-section. This procedure should be reserved for stage IA1 as well as select cases of IA2 and small IB1 Dz.

How should pts with preinvasive cervical cancer (HGSIL or CIN III) be managed?

Pts with preinvasive cervical cancer should be managed with **colposcopy → conization, LEEP, laser, cryotherapy, or simple hysterectomy.**

In which subset of cervical cancer pts is simple hysterectomy adequate as definitive management?

Pts with IA1 Dz can be treated with simple abdominal hysterectomy. Sometimes conization is also adequate for IA1, but there must be DOI <3 mm and no LVSI or dysplasia at the margin (*Van Nagell et al., Am J Obstet Gynecol 1983*). All other pts (≥IA2) should get radical hysterectomy with pelvic LND.

What is the difference between a class II and class III radical hysterectomy (Piver-Rutledge-Smith classification)?

In a class II modified radical hysterectomy (Piver-Rutledge-Smith classification), there is removal of the uterus, ureters are unroofed to remove parametrial and paracervical tissue medial to the ureters and 1–2 cm of vaginal cuff, and the uterine artery is ligated at the ureter. In a class III surgery, there is removal of parametrial and paravaginal tissue to the pelvic sidewall + pelvic LND, ligation of the uterine artery at the ureter, and removal of the upper half to two thirds of the vagina.

What stage of cervical cancer can be treated with brachytherapy alone?

Stage IA cervical cancer can be treated with brachytherapy alone with LDR 65–75 Gy or HDR 7 Gy × 5–6 fx), with LC of 97%. (*Grisby et al., IJROBP 1992*)

When treating cervical cancer pts with brachytherapy, is there a Dz control or toxicity difference between LDR and HDR?

This is **uncertain.** In *Teshima et al.* (*Cancer 1993*), pts with stage I–III cervical cancer were randomized to HDR cobalt-60 or LDR cesium-137 therapy. There was no statistically significant difference in 5-yr CSS between the 2 groups (stage I, 85%–93%; stage II, 73%–78%; stage III, 47%–53%). Moderate to severe complications were higher in HDR (10% vs. 4%).

Where is point A, and what should it correspond to anatomically?

Point A is **2 cm above the external cervical os and 2 cm lat to the central canal/tandem.** This should correspond to the paracervical triangle, where the uterine vessels cross the ureter.

Where is point B, and what should it correspond to anatomically? How does the dose to point B typically relate to the dose to point A?

Point B is **5 cm lat from the midline at the same level as point A** (2 cm above the external cervical os). It is supposed to represent the obturator nodes. The **dose to point B is usually one third to one fourth the dose to point A.**

Before CT-based planning, how were the bladder, rectum, and vaginal points defined for cervical cancer brachytherapy?

Before CT-based planning, the bladder point was 5 mm behind the post surface of the Foley balloon on a lat x-ray filled with 7 cc radiopaque fluid and pulled down against the urethra. The rectum point was 5 mm behind the post vaginal wall between the ovoids at the inf point of the last intrauterine tandem source or mid vaginal source. The vaginal point was the lat edge of the ovoids on AP film and mid ovoid on lat film. In the present age of CT planning, an alternative is to contour the organs and calculate the max dose to the organ using 3D planning.

What are the dose limits to the bladder, rectum, and vaginal points in cervical cancer brachytherapy?

In cervical cancer brachytherapy, typically the **max allowed dose to the rectal point is 75 Gy, the max bladder point dose is 80 Gy, and the max vaginal dose is 120 Gy.**

What RT dose can cause ovarian failure? What about sterility?

Ovarian failure can occur with **5–10 Gy** of RT. Sterility can occur **after 2–3 Gy.**

What are the typical LDR and HDR in cervical cancer Tx?

In cervical cancer brachytherapy, **LDR is usually 0.4–0.8 Gy/hr**, while **HDR is usually ~12 Gy/hr.**

What should be the dose to point A in RT for cervical cancer (sum of EBRT + brachytherapy)? Does it depend on the stage of Dz?

In cervical cancer radiotherapy, the cumulative dose to point A should be **65–75 Gy for stage IA Dz, 75–85 Gy for stage IB–IIB Dz, and 85–90 Gy for stage III–IVA Dz**, so **staging is a factor** in determining the dose.

What is the role for definitive surgery vs. definitive RT for the management of early stage (IB–IIA) cervical cancers? What study tested these 2 modalities?

In *Landoni et al.* (*Lancet 1997*), pts with stage IB and IIA cervical carcinoma were randomized to surgery (class III) vs. RT for definitive therapy. Adj RT was allowed for the surgery group based on preset criteria. 5-yr OS and DFS were equal (83% and 74%, respectively, for both groups). 64% of surgery pts rcv adj RT. Grade 2–3 morbidity was higher in the surgery arm (28% vs. 12%).

What are the benefits of surgery over RT for the Tx of early-stage cervical cancers?

Benefits of surgery over RT include **shorter Tx time, preservation of ovarian function, possibly better sexual functioning after Tx, and no 2nd malignancy risk.**

For pts with early-stage cervical cancer treated with radical or modified radical hysterectomy, what are 3 major indications for adj therapy?

For pts with early-stage cervical cancer treated with radical or modified radical hysterectomy, major indications for adj therapy include **+/close margin, LN mets, and microscopic parametrial invasion.** Other indications include tumor >4 cm, deep stromal invasion, or LVI.

What adverse features after surgery are indications for adj RT alone without chemo?	Cervical cancer pts after radical hysterectomy to −margins and negative nodal status but have ≥2 **risk features** (+LVSI, >4-cm tumors, more than one third stromal invasion) may benefit from PORT.

GOG 92 (*Rotman et al., IJROBP 2006*) enrolled 277 stage IB cervical cancer pts who underwent surgery and had −nodes but >1 adverse feature: more than one third stromal invasion, LVI, or tumor >4 cm. Compared to observation, there was a pelvic RT (46–50.4 Gy) RR of recurrence by 46% (21% → 14%, *p* = 0.007) and trend to OS benefit by ~10% (71% → 80%, *p* = 0.074).

When is adding chemo to adj RT after radical hysterectomy beneficial compared to RT alone for the surgical management of early-stage cervical cancer (IA2–IIA)?	In **GOG 109** (*Peters et al., JCO 2000*), high-risk pts (with at least 1 of the following features: +margin, +nodes, or microscopic parametrial invasion) with stage IA2, IB, and IIA cervical cancer treated with radical hysterectomy and pelvic lymphadenectomy were randomized to standard pelvic field RT (49.3 Gy) vs. RT + cisplatin/5-FU for 4 cycles. CRT was superior in both 4-yr OS (81% vs. 71%) and 4-yr PFS (80% vs. 63%).

What subset of pts from GOG 109 did not benefit from adding chemo to adj RT?	*Monk et al.* (*Gyn Onc 2005*) subset analysis of **GOG 109** demonstrated that pts with tumors ≤2 cm and only 1 +node did not benefit from CRT compared to RT alone.

For pts with bulky (>4 cm) early-stage cervical cancer, is there an advantage to adding adj hysterectomy to definitive RT?	In **GOG 71** (*Keys HM et al., Gyn Onc 2003*), pts with tumors >4 cm were randomized to RT alone vs. RT + adj hysterectomy. RT consisted of EBRT + brachytherapy (80 Gy to point A for the RT-alone group, and 75 Gy to point A for the surgery group). At median 9.6-yr follow-up, there was no difference in OS or severe toxicity. There was a trend to improved LR (26% vs. 14%, *p* = 0.08).

An option is to give upfront CRT and assess for response at 2 mos. If residual Dz is evident, then salvage surgery can be considered.

For stage IB2 cervical cancer pts, what is the advantage of preop CRT compared with preop RT alone?	In **GOG 123** (*Keys HM, NEJM 1999*), stage IB2 cervical cancer pts were randomized to preop RT vs. CRT → adj simple hysterectomy. RT was whole pelvis (WP) + brachytherapy to a point A dose of 75 Gy. CRT added weekly cisplatin 40 mg/m². CRT was superior in 3-yr pCR (52% vs. 41%), OS (83% vs. 74%), and pCR (52% vs. 41%). *Note:* Adj and immediate hysterectomy was included in this trial prior to the results of GOG 71 being available.

In stage IB cervical cancer, is there a role for neoadj chemo prior to surgery?

No. Currently, there is no role for neoadj chemo. **GOG 141** (*Eddy GL et al., Gyn Onc 2007*) looked at stage IB2 pts randomized to radical hysterectomy with nodal dissection +/− neoadj vincristine/cisplatin × 3 cycles. The study closed early, but there was comparable LC and OS in both groups, and PORT was needed in 45%–52% of pts.

EORTC 55994 is currently testing the question if preop CRT is better than preop chemo alone.

In locally advanced cervical cancer, what is the OS advantage of definitive CRT over RT alone?

The benefit of CRT over RT alone in locally advanced cervical cancer was evaluated in **RTOG 90-01** (*Eifel P et al., JCO 2004*). This study randomized stage IIB–IVA, large stage IB–IIA (>5 cm), or LN+ pts and randomized to RT to the pelvis and P-A nodes vs. pelvis RT + 3 cycles of cisplatin/5-FU. Both arms had brachytherapy with a point A dose of 85 Gy. 8-yr OS was 67% vs. 41%, benefiting the CRT.

What chemo agents are most effective in CRT for cervical cancer?

Weekly cisplatin at 40 mg/m^2 is the current standard to be given with definitive RT. **GOG 120** (*Rose et al., NEJM 1999*) randomized cervical cancer pts stage IIB–IVA to RT + 3 different chemo arms. RT was WP + brachytherapy (to 81 Gy at point A). Chemo was weekly cisplatin 40 mg/m^2, or hydroxyurea, or cisplatin/5-FU/hydroxyurea. Cisplatin arms had better 4-yr OS (65% vs. 47%) and reduced recurrence (34%–35% vs. 54%). Toxicity was less with cisplatin alone or hydroxyurea alone. The benefit of adding 5-FU is unknown b/c of the confounding effect of hydroxyurea.

To what subset of pts is adding P-A fields to the pelvic field beneficial in the definitive Tx of cervical cancer?

There are 2 indications where the P-A field should be added to the definitive management of cervical cancer pts: (1) pts with +P-A Dz and (2) pts with positive pelvic nodal Dz and not receiving CRT. 2 studies have addressed this:

RTOG 79-20 (*Rotman et al., JAMA 1995*) randomized 337 pts with IIB Dz without clinical or radiographic evidence of P-A Dz to the WP (45 Gy) alone vs. WP + P-A field (extended-field radiation therapy [EFRT]) (45 Gy). No chemo was given. Adding the P-A field improved 10-yr OS (55% vs. 44%) without improvement in LC or DM. However, there was slight increased toxicity with the P-A field (8% vs. 4%).

RTOG 90-01 (*Morris et al., NEJM 1999; Eifel P et al., JCO 2004*) randomized 386 pts with locally advanced cervical cancers (IIB–IVA or IB–IIA with ≥5 cm) or with a +pelvic LN (no P-A nodal Dz) to WP RT + chemo vs. WP + P-A field alone (EFRT). All pts were treated with post-EBRT brachytherapy to 85 Gy to point A. Chemo was cisplatin 75 mg/m² + 5-FU 1,000 mg/day × 4 days per 21-day cycle for 3 cycles. Pelvic CRT was superior to EFRT in 8-yr OS (67% vs. 41%), DFS (61% vs. 46%), LRF (18% vs. 35%), and DM (20% vs. 35%). There was a slight increase in P-A nodal failure in the CRT arm (8% vs. 4%, *p* = NSS).

Describe the borders of typical AP and lat fields in cervical cancer Tx.

In cervical cancer therapy, the typical borders of an AP field are sup to L4-5, inf to 3 cm below the most inf vaginal involvement or inf obturator foramen, and lat 2 cm from the pelvic rim. Lat beams would have the same sup and inf extent, with the ant edge to 1 cm ant of the pubic symphysis and post edge to include the entire sacrum. For common iliac nodal involvement, extend the field to cover up to L2. For P-A nodal involvement, extend the field to the top of T12. The borders can be tailored for early-stage vs. more advanced Dz. In the CT planning era, the alternative is to contour the organs and nodes of interest to ensure adequate coverage.

What is a typical EBRT prescription for cervical cancer?

Typically, cervical cancer pts treated with EBRT rcv RT to the WP to 45 Gy in 1.8 Gy fx. Sidewall boosts usually go to 50–54 Gy. Persistent or bulky parametrial tumors usually rcv 60 Gy. P-A nodes go to 45 Gy if treated. Bulky nodes go to 60 Gy with 3D-CRT or IMRT.

When should Tx of inguinal nodes be considered in cervical cancer?

In cervical cancer, Tx of inguinal nodes should be considered **if Dz involves the lower 3ʳᵈ of the vagina.**

Does overall Tx time in cervical cancer impact outcome? Ideally, how long should the RT Tx take?

Yes. Prolonged overall RT Tx time in cervical cancer is associated with poorer outcomes. Ideally, **EBRT and brachytherapy should be completed within 7 wks.** The effect is more notable in more advanced-stage pts (stage III–IV).

What are the common presenting signs and Sx of ovarian cancer?	The NCCN has released the following consensus guidelines for ovarian cancer Sx: **bloating, abdominal/pelvic pain, difficulty eating, early satiety, new urinary Sx (frequency/urgency >12 days/mo), palpable abdominal/pelvic mass, and ascites.** Identification of such Sx should prompt a workup for ovarian cancer.

▪ Workup/Staging

What is CA 125, and what is its utility in ovarian cancer?	CA 125 is a **mucinous protein encoded by the MUC16 gene and is used to assess response to Tx and predict prognosis after Tx for ovarian cancer.** Due to its low sensitivity and specificity as a diagnostic test, it is not used as a screening tool.
What is OvaSure, and can it be used as a diagnostic test for ovarian cancer?	OvaSure is a **serum-based test for leptin, prolactin, osteopontin, IGF II, macrophage inhibitory factor, and CA 125** being investigated as a screening tool for ovarian cancer. The Society of Gynecologic Oncologists has not yet endorsed its routine use due to lack of adequate clinical validation. (*Visintin I et al., Clin Cancer Res 2008*)
What are the initial steps in the workup of pts with an undiagnosed pelvic mass?	Pts with signs/Sx suspicious for ovarian cancer should undergo a full H&P, including a thorough family Hx and pelvic examination, CBC, CMP, CA 125, US, CT abdomen/pelvis, and CXR. Final staging is determined through surgical/pathologic evaluation of the abdomen and pelvis. (*NCCN 2010*)
What is the FIGO staging system for ovarian cancer?	**Stage IA:** limited to 1 ovary with capsule intact; no tumor on ovarian surface; no malignant cells in ascites or peritoneal washings **Stage IB:** limited to both ovaries with capsules intact; no tumor on ovarian surface; no malignant cells in ascites or peritoneal washings **Stage IC:** limited to 1 or both ovaries with any of the following: ruptured capsule, tumor on ovarian surface, malignant cells in ascites, or peritoneal washings **Stage IIA:** extension and/or implants on uterus and/or tube(s); no malignant cells in ascites or peritoneal washings **Stage IIB:** extension to and/or implants on other pelvic tissues; no malignant cells in ascites or peritoneal washings **Stage IIC:** pelvic extension and/or implants (T2a or T2b) with malignant cells in ascites or peritoneal washings **Stage IIIA:** microscopic peritoneal mets beyond pelvis (no macroscopic tumor)

Stage IIIB: macroscopic peritoneal mets beyond pelvis ≤2 cm in greatest dimension
Stage IIIC: peritoneal mets beyond pelvis >2 cm in greatest dimension and/or regional LN mets
Stage IV: DM (excludes peritoneal mets)

If a pt with ovarian cancer is found to have a liver met, what stage is she?

In ovarian cancer, the stage implications of a liver met depend on whether the met was on the liver capsule or in the parenchyma. **Liver capsule mets are T3/stage III,** and **liver parenchymal mets are M1/stage IV.**

What is the difference between the FIGO and AJCC TNM staging for ovarian cancer?

As of 2010, the **FIGO and AJCC staging systems do not differ for ovarian cancer.**

What % of pts with newly diagnosed ovarian cancer present with advanced-stage Dz?

~**70%** of all newly diagnosed ovarian cancer pts present with advanced-stage Dz (stage I, 20%; stage II, 12%; stage III, 45%; stage IV, 23%). Dx at earlier stages is difficult due to the location of the ovaries.

■ Treatment/Prognosis

What is the general Tx paradigm for ovarian cancer?

Ovarian cancer Tx paradigm: Pts with suspected ovarian cancer should undergo a comprehensive diagnostic and therapeutic laparotomy for surgical staging and cytoreduction, respectively. This should include peritoneal lavage; total abdominal hysterectomy with bilat salpingo-oophorectomy; and resection of suspicious LNs, including bilat pelvic/periaortic nodes in stage IIIB pts with a goal to cytoreduce to <1 cm of gross residual Dz.

Are there situations where unilat salpingo-oophorectomy may be considered in pts with ovarian cancer?

For a young woman with **early-stage Dz or a low malignant potential tumor wishing to preserve fertility,** a unilat salpingo-oophorectomy may be considered.

How should early-stage ovarian cancer be treated?

The gold standard for Tx of all stages of ovarian cancer is **surgery.** For stage IA-B, grade 1, non–clear cell tumors treated with cytoreductive staging laparotomy, 5-yr OS rates approach 95% and no adj therapy is indicated. All other stages of Dz should rcv adj chemo. (*Young RC et al., NEJM 1990; Trimbos JB et al., J Natl Cancer Inst 2003*)

What trials support the use of chemo in the postsurgical setting for pts with ovarian cancer?

The ICON1/ACTION trials randomized mostly stage I–II ovarian cancer pts (some advanced-stage pts in ICON1) to postsurgical platinum-based chemo (4–6 cycles) vs. chemo. Adj chemo significantly increased 5-yr OS (82% vs. 74%) and RFS (76% vs. 65%). (*Trimbos JB et al., J Natl Cancer Inst 2003*)

Describe the WAI fields used to treat ovarian cancer pts.

Pts being planned to rcv WAI should undergo CT simulation. An AP/PA open-field technique is historically used with borders as follows:

Superior: top of diaphragm
Inferior: obturator foramen
Lateral: peritoneal reflection

What dose is prescribed when treating ovarian cancer pts with WAI?

Pts being treated with WAI should rcv 30 Gy in 1.5 Gy/fx with a para-aortic boost to 45 Gy and pelvic boost to 50 Gy. Kidney and liver blocks should be applied at 15 Gy and 25 Gy, respectively.

What are the NCCN follow-up recommendations after Tx for ovarian cancer?

After surgery +/− chemo for Tx of ovarian cancer, pts should rcv full interval H&P (including pelvic exam) every 2–4 mos for the 1st 2 yrs, every 3–6 mos for 3 yrs, and annually thereafter. CA 125 should be checked at every visit if it was elevated at the time of Dx. Routine labs should be checked if there is an indication. Imaging should be ordered if clinically necessary.

How should pts with a rising CA 125 be managed following CR to initial therapy in the absence of clinical or radiographic evidence of Dz recurrence?

Pts who are chemo naive should be treated the same as newly diagnosed pts (**complete surgical staging +/− chemo, if appropriate**). Tx options for pts who have previously rcv chemo include observation until clinical relapse, hormonal therapy (e.g., tamoxifen), systemic therapy, or clinical trial enrollment.

What is the median time to clinically or radiographically detectable Dz after an isolated CA 125 relapse?

The median time to clinical relapse in the setting of a rising CA 125 is **3–6 mos.**

Are most relapses of ovarian cancer local or distant?

~80% of relapsed ovarian cancers are **local.**

How should ovarian cancer relapses be managed?

Pts with platinum-sensitive relapsed ovarian cancer (relapse ≥6 mos after initial chemo) should be treated with platinum-based combination chemo (*Fung Kee Fung M et al., Curr Oncol 2007*). In cases of platinum-resistant Dz, single agents such as docetaxel, gemcitabine, etoposide, pemetrexed, and others can be used (*Mutch DG et al., JCO 2007*). Response rates in the latter range from 20%–30%.

■ Toxicity

What is the most common severe toxicity experienced by ovarian cancer pts treated with WAI?

Grade 3–4 diarrhea occurs in ~30% of ovarian cancer pts treated with WAI. (*Chiara S et al., Am J Clin Oncol 1994*)

66
Endometrial Cancer
Kristin Janson Redmond and Fariba Asrari

Background

What is the incidence of endometrial cancer in the U.S.?

Endometrial cancer is the most common gyn malignancy in the U.S., with an incidence of ~**44,000 cases/yr** annually. It is the 2nd most common cause of gyn cancer deaths.

What are the 2 forms of endometrial cancer?

Forms of endometrial cancer:
1. <u>Type I</u>: endometrioid, 70%–80% of cases, estrogen related
2. <u>Type II</u>: nonendometrioid, typically papillary serous or clear cell, high grade, not estrogen related, aggressive clinical course

What are the risk factors for endometrial cancer?

Risk factors for endometrial cancer:
1. Exogenous unopposed estrogen
2. Endogenous estrogen (obesity, functional ovarian tumors, late menopause, nulliparity, chronic anovulation/polycystic ovarian syndrome)
3. Tamoxifen
4. Advancing age (75% postmenopausal)
5. Hereditary (HNPCC)
6. Family Hx
7. HTN

What are protective factors for endometrial cancer?

Protective factors for endometrial cancer include **combination oral contraceptives and physical activity.**

What is the most common clinical presentation of endometrial cancer?

Endometrial cancer presents with **abnl vaginal bleeding** in 90% cases.

What % of post-menopausal women with abnl vaginal bleeding have endometrial cancer?

Only **5%–20%** of postmenopausal women with abnl vaginal bleeding have endometrial cancer.

What are the 3 layers of the uterine wall?

The 3 layers of the uterine wall are the **endometrium, myometrium, and serosa.**

What is the primary lymphatic drainage of the uterus?

The primary lymphatic drainage of the uterus is to the **pelvic LNs** (parametrial, internal and external iliacs, obturator, common iliac, presacral). Also, direct spread to the para-aortic (P-A) nodes (from the fundus) can occur.

■ Treatment/Prognosis

What is the primary Tx modality for endometrial cancer?	**Surgery** is the primary Tx modality for endometrial cancer.
What is resected in a TAH?	TAH removes **the uterus and a small rim of vaginal cuff.**
What is resected in a modified radical hysterectomy?	Modified radical hysterectomy: 1. Removal of uterus and 1–2 cm of vaginal cuff 2. Wide excision of parametrial and paravaginal tissues (including median one half of cardinal and uterosacral ligaments) 3. Ligation of uterine artery at ureter
What is resected in a radical hysterectomy?	Radical hysterectomy: 1. Resection of uterus and upper vagina 2. Dissection of paravaginal and parametrial tissues to pelvic sidewalls 3. Ligation of uterine artery at its origin at internal iliac artery 4. Dissection of pelvic LNs
Pelvic and P-A lymphadenectomy is recommended in which pts with endometrial cancer?	Although controversial, LNs are commonly assessed at the time of initial surgery for endometrial cancer. Pelvic lymphadenectomy may not be indicated in women with Dz clinically confined to the uterus. The ASTEC trial randomized 1,408 pts with endometrial cancer that was clinically confined to the uterus to standard surgery (TAH + BSO, peritoneal washing, palpation of P-A nodes) vs. standard surgery + pelvic lymphadenectomy. Those at intermediate or high risk for recurrence (independent of nodal status) were further randomized to rcv pelvic RT or not. There was no benefit to pelvic lymphadenectomy in terms of OS or RFS. (*ASTEC Study Group et al., Lancet 2009*)
What is the risk of lymphedema following surgery for uterine malignancies?	According to an MSKCC retrospective review of 1,289 pts, the rate of lymphedema at a median follow-up of 3 yrs was 1.2%. When ≥10 LNs were removed, the rate of symptomatic lymphedema was 3.4%. (*Abu-Rustum NR et al., Gyn Onc 2006*)
What are considered negative prognostic factors for endometrial cancer?	Negative prognostic indicators for endometrial cancer: 1. LVSI 2. Age >60 yrs 3. Grade 3 4. Deep myometrial invasion 5. Tumor size 6. Lower uterine segment involvement 7. Anemia 8. Poor Karnofsky performance status

What adj therapy is indicated for completely surgically staged endometrial cancers limited to the endometrium?

No adj therapy is indicated for endometrial cancers limited to the endometrium, except for grade 3, where vaginal cuff brachytherapy is considered. In grade 3 tumors with adverse risk factors and incomplete surgical staging, pelvic RT is considered.

What adj therapy is indicated for completely surgically staged endometrial cancers that invade less than half of the myometrium?

Endometrial cancers that invade less than half of the myometrium could be **observed or treated with adj vaginal cuff brachytherapy.**

Note:
1. If the tumor is grade 3 with adverse risk factors, pelvic RT should be considered.
2. If the tumor is incompletely surgically staged and grade 1–2, consider observation or vaginal brachytherapy +/− RT.
3. Endocervical glandular involvement favors the use of vaginal brachytherapy.

What adj therapy is indicated for completely surgically staged endometrial cancers that invade half or more of the myometrium?

Endometrial cancers that invade half or more of the myometrium can be **observed or treated with adj vaginal cuff brachytherapy.**

Note:
1. If grade 3 or any grade with adverse prognostic factors, whole pelvic RT +/− brachytherapy should be considered.
2. If the tumor is incompletely surgically staged, consider pelvic RT + vaginal brachytherapy. For incompletely staged grade 3 tumors, consider chemo as well.
3. Endocervical glandular involvement favors the use of vaginal brachytherapy.

What adj therapy is indicated for completely surgically staged, stage II endometrial cancer?

Adj pelvic RT and vaginal brachytherapy is indicated for endometrial cancers that invade the cervical stroma. If grade 3, consider chemo.

What adj therapy is indicated for completely surgically staged, stage III endometrial cancer?

Adj chemo +/− RT should be given for stage III endometrial cancer. RT in addition to chemo is needed if there is gross residual Dz or unresectable Dz.

Describe the whole pelvic RT field for endometrial cancer. What total doses are typically prescribed?

Borders of the whole pelvis (WP) RT field for endometrial cancer:
    Superior: L4-5
    Inferior: bottom of obturator foramen
    Lateral: 1.5–2.0 cm lat to pelvic brim
    Anterior: front of pubic symphysis
    Posterior: split sacrum to S3

Treat to 45–50 Gy.

What is the border of an extended RT field for endometrial cancer, and when should extended fields be used?

The sup border of an extended RT field for endometrial cancer is **T10-11 or T11-12.** It should be used if there are **positive P-A LNs.**

According to the American Brachytherapy Society (ABS), what are the Tx site and depth for vaginal cuff brachytherapy for endometrial cancer?

According to the ABS, for endometrioid carcinoma of the endometrium, the proximal 3–5 cm of the vagina (approximately one half) should be treated. For CCC, UPSC, or stage IIIB, the target is the entire vaginal canal. Prescribe to 0.5 cm beyond the vaginal mucosa. (*Nag S, IJROBP 2000*)

What LDR and HDR are typically used for adj intracavitary RT alone for endometrial cancer?

For adj intracavitary RT therapy alone, the LDR is 50–60 Gy over 72 hrs (70–80 cGy/hr). The HDR is 21 Gy (7 Gy × 3) at 0.5 cm depth.

What are the LDR and HDR recommendations for adj intracavitary RT + WP RT for endometrial cancer?

When given in combination with WP RT, the LDR for endometrial cancer is 30 Gy, and the HDR is 15 Gy (5 Gy × 2 or 3) at 0.5 cm depth.

When should vaginal cuff brachytherapy begin relative to EBRT?

At the Johns Hopkins Hospital, the institutional practice is for vaginal cuff brachytherapy to begin **within a wk of completion of EBRT.** Give 2 Tx/wk.

How are nonbulky vaginal cuff recurrences treated in endometrial cancer pts with no prior RT?

For nonbulky vaginal cuff recurrences in pts with no prior RT, a **combination of pelvic RT and brachytherapy** is typically used. Treat to 45 Gy pelvic RT, and assess the response. If the residual is <0.5 cm, add HDR vaginal brachytherapy at 7 Gy × 3 to 0.5 cm depth of the vaginal mucosa. (*Nag S et al., IJROBP 2000*)

How are vaginal cuff recurrences that are bulky or within a previously irradiated field treated in endometrial cancer pts?

For endometrial cancer pts with vaginal cuff recurrences that are bulky (>0.5 cm thickness) or in a previously irradiated field, **consider interstitial brachytherapy.**

When do inguinal nodes need to be included in the RT fields for endometrial cancer?

In cases with **distal vaginal involvement,** the entire vagina and inguinal nodes need to be included in EBRT fields.

How should inoperable endometrial cancer be treated with RT?

Consider pelvic RT to 45 Gy → intracavitary RT boost using 2 tandem intrauterine applicators to 6.3 Gy × 3 prescribed to 2 cm depth (serosal surface). If pelvic RT is contraindicated, consider definitive intracavitary RT alone (7.3 Gy × 5 prescribed to 2 cm depth). (*Nag S et al., IJROBP 2000*)

Describe the design and results of PORTEC-1.

In **PORTEC-1**, 714 pts with more than one half myometrial invasion and grade 2–3 or one half or more myometrial invasion and grade 1–2 underwent TAH/BSO with washings *with no lymphadenectomy* and were randomized to adj EBRT (46 Gy) vs. observation. EBRT reduced LRR from 14% to 5% at 10 yrs. 75% of LRs were in the vaginal vault. There was no difference in 10-yr OS. Note that with central pathology review, there was a significant shift from grade 2 to grade 1. (*Scholten AN et al., IJROBP 2005; Creutzberg CL et al., Lancet 2000*)

Describe the design and results of GOG 99.

In **GOG 99**, 392 endometrial cancer pts with myometrial and/or occult cervical invasion underwent TAH/BSO, pelvic and P-A LN sampling, and peritoneal cytology and then were randomized to observation vs. WP RT (50.4 Gy). Inclusion criteria were revised during the trial to include only high-intermediate–risk pts defined as: (1) age >70 yrs with 1 risk factor (grade 2 or 3, LVI, outer one third myometrial invasion), (2) age >50 yrs with 2 risk factors, and (3) any age with 3 risk factors.

RT improved LR from 12% to 3%. The greatest benefit in LR was in high-intermediate–risk pts from 26% to 6% vs. low-intermediate–risk pts from 6% to 2%. There was no change in OS, but the study was not powered to detect this. *Conclusion:* Limit pelvic RT to high-intermediate–risk pts. The major flaw of this study is that grade 2 was grouped with grade 3 even though grade 2 Dz tends to behave more similarly to grade 1. (*Keys HM et al., Gyn Onc 2004*)

Describe the design and results of the Aalders Norwegian study.

The Aalders Norwegian study enrolled 540 pts with surgical stage I endometrial cancer s/p TAH/BSO (with no lymphadenectomy). *All pts rcv vaginal cuff brachytherapy (~40 Gy LDR at 0.5 cm or ~24 Gy HDR at 0.5 cm).* They were then randomized to no further therapy vs. pelvic RT (40 Gy with central shielding after 20 Gy). Overall, the pelvic RT arm had decreased 9-yr LR (7% to 2%) but more DM (5% vs. 10%). There was no difference in 9-yr OS. On subset analysis of pts with invasion of one half or more of the myometrium and grade 3 Dz, pelvic RT improved 9-yr OS (72% to 82%) and improved 9-yr LR (20% to 5%). There was no change in DM. There was no difference in OS, LR, or DM for pts with invasion of one half or more of the myometrium and grade 1–2 Dz. (*Aalders J et al., Ob Gyn 1980*)

Describe the design and results of GOG 122.

In **GOG 122,** 388 pts with endometrial tumors invading beyond the uterus (all histologies) underwent TAH/BSO and surgical staging with <2-cm residual tumor. P-A LNs were allowed, but mets to the chest or supraclavicular nodes were not allowed. Pts were randomized to whole abdomen irradiation (30 Gy AP/PA +15 Gy boost to pelvic +/− P-A LNs) vs. chemo (doxorubicin/cisplatin q3wks × 8 cycles). At 5 yrs, chemo had improved stage-adjusted OS (55% vs. 42%) and PFS (38% vs. 50%). Chemo had increased grade 3–4 heme toxicity (88% vs. 14%) and increased GI, cardiac, and neurologic toxicity. Note that results were questioned b/c though this was a randomized trial, the analysis was based on stage-adjusted results that may not be justified. (*Randall ME et al., JCO 2006*)

Describe the design and results of PORTEC-2.

PORTEC-2 randomized 427 pts with intermediate-high–risk endometrial cancer defined as:
1. Age >60 yrs and less than one half myometrial invasion and grade 3
2. Age >60 yrs and one half or more myometrial invasion and grades 1–2
3. Invasion of cervical glandular epithelium and grades 1–2
4. Invasion of cervical glandular epithelium and grade 3 with less than one half myometrial invasion

All pts were s/p TAH/BSO without pelvic LND and were randomized to EBRT (46 Gy) vs. vaginal brachytherapy alone (HDR 21 Gy in 3 fx or LDR 30 Gy). At median follow-up at 3.8 yrs, vaginal brachytherapy was similar to EBRT with respect to 5-yr outcomes: vaginal relapse (1.8% vs. 1.6%), isolated pelvic relapse (1.5% vs. 0.5%), LRR (5.1% vs. 2.1%), or OS (85% vs. 80%). However, there were significantly higher rates of acute grade 1–2 GI toxicity in the EBRT group. The authors concluded that vaginal brachytherapy should be standard in intermediate-high–risk endometrial cancer. (*Nout RA et al., Lancet 2010*)

Describe the design and results of the Finnish randomized trial comparing adj EBRT vs. interdigitated CRT in endometrial cancer.

The Finland trial included 156 endometrial cancer pts with (1) less than one half myometrial invasion and grade 3 or (2) one half or more myometrial invasion or extrauterine extension up to stage IIIA and any grade.

All were s/p TAH/BSO (with pelvic LAD in 80%) and randomized to split-course pelvic EBRT (28 Gy × 2 with a 3-wk break) vs. interdigitated CRT (28 Gy → chemo → 28 Gy → chemo, where chemo used was cisplatin/epirubicin/cyclophosphamide). There was no difference in 5-yr DFS, LR, or DM. Note the atypical Tx paradigms including split-course therapy. (*Kuoppala T et al., Gyn Onc 2008*)

Describe the design and results of the Japanese GOG (JGOG) 2033.	**JGOG 2033** enrolled 385 pts with more than one half myometrial invasion, including pts with stage II–III Dz. All were s/p TAH/BSO and surgical staging and were randomized to 40–50 Gy EBRT AP/PA vs. ≥3 cycles of chemo (cyclophosphamide/doxorubicin/cisplatin). At 5 yrs, there was no difference in PFS, OS, or toxicity. An unplanned subset analysis defined high-intermediate risk:

1. Stage I and age >70 yrs or grade 3 Dz
2. Stage II or +cytology

In this subset, chemo improved PFS (83.8% vs. 66.2%). The authors concluded that adj chemo is a reasonable alternative to RT in intermediate-risk endometrial cancer. (*Susumu N et al., Gyn Onc 2007*)

Describe the design and results of the Nordic Society of Gynaecological Oncology (NSGO)-EORTC trial that evaluated adj RT +/− chemo in high-risk endometrial cancer.	The NSGO-EORTC trial enrolled 367 endometrial cancer pts with surgical stage I–II, positive peritoneal fluid cytology or positive pelvic LNs. Most had ≥2 risk factors: grade 3, deep myometrial invasion, or DNA nondiploidy. Pts with serous, clear cell, or anaplastic carcinomas were eligible regardless of risk factors. Pts were randomized to RT vs. RT + chemo (various regimens allowed). RT was pelvic EBRT (44 Gy) +/− vaginal brachytherapy. 5-yr PFS favored the RT + chemo arm (82% vs. 75%). (*Hogberg T et al., ASCO abstract 2007*)
Describe the design and results of GOG 94—the study of UPSC and CCC.	**GOG 94** (*Sutton G, Gyn Onc 2006*) was a phase I–II trial enrolling 21 pts with UPSC or CCC of the uterus s/p TAH/BSO, pelvic/P-A nodal sampling, and peritoneal washing. Pts were treated with whole abdomen irradiation (30 Gy in 20 fx) and pelvic boost (19.8 Gy in 11 fx). At 5 yrs, >50% failures were within the RT field, and 5-yr PFS was 38% for UPSC and 54% for CCC. The authors concluded that chemo likely is necessary for these radioresistant histologies. (*Sutton G et al., Gyn Onc 2006*)

■ Toxicity

What are the RT tolerances of the mucosa of the upper, middle, and lower vagina?	The RT tolerance of the mucosa of the proximal vagina is 120 Gy and distal vagina is 98 Gy. (*Hintz BL et al., IJROBP 1980*)
At what RT dose does ovarian failure occur?	Ovarian failure occurs after **5–10 Gy.**
At what RT dose does sterilization occur in women?	Sterilization in women occurs after **2–3 Gy.**

Is there a benefit to postop pelvic RT for the management of uterine sarcomas?

The role of adj RT remains **controversial.** The issue has been addressed in at least 1 randomized trial and 2 important retrospective studies. In general, the data suggest an LC benefit for MMM but limited, if any, OS benefit with adj RT. The LC and OS benefits of adj RT in LMS are unclear.

EORTC 55874 (*Reed NS, Eur J Cancer 2008*) randomized 224 pts with stage I–II high-grade uterine sarcoma (46% LMS, 41% carcinosarcoma, 13% endometrial stromal tumor) s/p total abdominal hysterectomy/ BSO, washings (75%), and optional nodal sampling (25%) to either (1) observation or (2) pelvic RT to 50.4 Gy. The results suggest that pelvic RT improves LC but not OS or PFS for MMM; however, there is no benefit for LMS.

A SEER-based study found that adj RT offered survival benefits in pts with early MMM but not in LMS. (*Wright JD et al., Am J Obstet Gynecol 2008*)

A retrospective series from Mayo included 208 pts with uterine LMS. Pelvic RT had no impact on DSS ($p = 0.06$), but it was associated with a significant improvement in LR. (*Giuntoli R et al., Gyn Onc 2003*)

What is the role of whole abdomen irradiation (WAI) in MMM?

GOG 150 is a randomized trial of WAI vs. 3 cycles of cisplatin/ifosfamide/mesna (CIM) as postsurgical therapy in stage I–IV carcinosarcoma of the uterus.

Results: Neither Tx was particularly effective. Vaginal recurrence increased and abdominal recurrence fell in the chemo group. Serious late adverse events increased significantly in the group receiving WAI.

(*Wolfson AH et al., Gynecol Oncol 2007*)

For which pts with MMM is pelvic irradiation typically indicated?

Pelvic irradiation is typically recommended for MMM with **age >60 yrs, deep myometrial involvement, cervical involvement, high mitotic rate, nodal involvement, or residual Dz (micro- or macroscopic).**

For which pts with LMS is pelvic irradiation typically indicated?

Although controversial, pelvic irradiation should be considered **in pts with uterine LMS with micro- or macroscopic residual Dz,** particularly in the context of a clinical trial.

How do the RT fields for uterine sarcoma differ from those used for endometrial carcinoma?

The **RT fields are the same** for uterine sarcoma and endometrial carcinoma.

Does the prognostic index developed for soft tissue sarcomas apply to uterine sarcomas?

No. The prognostic index for soft tissue sarcomas does not apply to uterine sarcomas.

What is the role for adj chemo in uterine sarcoma?

The role of adj chemo for uterine sarcoma is **controversial.** Doxorubicin-based regimens appear to be most effective but have not resulted in significant improvements in OS. (*Sutton G, Gyn Onc 1996, 2005; Edmonson JH, Gyn Onc 2002; Long HJ III, Gyn Onc 2005*)

■ Toxicity

What are the expected acute and late toxicities associated with RT Tx for uterine sarcoma?

Acute toxicities: n/v, diarrhea, mucositis, fatigue, bladder irritation

Late toxicities: vaginal dryness and atrophy, pubic hair loss, vaginal stenosis and fibrosis (recommend vaginal dilators), urethral stricture, fistula formation, SBO

68

Vulvar Cancer

Charles H. Matthews and Daniel G. Petereit

■ Background

Approximately how many pts are affected by vulvar cancer per yr in the U.S.? What is the incidence of vulvar cancer in the U.S.?

~**3,500** pts are affected by vulvar cancer per yr in the U.S. The incidence is **1/100,000 people.**

Vulvar cancer accounts for what % of gyn malignancies? What % of all malignancies in women are vulvar malignancies?

Vulvar cancer represents **3%–5% of all gyn malignancies.** This comprises **1%–2% of all cancers in women.**

What are the risk factors for vulvar cancer?

Risk factors for vulvar cancer:
1. Increasing age
2. HPV
3. Vulvar intraepithelial neoplasia (VIN)
4. Bowen Dz (squamous cell CIS)
5. Paget Dz (lesions arising from Bartholin, urethra, or rectum)
6. Erythroplasia
7. Chronic vaginitis
8. Leukoplakia
9. Smoking
10. Employment in laundry facilities
11. Immune deficiency

What HPV subtypes are associated with vulvar cancer?

HPV subtypes associated with vulvar cancer include **6, 16, 18, and 33.**

What is the function of HPV-associated oncoproteins?

It is thought that HPV-associated oncoproteins **bind and inactivate tumor suppressor proteins** such as Rb, p53, and p21.

What are the 7 subsites of the vulva?

Subsites of the vulva:
1. Labia majora
2. Labia minora
3. Mons pubis
4. Clitoris
5. Vaginal vestibule
6. Perineal body
7. Posterior forchette

What are the most common presenting Sx of pts with vulvar cancer?

Common presenting Sx of vulvar cancer: pruritis, vulvar discomfort or pain, dysuria, oozing or bleeding, and difficulty with defecation

In which subsites does vulvar cancer most commonly arise?

70% of vulvar cancers arise from the **labia majora/minora.**

How is "locally advanced" vulvar cancer defined?

Locally advanced vulvar cancer is defined as **a vulvar tumor burden that cannot be resected without exenterative surgery.**

What % of vulvar cancers are locally advanced at Dx?

30% of vulvar cancers are locally advanced at Dx.

What are the 1ˢᵗ-, 2ⁿᵈ-, and 3ʳᵈ-echelon LN regions in vulvar cancer, and which subsite is associated with skip nodal mets?

LN regions in vulvar cancer:
  1ˢᵗ echelon: superficial inguinofemoral
  2ⁿᵈ echelon: deep inguinofemoral and femoral
  3ʳᵈ echelon: external iliac nodes

The **clitoris** can drain directly to the deep inguinofemoral or pelvic nodes.

What are the 2 strongest predictors of LN involvement in vulvar cancer?	The 2 strongest predictors of LN involvement in vulvar cancer are **tumor grade and DOI.**

Estimate the risk of inguinal LN involvement based on the DOI of a cervical tumor: <1 mm, 1–3 mm, 3–5 mm, and >5 mm.

LN involvement by cervical tumor DOI:
- <u><1 mm</u>: <5%
- <u>1–3 mm</u>: 8%
- <u>3–5 mm</u>: 27%
- <u>>5 mm</u>: 34%

(*Hacker NF et al., Cancer 1993*)

Estimate the risk of inguinal LN involvement based on the vulvar cancer FIGO stage.

LN involvement by the vulvar cancer FIGO stage:
- <u>Stage I</u>: 17%
- <u>Stage II</u>: 40%
- <u>Stage III</u>: 30%–80%
- <u>Stage IV</u>: 80%–100%

What histology constitutes the vast majority of vulvar cancers? Name 3 other histologies of tumors found on the vulva.

The most common vulvar histology is **squamous cell carcinoma** (80%–90%). Other histologies include **melanoma, basal cell, Merkel cell, sarcoma, and adenocarcinomas of the Bartholin glands.**

What % of vulvar cancers are multifocal?

~**5%** of vulvar cancers are multifocal.

■ Workup/Staging

What is the Bx approach for small (<1 cm) vulvar lesions?

For small (<1 cm) vulvar lesions, **excisional Bx with a 1-cm margin, including the skin, dermis, and connective tissue.**

What is the Bx approach for large (>1 cm) vulvar lesions?

For large (>1 cm) vulvar lesions, **wedge Bx including surrounding skin.** These should be taken from the edge of the lesion to include the interface between normal skin and the tumor to determine whether there is invasion of adjacent epithelium. (*Baldwin P et al., Curr Obst and Gyn 2005*)

What is the basic workup of vulvar cancer?

Vulvar cancer workup:
1. H&P
2. Labs: CBC (to check for anemia); UA (to r/o infection), HIV testing (to r/o immunodeficiency)
3. EUA with PAP smear, colposcopy, and directed Bx of the cervix, vagina, and vulva; cystoscopy and sigmoidoscopy if clinically indicated
4. DRE to r/o multifocal Dz
5. Imaging: CT abdomen/pelvis and CXR, but consider PET and MRI
6. Stage-specific inguinal nodal evaluation

Which pts with vulvar cancer do not require inguinal lymphadenectomy?

In vulvar cancer, all pts with clinically suspicious nodes require bilat inguinal lymphadenectomy unless there are bulky unresectable nodes. For pts with no clinically suspicious nodes, the need for inguinal lymphadenectomy depends primarily on DOI. If the DOI is <1 mm, a lymphadenectomy may not be needed unless there is LVI or a high grade. The use of sentinel node Bx instead of a full dissection is being studied.

In which pts with vulvar cancer is a unilat (instead of bilat) lymphadenectomy sufficient for workup?

Pts with a well-lateralized primary may undergo a unilat lymphadenectomy only.

Is the staging system for vulvar cancer surgical or clinical?

FIGO **surgical** staging is used for vulvar cancer.

Do imaging results affect the FIGO stage in vulvar cancer?

No. Imaging results are not included in FIGO staging.

Summarize the FIGO (2008) staging for vulvar cancer.

Stage IA: lesion ≤2 cm, confined to vulva or perineum with stromal invasion <1 mm, no nodal mets

Stage IB: lesion >2 cm or with stromal invasion >1 mm, confined to vulva or perineum, no nodal mets

Stage II: lesion of any size with extension to adjacent structures (lower 3rd of urethra, lower 3rd of vagina or anus), no nodal mets

Stage III: lesion of any size with or without extension to adjacent structures (lower 3rd of urethra, lower 3rd of vagina or anus) and positive inguinofemoral LN

Stage IIIA: 1 LN ≥5 mm or 1–2 LNs <5 mm

Stage IIIB: ≥2 LN ≥5 mm or ≥3 LNs each <5 mm

Stage IIIC: node(s) with extracapsular spread

Stage IVA1: lesion invades upper urethra and/or vaginal mucosa, bladder mucosa, rectal mucosa, or fixed to pelvic bone

Stage IVA2: fixed or ulcerated inguinofemoral LN

Stage IVB: DMs, including pelvic LNs

▌ Treatment/Prognosis

What is the Tx for vulvar CIS or VIN?

Pts with vulvar CIS or VIN can be treated with **superficial local excision.** If the labia minora or clitoris is involved, consider laser ablation.

How should the primary of a pt with FIGO stage I or II vulvar cancer be treated?

In a pt with stage I or II vulvar cancer, the primary can be resected via a **WLE,** which includes resection of the tumor + a 2-cm margin of normal tissue around it.

In a pt with a stage I or II vulvar cancer, does radical vulvectomy improve the LR rate over WLE?

No. In a pt with stage I or II vulvar cancer, radical vulvectomy and WLE have similar recurrence rates (~7%). (*Hacker NF et al., Cancer 1993*)

What is the next step if margins are positive following surgical resection of vulvar cancer?

Re-excise if possible; otherwise, give adj RT. Retrospective data suggests that adj RT improves LC and possibly survival (*Faul CM et al., IJROBP 1997*).

How are the inguinal nodes treated in vulvar cancer stage IA? Stage IB? Stage II?

Stage IA: Lymphadenectomy is not necessary (consider for high-grade lesions).

Stage IB: If the lesion is well lateralized, consider unilat dissection. If there is a midline lesion, then bilat groin nodal dissection is required.

Stage II: Bilat lymphadenectomy is recommended.

GOG 173 is an ongoing phase III trial examining the utility of sentinel LN mapping for stage I–II pts.

In which vulvar cancer pts is adj RT to the bilat groin and pelvis indicated? What RCT explored this question?

Adj RT to the bilat groin and pelvis is commonly recommended **in pts with ≥2 micromets in inguinal nodes, a single node >5 mm, or a single node with ECE.**

In **GOG 37,** 114 pts s/p radical vulvectomy + bilat inguinal lymphadenectomy were randomized to RT to the pelvis and bilat groin vs. pelvic node dissection if node+. The dose was 45–50 Gy. The 2-yr groin recurrence rate decreased with RT (5% vs. 24%), and there was an OS advantage for RT (68% vs. 54%). All the benefits of RT were for >1 +node. The survival benefit appeared to be due to improved control in the groin. In pts with only 1 +node on the dissection, surgery and RT outcomes were similar. (*Homesley HD et al., Obstet Gynecol 1986*)

In pts with N0 vulvar cancer, does groin RT eliminate the need for inguinal lymphadenectomy? What RCT explored this question?

The need for inguinal node dissection in N0 vulvar cancer prior to groin RT is **controversial**. In **GOG 88,** 58 pts with cN0 vulvar cancer s/p radical vulvectomy were randomized to bilat inguinal femoral and pelvic lymphadenectomy (+nodes rcv RT) vs. bilat groin-only EBRT (50 Gy). LR, PFS, and OS favored the lymphadenectomy arm. (*Stehman FB et al., Cancer 1992*)

What is the most common histology for vaginal cancer? What are 5 other rare vaginal cancer histologies?

Squamous cell carcinoma is the most common primary vaginal histology. **Melanoma, sarcoma, lymphoma, adenocarcinoma, and clear cell adenocarcinoma** are much more rare.

Increased risk for clear cell adenocarcinoma is linked with what exposure?

In utero exposure to the synthetic estrogen **diethylstilbestrol (DES)** is linked with an increased risk for clear cell adenocarcinoma.

What type of vaginal sarcoma is most common in adults? In children?

Adults: leiomyosarcoma
Children (<6 yo): embryonal rhabdomyosarcoma (i.e., sarcoma botryoides)

If an elderly woman has had a hysterectomy due to early-stage cervical cancer, is it reasonable to continue PAP smear screening of the vaginal vault?

Yes. Though the value of continued screening is not proven, PAP smears of the vaginal vault in elderly women who have had hysterectomy for invasive/preinvasive cervical cancer seems reasonable given the increased risk for vaginal cancer.

What is the nodal drainage of the upper two thirds of the vagina? Of the lower one third of the vagina?

The upper two thirds of the vagina drains to the obturator, internal, external, and common iliac nodes. The lower one third of the vagina may drain to the inguinofemoral nodes.

What are 4 common presenting Sx of vaginal cancer? What 2 additional Sx may suggest locally advanced Dz?

Vaginal cancer may present with **bleeding, discharge, pruritis, and dyspareunia. Pain or change in bowel/bladder habits may suggest locally advanced Dz.**

Where in the vagina is vaginal cancer most often located?

Vaginal cancer is most often found in the **post wall, sup one third** of the vagina (the speculum must be rotated to ensure exam of this region).

▌Workup/Staging

What staging exams/studies contribute to the FIGO stage?

Exams/studies that contribute to the FIGO stage include clinical exam of the pelvis and vagina (possibly under anesthesia), cystoscopy and proctosigmoidoscopy in women with locally advanced Dz, CXR, LFTs, and alk phos.

What imaging studies do not contribute to the FIGO stage?

Advanced imaging such as **CT, MRI, and PET** do not contribute to the FIGO stage (but still should be used to assess the Dz extent and plan therapy).

What is the FIGO (2008) staging for vaginal cancer?

Stage 0: CIS
Stage I: tumor limited to vaginal wall
Stage II: tumor invades paravaginal tissue but not pelvic sidewall
Stage III: tumor extends to pelvic sidewall
Stage IVA: tumor invades mucosa of bladder/rectum (bullous edema alone is not sufficient) and/or directly extends outside pelvis
Stage IVB: DMs

A vaginal cancer is never considered a vaginal primary if it involves either of what 2 structures?

Cancer involving the **vulva or cervix** is never considered to be a vaginal primary (even if the bulk of Dz lies in the vagina).

When working up a presumed vaginal cancer primary, what other 3 sites should be evaluated for cosynchronous in situ or invasive Dz?

When working up a presumed vaginal cancer primary, always evaluate for cosynchronous **cervical, vulvar, and/or anal Dz.**

■ Treatment/Prognosis

What are 3 appropriate Tx for vaginal intra-epithelial neoplasia (VAIN)?

Surgical excision, laser vaporization, and topical 5-FU are all appropriate Tx for VAIN.

VAIN is multifocal in what % of pts?

Up to 60% of pts with VAIN have multifocal Dz. Close follow-up is essential.

In general, what is the preferred definitive Tx modality for vaginal cancer?

Although surgery may be appropriate for early, stage I lesions, **definitive RT** is generally the preferred Tx modality (as morbidity is less compared with radical surgery).

What are the estimates of 5-yr pelvic Dz control and DSS for stage I, II, and III–IVA vaginal cancer managed with definitive RT?

For vaginal cancer managed with definitive RT, 5-yr pelvic Dz control is 86%, 84%, and 71% for FIGO stage I, II, and III–IVA, respectively. 5-yr DSS is 85%, 78%, and 58%, respectively. (*Frank SJ et al., IJROBP 2005*)

Is concurrent CRT a reasonable consideration in advanced-stage vaginal cancer?

Yes. Extrapolating from the cervical, vulvar, and anal cancer literature, concurrent CRT (typically cisplatin based) is reasonable to consider for advanced-stage vaginal cancer (i.e., stages III–IVA).

Is vaginal cylinder brachytherapy alone (without EBRT) appropriate in any vaginal cancer pts?

Possibly. While whole pelvis EBRT combined with brachytherapy is generally preferred, vaginal cylinder brachytherapy alone may be acceptable for pts with VAIN or very early stage I vaginal cancer <5 mm thick.

What brachytherapy technique is commonly required for stage II–III vaginal cancer (in addition to EBRT Tx)?

Interstitial brachytherapy needle implants are commonly required to achieve adequate brachytherapy dose coverage for stage II–III vaginal cancers (the depth-dose characteristics of intracavitary applicators are not favorable enough to treat deep lesions).

What are the typical field borders for vaginal cancer whole pelvis fields?

Typical whole pelvis vaginal cancer field borders:
Top: L5-S1
Bottom: entire vagina or 3 cm below Dz extent
Lateral: 2 cm beyond pelvic brim

If the lower 3rd of the vagina is involved, then treat inguinal nodes as well (as per vulvar or anal cancer).

What are the appropriate EB and cumulative (EB + brachytherapy) RT doses for vaginal cancer?

Whole pelvis (+/− inguinal nodes) EB doses are typically 45–50 Gy → brachytherapy boost to a total dose of 70–80 Gy.

Among pts who fail following definitive RT, what % have LR as a component of their relapse?

~**75%** of pts with relapse following definitive RT for vaginal cancer will experience LF. (*Frank SJ et al., IJROBP 2005*)

■ Toxicity

What are the 5- and 10-yr grade 3–4 toxicity rates following definitive RT for vaginal cancer?

Grade 3–4 toxicity rates are **10% and 17% at 5 and 10 yrs, respectively,** following RT for vaginal cancer. (*Frank SJ et al., IJROBP 2005*)

What are the 4 most common grade 3–4 late effects following definitive RT for vaginal cancer?

Following definitive RT for vaginal cancer, **proctitis (requiring transfusion), rectal fistula, SBO, and hemorrhagic cystitis** are the most common grade 3–4 toxicities.

What common late effect may limit sexual function as well as follow-up for vaginal cancer?

Vaginal stenosis is very common following RT for vaginal cancer. All pts should use a vaginal dilator.

70
Hodgkin Disease
Steven H. Lin and Eli Glatstein

Background

At what age does Hodgkin disease (HD) most commonly occur?

HD has a bimodal peak with peaks at **age 25 yrs and age 60–70 yrs.**

What are 2 broad histologic categories of HD? Which is more common?

Broad histologic categories of HD:
1. Classic (more common)
2. Nodular lymphocyte predominant Hodgkin lymphoma (NLPHL)

What are the subtypes of classic HD, and which is most common in the U.S.?

Subtypes of classic HD:
1. Nodular sclerosing (most common in the U.S.)
2. Mixed cellularity
3. Lymphocyte depleted
4. Lymphocyte rich

What are the 2 most commonly involved LN regions at the initial Dx of HD?

Most commonly involved LN regions at initial Dx of HD:
1. Cervical chains (70% of pts)
2. Mediastinum (50% of pts)

Pts who present with mediastinal LAD are most likely to have which subtype of HD?

Pts who present with mediastinal LAD are most likely to have **nodular sclerosing** HD.

In classic HD, what is the most common CD15, -30, -45, and -20 staining pattern?

In classic HD, tumors are typically **CD15 and -30 positive but CD45 and -20 negative.**

In NLPHL, what is the most common CD15, -30, -45, and -20 staining pattern?

In NLPHL, tumors are typically **CD15 and -30 negative but CD45 and -20 positive** (i.e., the reverse of classic HD).

Which HD subtype has the best prognosis?

Lymphocyte-rich HD has the best prognosis.

Which HD subtype has the worst prognosis?

Lymphocyte-depleted HD has the worst prognosis.

Which HD subtype is associated with older age or HIV+ pts?

Lymphocyte-depleted HD is associated with older age and HIV+ pts.

Pts with which subtype of HD are at greatest risk of developing a subsequent non-Hodgkin lymphoma?

Pts with **NLPHL** are at greatest risk of developing a subsequent non-Hodgkin lymphoma.

What are the "B Sx" of lymphoma?

B Sx include:
1. Fevers >38°C
2. >10% body weight loss in 6 mos
3. Drenching night sweats

How is bulky mediastinal Dz commonly defined?

Bulky mediastinal Dz is commonly defined as a **mass greater than one third of the intrathoracic diameter at T5-6 on upright PA film.**

How is bulky Dz defined outside of the mediastinum?

Outside of the mediastinum, bulky Dz is variably defined in clinical trials but **most often is either any mass >5 cm or any mass >10 cm.**

■ Workup/Staging

What kind of Bx is preferred for Dx of HD and why?

Excisional Bx is preferred for the Dx of lymphomas b/c **it shows LN architecture.**

What imaging studies are typically ordered as part of the workup of HD?

An **integrated PET/CT** is commonly used in the workup imaging for HD.

What lab work is required as part of the workup of HD?

The following labs have prognostic implications: ESR, CBC, albumin, and LDH.

Labs necessary for Tx planning are BUN, Cr, and a pregnancy test in women of childbearing age.

What are common indications for a BM Bx in the workup of HD?

Common indications for a staging BM Bx:
1. B Sx
2. Stages III–IV
3. Bulky Dz
4. >2 sites
5. Recurrent Dz

How is HD staged?

HD is staged using the **Ann Arbor system:**
Stage I: involvement of 1 LN region or localized involvement of a single extralymphatic organ or site (IE)
Stage II: involvement of ≥2 LN regions on same side of diaphragm or localized involvement of a single associated extralymphatic organ or site and its regional LN with or without involvement of other LN regions on same side of diaphragm (IIE)

> **Stage III:** involvement of LN regions on both sides of diaphragm that may also be accompanied by localized involvement of an associated extralymphatic organ or site (IIIE)
>
> **Stage IV:** multifocal involvement of ≥ 1 extralymphatic organ, with or without associated LN involvement, or isolated extralymphatic organ involvement with distant nodal involvement.

Note: Pts without B Sx are designated with an A, otherwise with a B. Pts with splenic involvement are designated with an S.

Involvement of what sites is considered stage 4 Dz?

Per the AJCC (7th edition), pts with involvement of the **BM, liver, pleura, and CSF** have stage IV Dz.

Name the 14 distinct LN regions as per the Rye classification.

LN regions per the Rye classification:
1. Waldeyer ring
2. Occipital, cervical, preauricular, and supraclavicular
3. Infraclavicular
4. Axillary
5. Epitrochlear
6. Mediastinum
7. Right hilum
8. Left hilum
9. Para-aortic
10. Spleen
11. Mesenteric
12. Iliac
13. Inguinofemoral
14. Popliteal

Is involvement of the Waldeyer ring and spleen considered extranodal?

No. Per the AJCC (7th edition), the Waldeyer ring and spleen are not classified as extranodal sites.

What does the Waldeyer ring include?

The Waldeyer ring includes:
1. Pharyngeal tonsil (adenoids)
2. Palatine tonsil
3. Lingual tonsil (base of tongue)

What are unfavorable factors for early HD?

Risk factors used to stratify early-stage HD in clinical trials vary.

Unfavorable factors for early HD:
1. Age ≥ 50 yrs
2. Bulky Dz
3. ≥ 4 sites
4. ESR >50 if no B Sx or >30 if B Sx
5. Presence of extranodal sites
6. Mixed-cellularity or lymphocyte-depleted histology

What are commonly used RT doses in HD after initial chemo?

Sites without bulky Dz are typically treated 30 Gy after chemo. Sites of initial bulky Dz are typically treated to 36 Gy after chemo.

Describe the evidence that suggests improved outcomes with CRT compared to RT alone in early-stage favorable HD.

In the 1990s, CRT vs. RT alone was evaluated in at least 4 major randomized trials:
1. **EORTC H7F** (*Noordijk EM et al., JCO 2006*)
2. **EORTC H8F** (*Ferme C et al., NEJM 2007*)
3. **German HD7** (*Engert A et al., JCO 2007*)
4. **SWOG S9133** (*Press OW et al., JCO 2001*)

While the chemo and RT techniques varied in these studies, long-term relapse rates consistently favored the CRT arms. In **EORTC H8F**, 10-yr OS was significantly improved with CRT, but long-term OS was not significantly different in the other studies.

Summarize the evidence for and against the elimination of consolidative RT in pts who achieve a CR after chemo in HD.

The outcomes after chemo alone in early and advanced HD have been evaluated in at least 3 major RCTs:

NCI-Canada/ECOG randomized unfavorable stage I–II nonbulky pts to ABVD × 4–6 cycles (4 if CR after 2nd cycle) vs. ABVD × 2 cycles + STNI. 5-yr freedom from progression favored the CRT arm (88% vs. 95%), but OS was not significantly different (95% ABVD alone vs. 92% CRT) (*Meyer RM et al., JCO 2005*). The authors suggested that lack of OS benefit was due to increased toxicity of the combined modality arm and that a difference favoring ABVD alone may be seen in the long term, given the known late RT toxicity profile.

Laskar et al. randomized a diverse cohort of pts in India (stage I–IV, +/− bulky Dz and/or B Sx, adults and children, all of whom had a CR after ABVD × 6 cycles) to IFRT or observation. A majority of pts had mixed cellularity histology (most common in India). IFRT improved 8-yr EFS (88% vs. 76%) and 8-yr OS (100% vs. 89%), especially in pts <15 yo, with B Sx, bulky Dz, and advanced stages. (*JCO 2004*)

Aleman et al. randomized stage III–IV HD who achieved a CR after 4 or 6 cycles of MOPP-ABV to IFRT or observation. Pts who had a CR after 2 cycles rcv 4 cycles, and those who had a CR after 4 cycles rcv 6 cycles. There was no difference in 8-yr EFS (observation, 77% vs. IFRT, 73%) or 8-yr OS (observation, 85% vs. IFRT, 78%). (*IJROBP 2007*)

EORTC H10 is an ongoing trial comparing ABVD alone in pts who have a PET CR after 2 cycles vs. ABVD + INRT.

Summarize the evidence to support the use of IFRT instead of more extensive RT in HD pts receiving CRT.

At least 4 RCTs have compared IFRT to more extensive RT in HD pts receiving CRT:

1. **Groupe Pierre-et-Marie-Curie (GPMC)** (*Zittoun R et al., JCO 1985*)
2. **German HD 8** (*Klimm B et al., Ann Oncol 2007*)
3. **Milan study** (*Banadonna G et al., JCO 2004*)
4. **EORTC H8-U** (*Ferme C et al., NEJM 2007*)

The 5–12-yr OS outcomes were similar in all of these studies, suggesting that more extensive RT than IFRT is not necessary.

Summarize the evidence to support the use of IFRT at 20 Gy after induction chemo in favorable stage I–II HD pts.

The use of <30 Gy in favorable stage I–II HD pts after initial chemo has been studied in at least 2 RCTs:

HD 10 from the German Hodgkin Study Group randomized pts to 2 vs. 4 cycles of chemo → 20 Gy vs. 30 Gy IFRT (2 × 2 factorial design). 5-yr PFS, freedom from Tx failure, and OS were similar between the chemo comparison and the RT dose comparison. (*Engert A et al., NEJM 2010*)

EORTC GELA H9F randomized favorable stage I–II HD pts with a CR after epirubicin/bleomycin/vinblastine/prednisone (EBVP) × 6 cycles to 36 Gy IFRT vs. 20 Gy IFRT vs. no RT. 4-yr EFS was similar between the 36 Gy and 20 Gy arms (87% vs. 84%, respectively) but was significantly lower in the no-IFRT arm (70%). (*Noordijk EM et al., ASCO abstract 2005*)

Summarize the evidence that suggests consolidative RT is more important in pts treated with Stanford V chemo compared to ABVD chemo.

2 RCTs have compared ABVD and Stanford V regimens for HD:

Gobbi et al. compared ABVD vs. Stanford V (vs. a 3rd regimen). RT was not mandatory and was used in only 66% of the Stanford V arm and 62% of the ABVD arm. 5-yr FFS significantly favored ABVD (78% vs. 54%). (*JCO 2005*)

Hoskin et al. randomized unfavorable stage I–II and stage III–IV HD pts to ABVD- or Stanford V–based regimens. Initially, IFRT was required to a site initially >5 cm, though in the latter part of the study, RT was optional for the ABVD arm. Ultimately, 53% in the ABVD arm and 73% in the Stanford V arm rcv IFRT. Despite the higher rate of consolidative RT, 5-yr PFS (ABVD, 76%; Stanford V, 74%) and OS (ABVD, 90%; Stanford V, 92%) were not significantly different. (*JCO 2009*)

Is there a relationship between clinical aggressiveness and curability of NHL?

Advanced-stage indolent NHL is rarely curable. Inter-mediate-grade NHL may be curable even in advanced stages.

Without Tx, what is the life expectancy for pts with NHL of varying aggressiveness?

Pts with indolent NHL have survival measured in yrs. Pts with aggressive NHL have survival measured in mos, and those pts with highly aggressive Dz have an expected survival of wks.

What % of NHL is indolent, and what are the most prevalent subtypes?

~**35%** of NHL is indolent by the WHO classification. 95% of indolent NHL are **follicular lymphoma** (FL) (grades 1–2; 65%), **small lymphocytic lymphoma** (SLL) (18%), and **marginal zone B-cell lymphoma or MALT lymphoma** (12%).

What are common cytogenetic abnormalities associated with indolent NHL?

t(14;18) is seen in 90% of FLs. This results in overexpression of antiapoptotic Bcl-2. **Chromosome 13 deletion**, t(14;19), and **trisomy 12** are associated with SLL and CLL. **Trisomy 3** (60%) and **t(11;18)** (25%–40%) are associated with MALT lymphoma.

How is FL graded?

FL demonstrates a mix of centrocytes (small, cleaved cells) and centroblasts (large, noncleaved cells). **Grade correlates to the density of centroblasts** (e.g., 0–5 centroblasts/high-power field (hpf), grade 1; >15 centroblasts/hpf, grade 3a).

What is SLL?

SLL is the same Dz entity as CLL but with a **predominant manifestation in the spleen, liver, or nodes** as opposed to peripheral blood or BM.

What is Richter syndrome? What is its rate of occurrence?

Richter syndrome is the **transformation of SLL or CLL into DLBCL.** It occurs in roughly **5% of cases.**

How is bulky mediastinal Dz commonly defined?

Bulky mediastinal Dz is commonly defined as a **mass greater than one third of the intrathoracic diameter at T5-6 on upright PA film.**

How is bulky Dz defined outside of the mediastinum?

Outside of the mediastinum, bulky Dz is variably defined in clinical trials but most often is **either any mass >5 cm or any mass >10 cm.**

■ Workup/Staging

What are the pertinent focused aspects of the physical exam in a person with suspected NHL?

The physical exam should include complete nodal assessment including epitrochlear and popliteal groups. Cervical adenopathy palpable above the hyoid bone should prompt an ENT exam. (The Waldeyer ring is more frequently involved in NHL than in HD.) Exam of extranodal at-risk sites including the liver, spleen, testicles, bones, abdomen, and flanks is appropriate.

What lab studies should be performed?

Laboratory studies should include: CBC with differential, CMP, LDH, β2-microglobulin, serum protein electrophoresis, HIV, hepatitis B virus (essential as it may reactivate with rituximab Tx), and hepatitis C virus. BM Bx should be performed for all lymphomas. LP should be performed for CNS Sx, testicular or paranasal sinus involvement, or immunodeficiency.

What imaging studies should be performed?

The imaging workup should include CT C/A/P. PET is appropriate in most cases. MRI brain should be performed for CNS Sx, testicular or paranasal sinus involvement, or immunodeficiency.

How is NHL staged?

NHL is staged similar to HD using the **Ann Arbor (AA) system:**

Stage 1: involvement of 1 LN region or localized involvement of 1 extralymphatic organ or site (IE)

Stage 2: involvement of $\geq$2 LN regions on same side of diaphragm or localized involvement of 1 associated extralymphatic organ or site and its regional LN, with or without involvement of other LN regions on same side of diaphragm (IIE)

Stage 3: involvement of LN regions on both sides of diaphragm, which may also be accompanied by localized involvement of an associated extralymphatic organ or site (IIIE)

Stage 4: multifocal involvement of $\geq$1 extralymphatic organ, with or without associated LN involvement, or isolated extralymphatic organ involvement with distant nodal involvement

Note: Pts without B Sx are designated with an A, otherwise with a B. Pts with splenic involvement are designated with an S.

What is a major limitation to the AA staging of NHL (as opposed to HD)?

NHL **typically spreads in a less contiguous fashion** compared to HD and thus stage I NHL is very rare (10%).

How is NHL practically staged?

NHL is practically divided into **limited stage and advanced stage.** Limited stage consists of AA stage I–II pts with $\leq$3 adjacent LN regions, no B Sx, and no bulky ($\geq$10 cm) lesions. Advanced stage includes all other pts. *For FL, practical division is between AA stage I–II, nonbulky, nonabdominal Dz, and all others.*

What are the basic Tx principles for stage III–IV, low-grade FL?	No Tx is considered curative. Several randomized trials have indicated that therapy can be deferred without reducing survival. Tx is reserved for the following: 1. Symptomatic Dz 2. Threatened end organ dysfunction 3. Cytopenias 4. Bulky Dz 5. Steady Dz progression 6. Clinical trial 7. Pt preference
What is the role of RT for stage III–IV, low-grade FL?	In advanced-stage indolent lymphomas, RT is reserved for **palliation of Sx.**
What is a typical RT Rx for symptomatic stage III–IV FL?	Traditionally, >**20 Gy.** A phase II study of RT for symptomatic local masses with indolent NHL demonstrated a 65% CR and 22% PR with a median duration of response of 22 mos with 2 Gy × 2 (*Johannsson J et al., IJROBP 2002*).
What is the role of RT in the Tx of SLL?	RT is used for **palliation of symptomatic lesions** in SLL. Consider 2 Gy × 2 regimens.
What is the role of RT in treating nodal marginal zone lymphomas?	RT is used for **palliation of symptomatic lesions** in advanced-stage nodal marginal zone lymphomas.
What is the most common initial multiagent chemo used in the management of intermediate-/high-grade NHL?	The most common initial multiagent chemo used in NHL is **R-CHOP,** which uses the following drugs: 1. Rituximab 2. Cyclophosphamide 3. Hydroxydaunomycin (Adriamycin) 4. Oncovin (vincristine) 5. Prednisone
What are the current indications for RT regarding early-stage, intermediate-/high-grade NHL?	The inclusion of RT in early-stage, intermediate-/high-grade NHL is very **institution dependent.** It may be included as consolidation after 3–4 cycles of R-CHOP in favorable Dz, in pts with a PR to chemo, or in pts with bulky Dz. The inclusion of rituximab to CHOP in advanced Dz has resulted in significant OS benefit, and the results of trials including rituximab in the management of localized Dz may obviate the inclusion of RT for most localized NHL. Alternatively, improved systemic control may further increase the importance of LC and thus RT in early-stage Dz.
What is the present Tx paradigm for advanced stage, intermediate-/high-grade NHL?	Advanced-stage, intermediate-/high-grade NHL Tx paradigm: R-CHOP × 6–8 cycles. IFRT may be considered for initially bulky sites.

Estimate the prognosis of limited-stage aggressive B-cell lymphoma treated with R-CHOP and IFRT.

Long-term outcomes with R-CHOP and IFRT are limited. **SWOG 0014** enrolled 60 pts with limited-stage aggressive NHL and at least 1 adverse risk factor and treated with R-CHOP × 3 + IFRT: 4-yr PFS was 88%, and OS was 92%. (*Persky DO et al., JCO 2008*)

What is the long-term DFS for pts with localized DLBCL treated with RT alone? What were the typical Tx doses used in clinical trials?

Using **45–50 Gy** to maximize LC, **only 40% of pts with localized DLBCL had long-term DFS** based on historical RT-alone data. (*Chen MG et al., Cancer 1979; Kaminski MS et al., Ann Intern Med 1986; Sweet DL et al., Blood 1981*)

What was demonstrated in the initial publication of the SWOG 8736 study comparing chemo alone to abbreviated CRT in localized intermediate-grade NHL?

In **SWOG 8736,** 401 pts with stage I or IE (including bulky Dz) and stage II or IIE (nonbulky) intermediate-grade NHL were randomized to CHOP × 8 cycles vs. CHOP × 3 + IFRT. RT doses of 40–55 Gy were employed. At 5-yr follow-up, PFS and OS favored the combined therapy group (OS: 82% vs. 72%). (*Miller TP et al., NEJM 1998*)

What was shown in the updated analysis of SWOG 8736 at median follow-up of 8.5 yrs?

In the updated analysis of **SWOG 8736,** published in abstract form in 2001, PFS curves overlapped at 7 yrs and OS curves overlapped at 9 yrs. There were excess late relapses and deaths from advanced lymphoma in the combined arm seen in yrs 5–10. Results are stratified by IPI criteria:

Stage I, no risk factors: 94% OS at 5 yrs
Stage II (nonbulky) and/or 1+ adverse risk factor: 71% OS at 5 yrs
3 risk factors (stage II may be 1 of them): 50% OS at 5 yrs

(*Miller TP et al., ASH abstract 3024 2001*)

What was demonstrated in the ECOG E1484 study randomizing postchemo complete responders to observation vs. IFRT?

In **ECOG E1484,** 352 pts with intermediate-grade, bulky stage I–IE or nonbulky stage II–IIE Dz were administered CHOP × 8 cycles. Complete responders (215 pts) were randomized to IFRT vs. observation. At 6 yrs, DFS favored IFRT (73% vs. 56%), but OS was equivalent. FFS was equivalent in partial responders administered IFRT and in CR pts. Failure at initial sites was greater in pts not given IFRT. (*Horning SJ et al., JCO 2004*)

What was demonstrated in the GELA LNH-93-1 study comparing aggressive chemo vs. standard chemo and RT in pts ≤60 yo?

In **GELA LNH-93-1,** 647 pts ≤60 yo with low-risk (IPI 0), stage I or II, intermediate-risk NHL (extranodal or bulky Dz allowed) were randomized to doxorubicin/cyclophosphamide/vindesine/bleomycin/prednisone (ACVBP) × 3, then methotrexate/etoposide/ifosfamide/cytarabine vs. CHOP × 3, then IFRT to 30–40 Gy. ACVBP improved EFS and OS regardless of the presence of bulky Dz. (*Reyes F et al., NEJM 2005*)

■ Treatment/Prognosis

What is the 1st-line therapy used for the Tx of MALT lymphoma?

If there is documented *H. pylori* infection, use **antibiotics against *H. pylori*** (triple therapy of Biaxin/Flagyl/proton-pump inhibitor [PPI] or Biaxin/amoxicillin/PPI).

If there is lymphoma but the pt is *H. pylori*–negative, consider RT as a primary therapeutic approach, especially if there are chromosomal abnormalities.

How is the eradication of *H. pylori* determined?

To determine the eradication of *H. pylori*, a **urea breath test should be done 1 mo after antibiotic use.** If there is persistence of tumor and *H. pylori* infection, switch to a different antibiotic regimen.

What response rate is expected from 1st-line Tx of MALT lymphoma?

75%–80% of pts have a CR. (*Wundisch T et al., JCO 2005*)

What is the typical response period to antibiotics in MALT lymphoma?

In MALT lymphoma, regression is slow and can take from a **median of 6 mos to 12–18 mos.**

How should response be assessed when using antibiotics for MALT lymphoma?

Response to antibiotics in MALT lymphoma is assessed by **EGD with visual inspection and Bx q3mos.** Dz should at least be stable or responding. If Dz if progressing, consider RT. If Dz is stable or regressing and the pt is asymptomatic, repeat the EGD in 3 mos.

What are 3 tumor characteristics that portend a poor response to the use of antibiotics for the Tx of MALT lymphoma?

Tumor characteristics that portend a poor response with antibiotics for MALT lymphoma include **t(11;18), trisomy 3, and DOI beyond the submucosa** (muscularis/serosa/adjacent organs) (*Sackmann M et al., Gastroenterology 1997*). There is an 86% CR with DOI < submucosa and 0% if invasion is beyond the submucosa.

What are the options for antibiotic-resistant MALT lymphomas?

Given the indolent nature of the Dz, there are many options. **Involved-field radiation therapy (IFRT) can be considered upfront or single-agent chemo such as rituxan or chlorambucil.** IFRT should be considered standard since the response is excellent and the pt can be potentially cured in the long term (~50% DFS at 10 yrs).

When should RT be considered for the Tx of MALT lymphoma?

RT for MALT lymphoma should be considered in the following situations:
1. *H. pylori*–negative with stage IAE lymphoma, with or without initial use of antibiotics, and pt has no documented response to Tx
2. t(11;18)
3. Invasion beyond submucosa (muscularis/serosa/adjacent organs)
4. Documented progression after initial use of antibiotics
5. Documented failure of 2nd course of antibiotics
6. Rapid symptomatic progression of Dz

What are some important prognostic factors for MALT lymphomas?

Important prognostic factors for MALT lymphomas:
1. Age
2. Histology
3. DOI
4. LN involvement
5. Tumor size, cytogenetics

What are the factors in the follicular lymphoma International Prognostic Index (FLIPI) used for predicting the prognosis in MALT?

FLIPI for predicting the prognosis in MALT:
Hgb <12 g/dL
Age >60 yrs
Stage III–IV Dz
Sites >3 nodal
LDH abnl

(Mnemonic: FLIPI is a **HASSL**)

Is there a benefit of adding chemo in low-risk (<1 FLIPI) MALT?

No. Trials have demonstrated no additional survival benefit. Thus, IFRT remains the standard 1st-line modality. Considerations are made with rituxan + IFRT or radioantibody therapy in the future.

What are some factors that would predict for poor response to RT alone?

Factors that predict for poor response to RT alone:
1. Stage II Dz
2. FLIPI >1 factor
3. B Sx
4. Tumor bulk
5. Age >60 yrs

How should pts with poor-risk MALT lymphoma be managed?

Pts with poor-risk MALT lymphoma should be managed with a combined modality, using **chemo + IFRT.**

What is the 3rd-line therapy for Tx of MALT lymphoma?

The 3rd-line therapy for MALT lymphoma is **chemo (rituxan, single-agent Cytoxan) or total gastrectomy + chemo.**

What is the Tx paradigm for DLBCL of the stomach?

DLBCL of the stomach Tx paradigm: rituximab/cyclophosphamide/hydroxydaunomycin (Adriamycin)/Oncovin (vincristine)/prednisone (R-CHOP) + IFRT

What % of plasma cell tumors are MM? Solitary plasmacytoma (SP)?	**MM constitutes 90%** of plasma cell tumors, while **SP constitutes 10%** of plasma cell tumors.
Is there a racial or gender predilection for MM?	**Yes,** with regard to race. The incidence of MM is **greater in blacks** than whites (2:1). However, the incidence is **similar among men and women.**
What is the avg decade of life in which pts present with MM?	On avg, pts present with MM in the **5th–6th decades of life.**
What environmental exposure is most strongly associated with MM?	**Ionizing RT** is strongly linked to MM, as seen in A-bomb survivors in Hiroshima.
What are the 2 forms of SP?	The 2 forms of SP are **solitary bone plasmacytoma** (SBP) and **solitary extramedullary plasmacytoma** (SEP).
What environmental or genetic alterations are consistently associated with MM?	There are **no strong genetic or environmental patterns associated with MM.** There may be a modest but increased risk of MM with exposure to RT (latency 20+ yrs) or the chemical alachlor, a commonly used pesticide.
What % of pts with SBP will progress to MM at 10 yrs?	SBP will progress to MM in **50%–80%** of pts at 10 yrs. (*Hu K et al., Oncology 2000*)
What % of pts with SEP will progress to MM at 10 yrs?	SEP will progress to MM in **10%–40%** of pts at 10 yrs. (*Hu K et al., Oncology 2000*)
What is the most common site of SEP?	The most common site of SEP is the **H&N** region (80% of SEP); the nasal cavity and paranasal sinuses are the most common subsites for SEP.
What is the relationship between secretory patterns in SBP vs. SEP?	Most pts with SBP have a secretory tumor, whereas most pts with SEP have a nonsecretory tumor.
What is the relationship between LN involvement in SBP vs. SEP?	SBP rarely involves LNs, but SEP will have LN involvement 30%–40% of the time.
What 3 lab abnormalities may prompt a clinician to evaluate for a plasma cell neoplasm?	Laboratory abnormalities that may prompt evaluation for a plasma cell neoplasm: 1. Unexplained normochromic/normocytic anemia 2. Unexplained renal insufficiency 3. Hypercalcemia

What lab tests are used for screening of a plasma cell abnormality?	**Serum protein electrophoresis** (SPEP) and **urine protein electrophoresis** (UPEP) are lab tests used to screen for a plasma cell abnormality. A positive screen on these tests results when a monoclonal population (or spike) is detected.
What is the common pattern of bone Dz in MM?	**Lytic bone lesions** are the most common bone abnormality seen on imaging of pts with MM.
What is monoclonal gammopathy of undetermined significance (MGUS), and how often will it transform to MM?	MGUS is a **condition with clonal proliferation of an immunoglobulin in the absence of clinical, radiographic, or lab evidence of MM.** The risk of transformation from MGUS to MM is 1%/yr.
What is 1 factor that predicts the risk of transformation from MGUS to MM?	The risk of transformation from MGUS to MM is predicted by the **initial size of the M-protein peak.**
What is the most common clinical Sx seen at Dx of MM or SP?	**Bone pain** is the most common clinical Sx seen at Dx of MM or SP. A subset of these pts will present with a pathologic fracture.
What is POEMS syndrome?	POEMS syndrome (polyneuropathy, organomegaly, endocrinopathy, M protein, and skin changes) is a **variant of MM with solitary or limited sclerotic bone lesions** that often responds to radiotherapy with a spontaneous improvement in neuropathy.

What 3 diagnostic criteria are required for MM?

Criteria requisite for Dx of MM (*all are required*):
1. Clonal plasma cells of ≥10% (on either BM Bx or a Bx from other tissue)
2. Monoclonal protein in serum or urine
3. Evidence of end organ damage

(*No author, Br J Haematol 2003*)

Name 7 factors that can be used as evidence of end organ damage in MM.

Factors that can be used as evidence of end organ damage in MM:
1. Hypercalcemia
2. Renal insufficiency
3. Anemia
4. Bone lesions
5. Frequent severe infections
6. Amyloidosis
7. Hyperviscosity syndrome

(*No author, Br J Haematol 2003*)

What is the difference between symptomatic MM and asymptomatic (smoldering) MM?

Smoldering (or asymptomatic) MM requires the presence of serum monoclonal protein ≥3 g/dL and/or bone marrow plasma cells ≥10% *but no evidence* of end organ damage attributable to plasma cell dyscrasia. (*No author, Br J Haematol 2003*)

What 3 criteria are necessary for the Dx of MGUS?

Criteria necessary for the Dx of MGUS:
1. Serum monoclonal protein <3 g/dL
2. BM plasma cell <10%
3. No end organ damage attributable to plasma cell dyscrasia

(*No author, Br J Haematol 2003*)

What 4 criteria are necessary for the Dx of SP?

Criteria necessary for the Dx of SP:
1. Solitary bone lesion on skeletal survery
2. Histologic evidence of plasmacytoma by Bx
3. <5% plasma cells on marrow aspirate
4. No other end organ damage attributable to plasma cell dyscrasia

(*No author, Br J Haematol 2003*)

■ Workup/Staging

What is β2-microglobulin (β2M)?

β2M is a component of major histocompatibility complex class 1 molecules. Increasing levels of β2M are associated with a worse prognosis in MM.

What are the 2 most commonly used staging systems for MM?

The 2 most commonly used staging systems for MM are the **Durie-Salmon Staging and the International Staging System** (ISS).

What 2 factors are used to stage pts in the ISS system, and how are they grouped?

The 2 factors used in the ISS system are **β2M and albumin.** They are used to stage pts as follows:
Stage I: β2M <3.5 mg/L, albumin ≥3.5 g/dL
Stage II: β2M <3.5 mg/L, albumin <3.5 g/dL, or β2M ≥3.5 and <5.5
Stage III: β2M ≥5.5

What is the MS of MM by ISS stage?

MS of MM by ISS stage:
<u>Stage I</u>: 62 mos
<u>Stage II</u>: 44 mos
<u>Stage III</u>: 29 mos

(*Greipp PR et al., JCO 2005*)

What is the Durie-Salmon staging scheme for MM?

Durie-Salmon staging scheme for MM:
Stage I: all of the following are required:
   a. Hgb >10 g/dL
   b. normal calcium
   c. skeletal survey with no lytic bone lesions
   d. serum paraprotein level <5 if IgG (<3 if IgA)
   e. urinary light chain excretion <4 g/24 hrs

Stage II: not fitting stage I or III
Stage III: 1 or more of the following:
   a. Hgb <8.5 g/dL
   b. calcium >12
   c. skeletal survey with ≥3 lytic lesions
   d. serum paraprotein level >7 if IgG (>5 if IgA)
   e. urinary light chain excretion >12 g/24 hrs

The Durie-Salmon staging system gives a subclassification of A or B based on what factor?

Durie-Salmon staging subclassification distinguishes pts based on **serum Cr:** A, Cr <2 mg/dL; B, Cr ≥2 mg/dL.

Besides a careful H&P, what lab and radiographic studies are necessary to evaluate a pt with newly diagnosed or suspected MM?

The lab and radiographic workup of MM includes CBC with differential, LDH, calcium and albumin levels, β2M, 24-hr total protein, SPEP/UPEP, skeletal survey, and unilat BM aspirate and Bx (with BM flow cytometry or immunohistochemistry). Other studies that may be helpful in select cases include MRI for suspected vertebral compression or tissue BM to Dx an SP.

What is the role of a bone scan in the workup and staging for plasma cell neoplasms?

There is **no role for routine staging** with a bone scan in pts with plasma cell neoplasms b/c the lesions are primarily lytic with little evidence of bone repair and consequent low isotope uptake.

■ Treatment/Prognosis

What is the recommended management of smoldering (asymptomatic) MM?

The recommended management of smoldering MM is **close observation** (expectant management).

What is the recommended management of SBP?

The recommended management of SBP is **involved-field RT to ≥45 Gy.**

What is the recommended management of SEP?

The recommended management of SEP is either **involved-field RT to ≥45 Gy, surgery, or surgery + RT.**

In what subgroup of pts with SEP may combined modality therapy (surgery → RT) be preferred?

In 1 study of **pts with SEP in the upper aerodigestive tract,** surgery → RT yielded improved OS in retrospective comparison of surgery or RT alone. (*Alexiou C et al., Cancer 1999*)

What is the role of RT in the Tx of MM, and what dose should be given?

The role of RT in the management of MM is for the **palliation of symptomatic bone mets, prevention of pathologic fractures, and the relief of cord compression.** The dose of RT given in MM is generally **20–36 Gy in 1.5–2 Gy/fx.**

What are the clinical presentations/phases of MF?

Clinical presentations/phases of MF:
1. Premycotic (erythematous macule) phase
2. Patch phase
3. Plaque phase
4. Tumor phase
5. Erythroderma (>80% surface area involvement)

When MF progresses from patch to plaque, what is seen under the microscope?

When MF progresses from patch to plaque, it is apparent that the **lymphoid clones begin to invade deeper into the dermis** and the **Pautrier abscesses are seen.**

What % of MF pts have LN involvement of Dz?

~**15%** of MF pts have LN involvement of their Dz.

What is a Sézary cell?

Sézary cells are defined as malignant **T cells with hyperconvoluted cerebriform nuclei.**

What is Sézary syndrome?

Sézary syndrome is an aggressive T-cell lymphoma with the presence of erythroderma + a Sézary cell count ≥100 cells/μL, CD4 to CD8 ratio ≥10, chromosomal T-cell clones that are abnl, T-cell clone detected in the bloodstream with an abnl T-lymphocyte count, and abnl expression of pan T-cell markers (CD2, -3 ,-4, -5). It sometimes is considered a leukemic form of Dz.

▇ Workup/Staging

What is the workup of MF?

MF workup: Hx with focus on B Sx, duration, distribution, and changes in any lesions, with presence or absence of pain or pruritis of lesions; physical exam with focus on the entire skin, including soles, perineum, nails, and auditory canals. Delineate skin involvement with photographs. Pathologic evaluation should include T-cell receptor gene analysis. Obtain a Sézary cell count and a T-cell receptor gene analysis in the peripheral blood. Obtain a CBC, CMP, LFTs, and PET/CT to assess for extracutaneous manifestations. Consider LN and BM Bx.

Describe the T classification system for MF.

T1: limited patch/plaque (<10% total skin surface): (a) patch only; (b) plaque +/− patch
T2: generalized patch/plaque (>10% total skin surface): (a) patch only; (b) plaque +/− patch
T3: tumor(s) ≥1 cm in diameter
T4: generalized erythroderma covering ≥80% of body surface area

Describe the N and M classification system for MF.

N0: uninvolved
N1: clinically abnl peripheral LN, histopathologically Dutch grade 1 or NCI LN 0-2: (a) T-cell clone negative; (b) T-cell clone positive

N2: clinically abnl peripheral LNs, histopathologically Dutch grade 2 or NCI LN 3: (a) T-cell clone negative; (b) T-cell clone positive

N3: clinically abnl peripheral LN, histopathologically Dutch grades 3–4 or NCI LN 4, clone positive or negative

M0: no visceral involvement

M1: visceral involvement

Describe the B classification of MF.

B0: ≤5% of peripheral blood lymphocytes are Sézary cells: (a) T-cell clone negative; (b) T-cell clone positive

B1: >5% of peripheral blood lymphocytes are Sézary cells, but pt not B2: (a) clone negative; (b) clone positive

B2: >1,000/μL Sézary cells with a positive T-cell clone

Describing the stage grouping of MF.

Stage IA: T1, N0, M0, B0-1
Stage IB: T2, N0, M0, B0-1
Stage IIA: T1-2, N1-2, M0, B0-1
Stage IIB: T3, N0-2. M0, B0-1
Stage IIIA: T4, N0-2, M0, B0
Stage IIIB: T4, N0-2, M0, B1
Stage IVA1: any T, N0-2, M0, B2
Stage IVA2: any T, N3, M0, any B
Stage IVB: any T, any N, M1, any B

If MF involves <10% of the body surface area, what T stage is this?

A **T1** MF lesion involves <10% of the body surface area.

How would erythroderma be staged for MF?

Erythroderma constitutes a **T4 lesion** for MF.

What constitutes stage I Dz in MF?

A pt with **T1 or T2, N0, M0, B0-1** would be stage I in MF.

What constitutes stage III Dz in MF?

A pt with a **T4 lesion with N0-2, M0, B0-1** Dz constitutes stage III in MF.

■ Treatment/Prognosis

What are the Tx options for MF that are limited to the skin?

Tx options for MF limited to skin:
1. Topical nitrogen mustard
2. Topical carmustine
3. Topical steroids
4. PUVA
5. UVB therapy
6. Local or total skin electron beam therapy (TSEBT)

75

Transplant/Total Body Irradiation

Bronwyn R. Stall and Deborah E. Citrin

Background

Define *hematopoietic stem cell transplantation* (HSCT).

HSCT is a **procedure to infuse hematopoietic cells** in order to restore normal hematopoiesis and/or to treat cancer.

What is the difference between *allogeneic* and *autologous*?

Allogeneic: stem cells from another person
Autologous: stem cells from the affected pt

What is a syngeneic transplant?

A syngeneic transplant uses an **identical twin as the donor.**

Name 3 sources of stem cells.

Umbilical cord blood, BM, and peripheral blood are 3 sources of stem cells.

What source of stem cells is most often used for transplant?

Most stem cells for transplant are obtained from **peripheral blood.**

What is a mini-transplant?

A mini-transplant, also known as nonmyeloablative or reduced-intensity transplant, **employs less toxic preparatory regimens, targeted to host T cells to facilitate engraftment.**

Name 4 malignancies routinely treated with autologous transplant.

Malignancies routinely treated with autologous transplant:
1. Recurrent Hodgkin Dz
2. Multiple myeloma
3. Chemosensitive aggressive non-Hodgkin lymphoma
4. Refractory testicular cancer

Which type of transplant is associated with a graft vs. tumor effect?

Allogeneic transplants may have graft vs. tumor effect.

Why is there decreased mortality with an autologous transplant in comparison to an allogeneic transplant?

The mortality rate with autologous transplant is lower due to the **absence of graft-versus-host disease** (GVHD).

What limits the use of allogeneic transplant?	The use of allogeneic transplant is limited by **availability of donors.**
What is the most important risk associated with autologous transplant?	The major risk of autologous transplant is **relapse.**
Allogeneic transplant is used most commonly in what type of malignancy?	Allogeneic transplant is most commonly used to treat **acute leukemias.**
What is a conditioning regimen?	A conditioning regimen is a **Tx used to prepare pts for infusion of hematopoietic cells,** which may be chemo alone or CRT.

Workup/Staging

What evaluations should be done prior to total body irradiation (TBI)?	TBI evaluation: complete H&P, PFTs, LFTs, serum Cr, and fertility counseling to include potential cryopreservation. A dental evaluation should also be done.

Treatment/Prognosis

What randomized data supports the use of fractionated rather than single-Tx TBI?	A **French (Institut Gustave Roussy) study** of single vs. hyperfractionated TBI randomized 160 pts with various hematologic malignancies to 10 Gy single dose or 14.85 Gy/11 fx. OS at 8 yrs was nonsignificantly higher in the hyperfractionated arm (45% vs. 38%) as well as CSS (77% vs. 63.5%). The rate of interstitial pneumonitis was similar between the 2 arms (14% and 19%); however, the rate of liver veno-occlusive Dz was significantly higher with a single fx (4% vs. 14%). (*Girinsky T et al., J Clin Oncol 2000*)
What is the main site of recurrence after transplant for lymphoma?	Following transplant for lymphoma, **local tumor** recurrence is the main cause of failure.
In pts receiving BMT for refractory lymphoma, is it safe to give local RT prior to transplant?	**Yes.** In the Johns Hopkins Hospital dose-escalation study of locoregional RT prior to Cytoxan/TBI for pts with refractory lymphoma, 21 pts with chemorefractory Dz rcv RT to current or previous sites of Dz to total doses from 1,000–2,000 cGy (all in 5 fx at an LDR of 10–20 cGy/minute) → TBI to 1,200 cGy in 4 daily fx. 3 of 6 pts at the 2,000-cGy level had acute grade 3 toxicity. It was concluded that LDR locoregional RT has acceptable toxicity up to 1,500 cGy/5 fx → Cytoxan/TBI. (*Song D et al., IJROBP 2003*)
What 2 pt positions are used for TBI?	TBI pt Tx positions include **supine, lateral recumbent or standing.**
Why are beam spoilers used for TBI?	Beam spoilers are used **to ensure adequate dose buildup in the skin;** a screen of tissue-equivalent material is positioned between the pt and the beam.

What variation in homogeneity is considered acceptable for TBI?	Homogeneity +/− **5%** is considered ideal for TBI.
Why is the dose rate lowered in TBI?	A lower dose rate is used in TBI **to decrease the incidence of interstitial pneumonitis.**
What compensators are often used in TBI?	**H&N compensators** are often used in TBI to improve homogeneity.
What organs are most frequently blocked in TBI?	The **lungs** are most frequently blocked in TBI.
What areas may be boosted in TBI?	When using TBI for lymphomas, the **site of residual Dz** may be boosted to decrease the chance of LR.

■ Toxicity

What is the major complication of allogeneic transplants?	The major complication of allogeneic transplants is **GVHD.**
What is acute GVHD?	Acute GVHD is the syndrome of **hepatitis, enteritis, and dermatitis occurring secondary to allogeneic transplant.**
What predicts the risk of GVHD and graft rejection?	GVHD and graft rejection risk increase with **human leukocyte antigen disparity.**
What is chronic GVHD?	The chronic form of GVHD **occurs >3 mos after transplant** and can affect many organs such as the GI tract, skin, liver, lungs, and eyes.

Name acute toxicities from TBI.

Most common acute toxicities from TBI:
1. N/v
2. Diarrhea
3. Xerostomia
4. Parotitis
5. Mucositis
6. Fatigue

What is the most common acute side effect?

The most common acute side effects from TBI are **n/v.**

Name 9 chronic toxicities from TBI.

Chronic toxicities from TBI:
1. Cataracts
2. Change in cognitive function
3. Endocrinopathies
4. Interstitial penumonitis
5. Hepatic dysfunction
6. Renal dysfunction
7. Growth retardation
8. Infertility
9. 2nd malignancies

PART XI Bone

76

Osteosarcoma

Russell K. Hales and Deborah A. Frassica

Background

Name the 2 most common types of malignant bone tumors in the pediatric population.

The 2 most common types of malignant bone tumors in the pediatric population are **osteosarcoma and Ewing sarcoma.**

Osteosarcoma is associated with what other pediatric tumor?

Pts with **retinoblastoma** have an increased risk of osteosarcoma, both within and outside the irradiated tissue.

Describe the distribution of osteosarcoma cases as a function of population age.

Osteosarcoma has a **bimodal distribution** as a function of age, with cases arising during the teenage years as well as cases associated with other conditions (Paget Dz, fibrous dysplasia) that arise in an older (age >65 yrs) population.

What is the incidence of osteosarcoma in the U.S. population?

400 cases/yr of osteosarcoma are diagnosed in the U.S. population, and most occur during the teenage years. Osteosarcoma is ~2 times more common than Ewing sarcoma.

What are the most common risk factors associated with the development of osteosarcoma?

High rate of bone production and turnover (as in puberty) are associated with the development of osteosarcoma.

Describe sex and ethnic factors associated with osteosarcoma.

Osteosarcoma is more common in **boys** (> girls) and in **blacks** (> whites).

What is another name for the shaft of the bone? End of the bone?

The **diaphysis is the shaft** of the bone. The **epiphysis is the end** of the bone, and the growth plate is located in this region. The conical area of bone between the diaphysis and epiphysis is the metaphysis.

Osteosarcoma is most likely to develop in what part of the bone?

Osteosarcoma arises most frequently in the **appendicular skeleton** (80% of cases) at the metaphyseal portions of the femur, tibia, and humerus.

Osteosarcoma most commonly arises in which bone?

The **femur** is the bone in which osteosarcoma most commonly arises.

Describe the histologic defining feature of osteosarcoma.

Production of osteoid bone is the defining feature of osteosarcoma.

Describe 2 genetic syndromes associated with osteosarcoma.

Osteosarcoma is associated with **Li-Fraumeni syndrome** as well as **retinoblastoma.**

What is the difference between conventional osteosarcoma and juxtacortical osteosarcoma?

Conventional (sometimes called *classic*) osteosarcoma refers to the most common (75% of all cases) variant of osteosarcoma, which typically presents within areas of rapidly proliferating skeletal bone. Juxtacortical osteosarcoma refers to a set of more rare osteosarcoma variants that arise adjacent to the outer surface of cortical bone.

Conventional osteosar-coma is usually what grade?

Conventional osteosarcoma is usually **high grade.**

Describe juxtacortical osteosarcoma in terms of pathologic grade and prognosis.

Juxtacortical osteosarcoma are usually **low grade** and rarely metastasize. They are **highly curable** with surgery alone and usually are located in the popliteal fossa.

What % of osteosarcoma pts have localized Dz at Dx?

90% of pts with osteosarcoma have localized Dz at Dx.

What % of osteosarcoma pts with localized Dz will develop DMs without chemo?

90% of pts with localized Dz will develop mets without chemo. (*Link M et al., Clinical pediatric oncology 1991*)

What are the 2 most common presenting Sx of osteosarcoma?

Pts with osteosarcoma typically present with **localized bone pain** (often associated with an injury) of several mos duration and a **soft tissue mass.**

■ Workup/Staging

Define the lab and radiographic studies used in the workup and staging of osteosarcoma.

Osteosarcoma workup: basic labs (CBC, CMP) as well as alk phos, LDH, and ESR. After plain films of the affected bone are obtained, MRI of the primary site is needed. PET or bone scan may be used for systemic staging of the Dz.

Define 3 principles used in the Bx of a suspected bone tumor.

Principles used in the Bx of a suspected bone tumor:
1. Bx should be performed at the same institution where the definitive resection will take place, preferably by the same surgeon who will undertake the definitive resection.
2. Bx should be placed carefully to avoid contamination of other areas, as may happen with a hematoma formation.
3. The Bx should not increase the extent of subsequent surgery.

What 3 lab values are most likely to be elevated in osteosarcoma?

Elevated **alk phos, LDR, and ESR** are the most likely lab abnormalities associated with osteosarcoma.

What radiographic features distinguish osteosarcoma from Ewing sarcoma?

Osteosarcoma is usually sclerotic, involves the metaphysis, and has periosteal new bone formation (sunburst pattern), whereas Ewing sarcoma is usually lytic, located in the diaphysis, and displays an onion skin effect. (*Lee B et al., Handbook of radiation oncology 2007*)

What is the most common site of mets from osteosarcoma?

The **lung** is the most common site of osteosarcoma mets.

What are the AJCC 7th edition (2009) TNM stage categories for bone tumors?

T1: ≤8 cm
T2: >8 cm
T3: discontinuous tumors in primary bone site
N0: no regional LN mets
N1: regional LN mets
M0: no DMs
M1a: DMs to lung
M1b: DMs to nonpulmonary sites

What is the AJCC stage grouping for bone tumors?

Stage Ia: T1N0, low grade
Stage Ib: T2-3N0, low grade
Stage IIa: T1N0, high grade
Stage IIb: T2N0, high grade
Stage III: T3N0, high grade
Stage IVa: M1a
Stage IVb: N1 or M1b

Define the Musculoskeletal Tumor Society (MSTS) staging system for bone sarcomas.

The MSTS staging system for bone sarcomas is as follows: stage I (low grade) vs. stage II (high grade), with A vs. B for anatomic extent (A, intracompartment vs. B, extracompartment). DMs are classified as stage III. Compartmental status is defined by whether the tumor extends though the cortex of the involved bone.

▪ Workup/Staging

What are 3 imaging tests commonly ordered for the workup of a possible chondrosarcoma?	**Plain radiographs, MRI, and CT** are commonly ordered for the workup of a possible chondrosarcoma. CT is best for examining tumor matrix mineralization, while MRI is best for assessing marrow and soft tissue involvement. In addition (especially for pts >40 yrs of age), CT C/A/P and other appropriate tests are often performed during the workup (to evaluate for possible metastatic Dz from an undiagnosed primary).
What is the characteristic plain film appearance of chondrosarcoma?	Although chondrosarcoma has a variable plain radiograph appearance, mineralization of chondroid matrix may produce a **punctate or ring-and-arc pattern of calcification.**
What 2 subspecialty referrals/workups should be performed prior to Tx of skull base chondrosarcoma?	**Baseline neuro-ophthalmology and endocrinology** workup is indicated for skull base chondrosarcoma.
What is the most common site for metastatic chondrosarcoma?	Although most chondrosarcomas have low metastatic potential, the **lung** is the most common site of metastatic Dz.
What are the AJCC 7th edition (2009) TNM stage categories for bone tumors?	**T1:** ≤8 cm **T2:** >8 cm **T3:** discontinuous tumors in primary site **N0:** no regional LN mets **N1:** regional LN mets **M0:** no DMs **M1a:** DMs to lung **M1b:** DMs to nonpulmonary sites
What is the AJCC stage grouping for bone tumors?	**Stage Ia:** T1N0, low grade **Stage Ib:** T2-3N0, low grade **Stage IIa:** T1N0, high grade **Stage IIb:** T2N0, high grade **Stage III:** T3N0, high grade **Stage IVa:** M1a **Stage IVb:** N1 or M1b
How is chondrosarcoma definitively diagnosed?	Chondrosarcoma is diagnosed by **percutaneous core-needle Bx** (which should be performed at the treating institution).

▌Treatment/Prognosis

What type of surgical resection is typically recommended for chondrosarcoma?

WLE (i.e., removal of tumor and a cuff of normal tissue) is typically recommended for definitive surgical Tx of chondrosarcoma. For low-grade chondrosarcoma confined to the bone, some surgeons attempt to minimize morbidity by performing marginal excision (i.e., intralesional curettage) → phenolization/cryotherapy, then cementing/bone grafting (though this may cause increased risk of LR, it may be acceptable given the lesion's low metastatic potential).

When is RT recommended for chondrosarcoma? What are typical doses?

RT is typically recommended for **unresectable chondrosarcoma or following margin+ resection of recurrent or high-grade lesions**. Doses **>65 Gy** are commonly recommended.

What is the recommended definitive Tx for skull base chondrosarcoma?

Surgical resection/debulking is recommended for skull base chondrosarcoma.

Why is PORT often recommended for skull base chondrosarcoma?

B/c gross total resection is often morbid for skull base chondrosarcoma (tumor resection is often piecemeal, and there may be adherence to critical structures), PORT is frequently recommended due to **+margins or gross residual Dz.**

What adj RT doses are necessary for control of skull base chondrosarcoma? What delivery methods are recommended?

Adj RT doses **>65 Gy** are needed for control of skull base chondrosarcoma. **IMRT or proton therapy** may be required to deliver this dose while respecting normal tissue tolerances.

When treated with surgical resection and adj RT, what control rates can be expected for skull base chondrosarcoma?

When treated with surgical resection and adj RT (to doses >65 Gy), control rates **>90%** can be expected for skull base chondrosarcoma (better than chordoma). (*Rosenberg AE et al., Am J Surg Pathol 1999*)

In general, is chemo recommended for chondrosarcoma?

No. Chemo is not generally recommended for chondrosarcoma (except for the dedifferentiated and mesenchymal subtypes, which according to NCCN category 2B recommendations can be treated as osteosarcoma and Ewing sarcoma, respectively).

What is a reasonable follow-up schedule for low- and high-grade chondrosarcoma?

According to the NCCN, a reasonable follow-up schedule for chondrosarcoma includes exam, local imaging, and chest imaging q6–12mos for 2 yrs, then annually. For high-grade lesions, recommendations include exam, local imaging, and chest imaging q3–6mos for 5 yrs, then annually for at least 10 yrs (as late recurrences may be seen).

Is conventional fractionated RT an effective Tx for chordomas?

Yes. Conventional fractionated RT is effective for palliating chordomas. Retrospective series of skull base chordomas demonstrated that with 50 Gy (photons only), 85% of pts achieved useful and prolonged pain palliation. However, LC was ~27%, 5-yr PFS was ~23%, and MS was ~62 mos (*Catton C et al., Radiother Oncol 1996*). Larger total doses are not achievable with conventional fractionated RT without causing undue toxicities.

What RT modality is preferred for the management of skull base chordomas?

Charged-particle RT (protons or carbon ions) allows high doses of RT to be delivered while limiting the dose to surrounding normal structures. Doses of 70–80 Gy can be achieved. In the largest series of 195 pts with chordomas treated at the Massachusetts General Hospital from 1974–1995, with a mean dose of 67.8 cobalt Gray equivalents (CGE; 63–79.2 CGE), the 5- and 10-yr PFS was 70% and 45%, respectively. (*Debus J et al., IJROBP 1997*)

What factor determines the risk for recurrence after Tx with proton beam therapy?

The **volume of residual Dz after surgical resection** determines the risk of recurrence after Tx with proton beam therapy.

In a series from Loma Linda (*Hug EB et al., J Neurosurg 1999*), for residual tumors abutting the brain stem or >25 cc, the control rate was about 50% in the follow-up period (mean, 33 mos); those not abutting the brain stem or <25 cc residual Dz did not have recurrence.

What is the pattern of recurrence of chordomas after Tx?

LR is most common (95%), while 10%–20% of the pts who recur also develop nodal or distant Dz. The most common sites of distant Dz are lung and bone. (*Fagundes MA et al., IJROBP 1995*)

What is the typical LC and OS for chordomas compared to chondrosarcomas after 70 CGE of proton beam therapy?

In the Loma Linda series of 58 pts (33 chordomas and 25 chondrosarcomas), with a mean follow-up of 33 mos, LC was 76% for chordoma and 92% for chondrosarcoma. The 5-yr OS rates were 79% for chordoma and 100% for chondrosarcoma. (*Hug EB et al., J Neurosurg 1999*)

What is the role of SRS in the management of chordomas?

FSR and SRS are feasible options but with less of a track record compared with charged-particle therapy. The LC and survival rates are promising.

In 1 series using FSR (*Debus J et al., IJROBP 2000*), achieving a median dose of 66.6 Gy at the isocenter, the 2- and 5-yr LC rates were 82% and 50%, and the 2- and 5-yr OS were 97% and 82%, respectively.

In a series from Pittsburgh using SRS to 16 Gy × 1 fx (in mainly recurrent chordoma), the 5-yr LC was 63%. (*Martin JJ et al., J Neurosurg 1987*)

What is the role of brachytherapy in the management of chordomas?	Small series have shown that recurrent chordomas of the skull base and spine can be successfully managed with interstitial iodine-125 in select cases. (*Gutin PH et al., J Neurosurg 1987*; *Kumar PP et al.. J Neurosurg 1988*)
What is the role of chemo or molecularly targeted agents in the management of chordomas?	In chordomas, cytotoxic chemo has not shown clinically significant activity. Imatinib (Gleevac) is currently being evaluated in the phase II setting. In addition, preclinical work suggests potential for the inhibition of PI3K/ MTOR pathways (*Schwab J et al., Anticancer Res 2009*).
What is the survival of pts with recurrent Dz who rcv salvage Tx compared to supportive care?	The outcomes after recurrence are **generally poor**, but salvage Tx (surgery + RT) can be used after recurrence, with 2-yr survival of 63% vs. 21% with supportive care. However, most pts die even with therapy, with 5-yr survival only 6% after recurrence. (*Fagundes MA et al., IJROBP 1995*).
	Definitive proton beam can salvage some pts, with a 2-yr actuarial LC rate of 33%. (*Berson AM et al., IJROBP 1988*)
What are 5 poor prognostic factors for chordomas?	Poor prognostic factors for chordoma:

1. Recurrent Dz
2. Base of skull tumors
3. Female sex
4. Presence of tumor necrosis in pre-Tx Bx
5. Large tumors (>70 cc in 1 series)

▇ Toxicity

What are some common late toxicities that manifest after the Tx of skull base chordomas?	~26% of skull base chordoma pts develop **endocrine abnormalities,** while 5%–10% of pts develop **vision loss, brainstem injury, or temporal lobe injury** in 2–5 yrs. (*Berson AM et al., IJROBP 1988*; *Santoni R et al., IJROBP 1998*)

79

General and Extremity Soft Tissue Sarcoma

Kristin Janson Redmond and Deborah A. Frassica

Background

What is the most common type of sarcoma?

The most common type of sarcoma is **soft tissue sarcoma** (STS).

Approximately how many cases of STS are diagnosed annually in the U.S.? How many deaths occur?

~**9,000 cases/yr** of STS are diagnosed in the U.S., with ~**3,500 deaths/yr.**

What is the median age at Dx of STS?

The median age at Dx of STS is **45–55 yrs.**

What are the 3 most common sites of STS?

The 3 most common sites of STS are the **extremity** (60%), **trunk** (30%), and **H&N** (10%). The retroperitoneal site comprises 10%–15%.

What % of extremity STS involves the lower extremity?

75% of extremity STS involves the lower extremity.

What % of lower extremity STS is at or above the knee?

75% of lower extremity STS is at or above the knee.

What is the most common presentation of STS?

The most common presentation of STS is a **painless mass.**

What is the DDx of a painless mass of the extremity?

Painless mass of the extremity DDx: STS, primary or metastatic carcinoma, lymphoma, desmoids, and benign lesions (lipoma, lymphangioma, leiomyoma, neuroma)

What are the 5 most common types of STS?

Most common types of STS:
1. High-grade undifferentiated pleomorphic sarcoma (previously called *malignant fibrous histiocytoma*) (20%–30%)
2. Liposarcoma (10%–20%)
3. Leiomyosarcoma (5%–10%)
4. Synovial sarcoma (5%–10%)
5. Malignant peripheral nerve sheath tumors (5%–10%)

How many different histologic subtypes of STS have been identified?

>**50** histologic subtypes of STS have been identified.

What are the chromosomal translocations seen for (1) synovial sarcoma, (2) clear cell sarcoma, (3) Ewing sarcoma/PNET, and (4) alveolar rhabdomyosarcoma?

Chromosomal translocations:
1. Synovial sarcoma: t(X,18)
2. Clear cell sarcoma: t(12,22)
3. Ewing sarcoma/PNET: t(11,22)
4. Alveolar rhabdomyosarcoma: t(2,13), t(1,13)

Name 4 genetic syndromes associated with sarcoma and the type of sarcoma associated with each of these syndromes.

Genetic syndromes associated with sarcoma and their type:
1. Gardner (desmoid tumors)
2. Retinoblastoma (bone and STS)
3. NF-1 (benign neurofibromas and malignant peripheral nerve sheath tumors)
4. Li-Fraumeni (bone and STS)

Name 6 environmental risk factors for STS.

Environmental risk factors for STS:
1. RT
2. Thorotrast
3. Chlorophenols
4. Vinyl chloride
5. Arsenic
6. Herbicides

What is Stewart-Treves syndrome?

Stewart-Treves syndrome is an **angiosarcoma that arises from chronic lymphedema,** most often as a complication of mastectomy +/− radiotherapy for breast cancer.

Where does STS originate?

STS originates from the **primitive mesenchyme of the mesoderm,** which gives rise to muscle, fat, fibrous tissues, blood vessels, and supporting cells of the peripheral nervous system.

What % of STS have +LNs at Dx?

5% of STS have +LNs at Dx.

Which 5 types of STS have an increased risk of LN mets?

STS types that have an increased risk of LN mets:
1. **S**ynovial sarcoma (14%)
2. **C**lear cell sarcoma (28%)
3. **A**ngiosarcoma (23%)
4. **R**habdomyosarcoma (15%)
5. **E**pithelioid sarcoma (20%)

(Mnemonic: **SCARE**)

With the exception of myxoid liposarcoma, what is the most common site of DM from STS?

The most common site of DM from STS is to the **lung** (70%–80%), except for myxoid liposarcoma, which spreads to nonpulmonary sites in 60% of mets.

Name 5 factors associated with an increased risk of LR in pts with STS.

Factors associated with an increased risk of LR in pts with STS:
1. Age >50 yrs
2. Recurrent Dz
3. Positive surgical margins
4. Fibrosarcoma (including desmoid)
5. Malignant peripheral nerve sheath tumor

Name 5 factors associated with an increased risk of DM in pts with STS.

Factors associated with an increased risk of DM in pts with STS:
1. High grade
2. Size >5 cm
3. Deep location
4. Recurrent Dz
5. Leiomyosarcoma

▓ Workup/Staging

What is an appropriate workup for a painless mass?

Painless mass workup: H&P, careful exam of the primary site and draining LN regions, basic labs (CBC/BMP/LFTs), CXR, CT/MRI primary site, and a schedule for core Bx or incisional Bx

What is the AJCC 7th edition (2009) TNM classification for STS?

T1: tumor ≤5 cm
T1a: superficial to superficial fascia
T1b: deep to superficial fascia
T2: tumor >5 cm
T2a: superficial to superficial fascia
T2b: deep to superficial fascia
N1: regional LN mets
M1: DMs

Note: The retroperitoneal location is always considered deep.

What grading system is used by the AJCC for STS, and how many grades are there in this system?

Historically, the AJCC used a 4-grade system but switched to the **French 3-grade system** in their 7th edition (2009).

What are the AJCC 7th edition (2009) stage groupings with TNM and grade for STS?

Stage IA: T1a-bN0M0, grade 1
Stage IB: T2a-bN0M0, grade 1
Stage IIA: T1a-bN0M0, grades 2–3
Stage IIB: T2a-bN0M0, grade 2
Stage III: T2a-bN0M0, grade 3, or anyTN1M0, any grade
Stage IV: M1

What 2 imaging studies should be used to evaluate a potential STS?	According to NCCN 2010 guidelines, a pt with a potential STS should have MRI +/− **CT scan of the primary site and chest imaging. Other imaging is optional.**
What type of Bx should be done to evaluate a concerning soft tissue mass?	According to NCCN 2010 guidelines, soft tissue masses should be diagnosed using either a **core needle Bx** or an **incisional Bx** oriented so that it may be excised during the definitive surgery. Either Bx should be done by or in coordination with the surgeon who will be performing the definitive surgery.
According to NCCN 2010 guidelines, under what certain circumstances are PET, CT, or MRI useful in the workup of STS?	<u>FDG-PET</u>: may be useful for prognostication and grading as well as to determine response to chemo <u>CT abdomen/pelvis</u>: myxoid liposarcoma, epithelioid sarcoma, angiosarcoma, and leiomyosarcoma <u>MRI spine</u>: round cell liposarcoma
What is the LC of STS after excisional Bx alone?	The LC of STS after excisional Bx alone is ~**20%.**

■ Treatment/Prognosis

What is the primary Tx modality for STS?	**Surgery** is the primary Tx modality for STS.
What is the LR rate after surgery alone for STS?	LR after surgery alone **depends on the extent of resection.** LR is 90% after simple excision, 40% after wide excision, 25% after soft part excision, and 7%–18% after amputation.
What is the LR rate and DFS after primary RT alone for STS?	**2-yr LR is 66% and 2-yr DFS is 17%** after primary RT alone for STS. (*Lindberg RD et al., Proceedings National Cancer Conf 1972*)
Surgery alone is adequate for which pts with STS of the extremity?	According to the NCCN, pts with low-grade extremity STS **(stage I)** s/p surgical resection with >**1-cm margins** do not require adj therapy. Consider RT if the margin is ≤1 cm.
What are the management options for a pt with stage II or III resectable STS?	Stage II or III resectable STS management options: 1. Surgery → RT +/− chemo 2. Preop RT → consideration of postop chemo 3. Preop chemo or CRT

What studies support the use of adj RT following limb-sparing surgery in high- and low-grade STS?

There have been 2 RCTs that have evaluated the impact of adj RT after limb-sparing surgery in STS:

Yang et al., from the NCI, randomized pts with high- and low-grade STS of the extremity treated with limb-sparing surgery to adj EBRT (63 Gy) or no RT. Pts with high-grade STS rcv concurrent Adr/cyclophosphamide with EBRT. For high-grade pts, 10-yr LC significantly favored RT (100% vs. 78%), but there was no difference in 10-yr DMFS or OS. For low-grade pts, LC favored the RT arm, but there was also no difference in DMFS or OS. (*JCO 1998*)

Pisters et al. randomized (in the operating room) pts with high- and low-grade STS who had a complete resection to iridium-192 brachytherapy implant (42–45 Gy) over 4–6 days or no RT. For high-grade pts, 5-yr LC favored the RT arm (89% vs. 66%), but there was no OS difference. For low-grade pts, LC and OS were not significantly impacted by RT. (*JCO 1996*)

What RCT compared preop RT vs. PORT for extremity STS, and what did it show?

The **NCI Canada trial** randomized pts with extremity STS to preop RT (50 Gy in 25 fx + a 16–20 Gy boost for positive surgical margins) vs. PORT (50 Gy in 25 fx + a 16–20 Gy boost). The initial field was a 5-cm proximal and distal margin, and boost was a 2-cm proximal and distal margin. The primary endpoint was major wound complications. The trial closed after accruing 190 of the planned 266 pts b/c of significantly greater wound complications with preop RT (35%) vs. PORT (17%), with the highest rates of complications in the upper leg (45% vs. 38%). 6-wk function was better with PORT (*O'Sullivan B et al., Lancet 2002*). At median follow-up of 6.9 yrs, there was no difference in LC (93% preop RT vs. 92% PORT), RFS (58% vs. 59%), or OS (73% vs. 67%). Predictors for outcome included surgical margin status for LC and size and grade for RFS and OS (*O'Sullivan B et al., Proceedings ASCO 2004*). The decision regarding preop vs. postop therapy was driven by toxicity profiles. In the long term, **PORT was associated with worse fibrosis and joint stiffness** (grade 2 fibrosis was 31% vs. 48%, $p = 0.07$) (*Davis AM et al., Radiother Oncol 2005*).

What are the advantages of preop RT compared to PORT for the management of extremity STS?

Advantages of preop RT for Tx of extremity STS:
1. Lower RT dose
2. Smaller Tx volume
3. Improved resectability
4. Margin-negative resections
5. Better oxygenation of tumor cells
6. Fewer long-term toxicities

What is the evidence that a limb-sparing approach of local excision with PORT yields equivalent outcomes compared to amputation alone in the management of high-grade extremity STS?

The **NCI trial** randomized 43 pts with high-grade extremity STS to amputation at the joint proximal to the tumor vs. limb-sparing resection + RT. Randomization favored limb sparing (2:1). RT was 45–50 Gy → a boost to 60–70 Gy with concurrent Adr/Cytoxan → high-dose methotrexate. 4 of 27 pts in the RT group had +margins. There was no difference in 5-yr DFS (78% amputation vs. 71% RT) or OS (88% vs. 83%). There was increased LR with limb sparing (0% vs. 20%). (*Rosenberg SA et al., Ann Surg 1982*)

What is the benefit of adding adj chemo for high-grade extremity STS after surgery?

Based on the NCI trial that randomized 65 pts with extremity STS to surgery alone (either limb sparing or amputation) vs. surgery + adj chemo. There was improved DFS (92% chemo vs. 60%) and OS (95% vs. 74%) both for pts treated with limb-sparing surgery and with amputation. (*Rosenberg SA et al., Ann Surg 1982*)

Which STS pts appear to benefit most from adj chemo?

The British STS adj chemo meta-analysis included 1,568 pts with STS s/p WLE +/− adj doxorubicin-based chemo. Chemo improved LC (absolute 6%), DMFS (10%), RFS (10%), and OS (4%, NSS). The largest benefit was found in pts with **high-grade extremity** STS. (*Tierney et al., Br J Cancer 1997*)

Should adj chemo be used in all high-grade STS pts?

This is **controversial.** Adj chemo should not be adopted as standard practice, regardless of histology or tumor size. Rather, it should be considered on a pt-by-pt basis, taking into account pt performance status and Tx toxicities.

Which pts with extremity STS should be treated with neoadj therapy?

According to the NCCN, neoadj RT, chemo, or CRT are reasonable options for all pts with **stage II or III extremity STS,** though surgery → adj therapy is also an option for these pts. Neoadj therapy is the *preferred* option in pts with stage II or III extremity STS when Dz is only potentially resectable or the risk of adverse functional outcomes is high (e.g., in pts who require extensive resection such as disarticulation, amputation, or hemipelvectomy).

Cite 2 studies that demonstrate the efficacy of neoadj CRT for large extremity STS.

The **Harvard retrospective study and RTOG 9514** are 2 studies that demonstrate the efficacy of neoadj CRT for large extremity STS.

What were the results of the Harvard retrospective study for STS?

The Harvard retrospective study of neoadj CRT for large STS reviewed 48 pts with >8-cm extremity STS. Pts were treated with interdigitated sequential CRT as follows:

mesna/doxorubicin/ifosfamide/dacarbazine (MAID) → RT (22 Gy in 11 fx) → MAID → RT (22 Gy in 11 fx) → MAID → surgery → MAID × 3. If surgical margins were positive, pts rcv an additional 16 Gy boost postop. **5-yr LC was 92%, DFS was 86%, and OS was 44%.** Compared with historical controls, there was a significant decrease in DM and a significant increase in DFS and OS. There were 29% wound complications and 2% Tx-related deaths. (*DeLaney TF et al., IJROBP 2003*)

What were the results of RTOG 9514 for STS?

RTOG 9514 was a phase II trial enrolling 64 pts with ≥8-cm grade 2 or 3 STS of the extremity or torso with expected R0 resection. 44% had malignant fibrous histiocytoma, 13% had leiomyosarcoma, and 88% had STS of the extremity. Pts were treated with MAID → RT (22 Gy in 11 fx) → MAID → RT (22 Gy in 11 fx) → MAID → surgery → MAID × 3 → a 14 Gy postop boost if necessary. 91% were R0 resections, and 59% rcv the full chemo course. 3-yr LRF was 18% (if amputation was considered a failure and 10% if not). **3-yr DFS was 57%, distant DFS was 64%, OS was 75%, and there was a 92% amputationfree rate.** There were 5% Tx-related deaths (mostly secondary acute myeloid leukemia), and 84% of pts had grade 4 toxicity (mostly hematologic).

The authors concluded that the regimen is effective, but substantial toxicity makes this approach controversial (*Kraybill WG et al., J Clin Oncol 2006*). Note that RTOG 9514 used a more intense version of MAID than was used in the Harvard study, which probably worsened toxicity.

What were the results of the EORTC STBSG 62871 trial regarding neoadj chemo for STS?

EORTC STBSG 62871 was a randomized phase II trial enrolling 134 pts with STS ≥8 cm or grade 2 or 3. Pts were randomized to surgery alone vs. neoadj doxorubicin/ifosfamide. PORT was given for marginal surgery, positive surgical margins, or LR. There was no difference in 5-yr DFS (52% vs. 56%) or OS (64 vs. 65%), but the study was not sufficiently powered to detect a difference. (*Gortzak E et al., Eur J Cancer 2001*)

What were the results of EORTC 62961 regarding hyperthermia + neoadj chemo for STS?

EORTC 62961 randomized 341 pts with ≥5-cm, grade 2 or 3, deep and extracompartmental STS to neoadj etoposide/ifosfamide/Adriamycin (EIA) vs. neoadj EIA + deep wave regional hyperthermia. Hyperthermia resulted in improved median LRC (3.8 yrs vs. 2 yrs) and median DFS (2.6 yrs vs. 1.4 yrs). (*Issels RD et al., Proc ASCO 2007*)

What were the results of the MSKCC retrospective review regarding IMRT for extremity STS?

The MSKCC reported a retrospective review of 41 pts with extremity STS treated with limb-sparing surgery and IMRT. 51% had close or positive surgical margins. IMRT was used preop in 7 pts (mean dose, 50 Gy) and postop in 21 pts (mean dose, 63 Gy). At median follow-up at 2.9 yrs, 5-yr LC was 94% regardless of margin status, DMFS was 61%, and OS was 64%. (*Alektiar KM et al., J Clin Oncol 2008*)

How long after surgery should adj RT for STS begin?

According to the NCCN, PORT for STS should begin **after healing is completed, by 3–8 wks post surgery.**

What dose is recommended for adj RT for STS?

According to the NCCN, adj RT for STS should be 50 Gy in 2 Gy/fx → a 10–16 Gy boost for –margins, a 16–20 Gy boost for microscopically positive margins, and a 20–26 Gy boost for grossly positive margins.

Surgery should take place approximately how long after completion of neoadj RT for STS?

According to the NCCN, surgery should take place **3–6 wks after completion of neoadj RT** in order to decrease the risk of wound complications.

What dose is recommended for neoadj RT for extremity STS?

According to the NCCN, neoadj RT for extremity STS should be to **50 Gy in 2 Gy/fx.** If postop margins are close or positive, consider a boost using IORT (single 10–16 Gy), brachytherapy (12–20 Gy), or EBRT (10–14 Gy for close margins, 16–20 Gy for microscopically positive margins, and 20–26 Gy for grossly positive margins).

What are the initial and boost RT Tx volumes for STS in the adj setting?

The **initial** RT Tx volume for STS in the adj setting includes the tumor, scar, and drainage sites + a 5–7-cm margin longitudinally and a 2–3-cm margin perpendicularly to the block/field edge. The **boost** volume is the surgical bed + a 2-cm margin to the block/field edge. Try to spare a 1.5- to 2-cm strip of skin.

How is postop brachtherapy performed for the Tx of high-grade STS of the extremity?

Catheters are placed in the operating room after tumor resection, 1 cm apart, with a 2-cm longitudinal and 1–1.5-cm circumferential margin on the tumor bed. Tx begins on or after the 6th postop day to allow for wound healing.

Low dose rate: 45–50 Gy to tumor bed over 4–6 days
High dose rate: 3.4 Gy bid × 10 fx (34 Gy in 5 days)

How should pts with unresectable STS be managed?	**Consider preop RT, chemo, or CRT.** If still deemed unresectable, consider definitive RT, chemo, palliative surgery, observation, or the best supportive care. (*NCCN 2010*)
What dose of RT is recommended for unresectable STS?	If possible, the dose should be ≥**70–80 Gy** using sophisticated Tx planning (IMRT or proton beam).

▋ Toxicity

What are the short- and long-term toxicities associated with RT for STS of the extremity?	Toxicities associated with RT for extremity STS: Short term: wound complications (5%–15% with PORT, 25%–35% with preop RT), dermatitis, recall reactions with doxorubicin and dactinomycin, epilation Long term: Abnl bone and soft tissue growth and development, leg length discrepancy, permanent weakening of bone with the greatest risk of fracture within 18 mos of completion of therapy, fibrosis leading to decreased range of motion, lymphedema, skin discoloration, telangiectasias, 2nd malignancy (≤5%)
What is the recommended follow-up after Tx of STS?	STS Tx follow-up per the NCCN: evaluation by occupational/physical therapy for functional restoration, H&P and chest imaging (CXR or CT chest) q3–6mos × 2–3 yrs, then q6mos for the next 2 yrs, then annually. Consider periodic imaging of the primary site (MRI, CT, or US) to assess LR.

80

Hemangiopericytoma

Steven H. Lin and Ramesh Rengan

▋ Background

Are hemangiopericytomas benign or malignant lesions?	Hemangiopericytomas are **malignant** lesions (sarcomatous lesions of vessels).
What is the cell of origin of hemangiopericytomas?	Hemangiopericytomas were originally thought to originate from pericytes of the smooth muscle cells of vessels but are now felt to be of **fibroblastic** origin.

From which other tumor is a hemangiopericytoma of the meninges difficult to distinguish?

Solitary fibrous tumor. The consensus view is that solitary fibrous tumors and hemangiopericytomas belong to the same spectrum of tumors of fibroblastic origin.

What is the most common location of hemangiopericytoma?

The most common location for hemangiopericytomas is in the **lower extremity** (femur and proximal tibia). Other sites are the H&N, retroperitoneum, and brain (least common). If in the brain, it is a meningeal location, particularly the base of the skull.

What are the incidence and sites of DM in pts with hemangiopericytoma?

~**25%** (10%–60%) of hemangiopericytoma pts develop hematogenous DMs, with the majority traveling to the **lungs > bone > liver** (rarely the nodes).

What is the prognosis of hemangiopericytoma as it relates to the location of the tumor?

The prognosis of hemangiopericytoma **varies** based upon the ability to achieve complete surgical excision.

▪ Workup/Staging

What are the typical presenting Sx of a pt with hemangiopericytoma?

Pts with hemangiopericytomas present with a **firm, painless, localized mass,** typically in the extremities.

How do hemangiopericytomas appear on imaging (CT, MRI)?

Hemangiopericytomas typically appear to be **hypervascular lesions with diffuse contrast enhancement** on CT or MRI.

▪ Treatment/Prognosis

What is the Tx paradigm for managing hemangiopericytoma?

Hemangiopericytoma Tx paradigm: **Complete surgical resection** is the mainstay of therapy **+ adj or neoadj RT, chemo, or CRT**. Unresectable cases can be treated with either radiotherapy alone or chemoradiotherapy with a less favorable outcome.

Is there a role for chemo in the management of hemangiopericytoma?

Yes. Chemo may be used either preoperatively or adjuvantly. Antiangiogenic therapy is currently being explored, as these are highly vascularized tumors.

What is the typical PORT dose used for treating hemangiopericytoma after surgery?

The typical PORT dose is **50–60 Gy** to the surgical bed with the margin varying by site.

What is the 5-yr OS for hemangiopericytoma of the meninges?

5-yr OS is ~**70%** with complete surgical resection. (*Guthrie BL et al., Neurosurgery 1989*)

For what type of pts is nonoperative initial management of DT recommended?

Pts with intra-abdominal DTs that are large, slow growing, involve the mesentery, or encase vessels and/or organs should be treated upfront with nonsurgical approaches according to the American Society of Colon and Rectal Surgeons. (*DeLaney T et al., Up to date 2009*)

What is the recurrence rate after margin− surgery vs. margin+ surgery for DT in pts who do not get adj therapy?

In DT Tx with surgery alone, **LR is 13% for −margin resection**, and **LR is 52% for +margin resection**. (*Ballo MT et al., IJROBP 1998*)

Estimate the LR rate by margin status for DT pts who are treated with surgery and then adj RT.

The LR rate for DT treated with surgery and then adj RT is **7% in margin− pts and 26% in margin+ pts**. (*Ballo MT et al., IJROBP 1998*)

What group of pts with DT should not be offered routine adj RT?

Pts with DT who have a **margin− resection** should not be offered routine adj RT; however, according to NCCN guidelines, PORT can be considered for large lesions.

What 2 factors should be considered when determining whether or not a pt with a margin+ DT needs adj RT?

Factors to consider whether a margin+ DT pt needs adj RT:

1. Salvage options should be identified for a subsequent recurrence.
2. The risk of significant morbidity if the tumor recurs should be considered in determining whether a margin+ resection of DT needs adj RT.

Note: If the lesion is amenable to salvage repeat resection at the time of recurrence and is not likely to produce significant morbidity if the tumor recurs, then observation may be appropriate.

According to NCCN guidelines, what type of DT is usually not treated with RT?

According to NCCN guidelines, RT is not generally recommended for a DT that is **retroperitoneal/intra-abdominal.**

What is the LR rate for DT treated with RT alone?

The LR rate for DT treated with RT alone is **22%.** (*Nuyttens JJ et al., Cancer 2000*)

What dose of RT is needed to control DT with RT alone?

A dose >**50 Gy** is needed to treat DT with RT alone. The recommended dose for gross Dz is 50–56 Gy. The LR for pts treated with RT alone is 60% with doses <50 Gy and ~15% with doses >50 Gy. (*Nuyttens JJ et al., Cancer 2000*)

What dose of RT is recommended after an R1 resection of DT in a pt who cannot be salvaged with repeat resection?

A pt treated with adj RT after an R1 resection should be treated to a dose of **50 Gy in 1.8–2 Gy/fx.**

Define the target volume for RT in the management of DT.	The target volume to include when treating DT with RT includes the tumor bed (and/or gross tumor), a portion of the muscle compartment to cover fascial planes, or neurovascular structures along which tumor may track with a 3–5-cm margin longitudinally.
Define 4 nonsurgical, non-RT approaches to DT Tx.	Nonsurgical, non-RT approaches to DT Tx: 1. Hormone ablation (tamoxifen) 2. NSAIDs (sulindac) 3. Low-dose cytotoxic chemo (methotrexate or doxorubicin based) 4. Targeted therapy (imatinib)
Define 2 pt populations in which radiotherapy for DT should be avoided.	RT should be avoided in **intra-abdominal DT** or in **children** with DT. RT is avoided in skeletally immature pts to prevent RT effects associated with growth delay. **However, in refractory cases, RT may be used in both cases.**
Name 1 prognostic classification system for FAP-associated DT.	The **Cleveland Clinic** devised a prognostic stratification system for FAP-associated DT: **Stage I:** asymptomatic, ≤10 cm in max diameter, not growing **Stage II:** mildly symptomatic, ≤10 cm, not growing **Stage III:** moderately symptomatic or bowel/ureteric obstruction of 10–20 cm in max diameter, slowly growing **Stage IV:** severely symptomatic or >20 cm, rapidly growing In a series by *Church et al.*, there were no deaths for stages I–II, but there was a death rate of 15% for stage III and 44% for stage IV. (*Dis Colon Rectum 2008*)

■ Toxicity

Define 6 late complications associated with RT Tx to the extremity.	Late complications associated with RT to the extremities: 1. Fibrosis 2. Edema 3. Fracture 4. 2nd malignancy 5. Joint stiffness 6. Neuropathy
Define the dose of RT associated with premature closure of the epiphysis.	The dose of RT associated with premature closure of the epiphysis is **>20 Gy.**
What dose of RT is associated with an increased risk of late complications in Tx of DT of the extremity?	The risk of late complications for pts with DT of the extremity treated with RT is **30% with doses >56 Gy vs. 5% with doses <56 Gy.** (*Ballo MT et al., IJROBP 1998*)

82

Retroperitoneal Soft Tissue Sarcoma

Kristin Janson Redmond and Deborah A. Frassica

Background

What is the median age at Dx of retroperitoneal soft tissue sarcoma (STS)?

The median age at Dx of retroperitoneal STS is **65 yrs.**

What % of STS are retroperitoneal?

10%–15% of STS are retroperitoneal.

What is the typical presentation of pts with retroperitoneal STS?

Pts with retroperitoneal STS typically present with **vague abdominal complaints.**

What is the median diameter of retroperitoneal STS at presentation?

The median diameter of retroperitoneal STS is **15 cm.**

What % of retroperitoneal STS occur in the abdomen vs. the pelvis?

With regard to retroperitoneal STS, **70% occur in the abdomen and 30% in the pelvis.**

What are the boundaries of the retroperitoneal space?

Boundaries of the retroperitoneal space:
  Superior: diaphragm
  Inferior: pelvic diaphragm
  Lateral: lat edge of quadratus lumborum, but lat edge of 12th rib is also considered since it corresponds to origin of transversus abdominus aponeurosis
  Anterior: parietal peritoneum
  Posterior: psoas, quadratus lumborum muscles in abdomen; iliacus, obturator internus, and pyriformis in pelvis

Which organs are retroperitoneal?

Retroperitoneal organs include the **pancreas, kidneys, adrenal glands, and ureters.**

What is the DDx of a retroperitoneal soft tissue mass?	The DDx of a retroperitoneal mass includes **either malignant or benign tumors.** Malignant etiology includes: 1. Sarcoma 2. GI stromal tumor 3. Lymphoma 4. Germ cell tumor Benign etiology includes: 1. Desmoid tumor 2. Lipoma 3. Benign peripheral nerve sheath tumor (schwannoma, neurofibroma) 4. Teratoma 5. Paraganglioma
What are the 2 most common histologies of retroperitoneal sarcoma in adults?	The 2 most common histologies for retroperitoneal sarcoma in adults include **liposarcoma and leiomyosarcoma.**
What is the most common histology of retroperitoneal sarcoma in children?	The most common histology of retroperitoneal sarcoma in children is **rhabdomyosarcoma.**

■ Workup/Staging

How does staging for retroperitoneal sarcoma differ from the general STS AJCC staging?	Staging for retroperitoneal STS is according to the AJCC staging for STS except the retroperitoneal location is always considered deep.
Do all pts with suspected retroperitoneal sarcoma require a preop Bx?	**No.** According to the NCCN, preop Bx is not required if the suspicion for retroperitoneal sarcoma is high. However, CT-guided core Bx is necessary in pts undergoing neoadj chemo or RT.
What imaging studies should be performed to stage retroperitoneal sarcoma?	According to the NCCN, staging studies for retroperitoneal sarcoma include **CT abdomen/pelvis with contrast, chest imaging, and optional MRI.**

■ Treatment/Prognosis

What is the primary Tx modality for retroperitoneal sarcoma?	**Surgery** (en bloc resection of the tumor + involved organs) is the primary Tx modality for retroperitoneal sarcoma.

What are the Tx paradigms for retroperitoneal STS?

Retroperitoneal STS Tx paradigms:

1. Surgery alone
2. Surgery → adj RT and/or chemo
3. Neoadj RT and/or chemo → surgery

Note: If RT will be included in the Tx, the authors' strong institutional preference is for neoadj RT given the substantial morbidity of adj RT and the limited data supporting this approach.

What % of retroperitoneal sarcomas are amenable to a GTR?

~**50%** of retroperitoneal sarcomas are amenable to a GTR.

Is recurrence after surgery for retroperitoneal sarcoma more likely to be local or distant?

Most recurrences after surgery for retroperitoneal sarcoma are **local.**

What is the LR rate after GTR (R0 or R1) for retroperitoneal sarcoma?

LR ranges from **50%–95%** in pts who have undergone GTR for retroperitoneal sarcoma.

Is preop RT or PORT believed to be superior for retroperitoneal sarcoma? Why?

Preop RT is believed to be superior to PORT for retroperitoneal sarcoma b/c of better tumor volume definition, displacement of normal viscera by tumor (therefore less normal tissue in Tx volume), smaller Tx fields, and the potential radiobiologic advantage of having normal vasculature/oxygenation in place. While there is no RCT comparing preop RT vs. PORT, *Bolla et al.* found significantly worse 5-yr RT-related complication rate with PORT (23% vs. 0%) (*IJROBP* 2007).

Is there a benefit of adding IORT with postop EBRT after the surgical management of retroperitoneal sarcoma? What evidence (randomized trial and retrospective review) supports its use?

Yes. IORT improves LC. An **NCI trial** (*Sindelar WF et al., Arch Surg 1993*) compared IORT + PORT to PORT alone for retroperitoneal STS. 35 pts were randomized to IORT (20 Gy) + postop EBRT (35–40 Gy) vs. PORT (50–55 Gy). Both groups rcv chemo (doxorubicin/cyclophosphamide/methotrexate). At a min follow-up of 5 yrs, there was no difference in OS between the groups (MS was 3.7 yrs with IORT vs. 4.3 yrs with PORT). There was a significant improvement in LR with IORT (40% IORT vs. 80% PORT). RT enteritis occurred in 13% of pts with IORT and 50% of pts with PORT. Peripheral neuropathy was found in 60% of pts with IORT vs. 80% of pts with PORT.

A **Massachusetts General Hospital retrospective review** included 29 pts: 16 treated with IORT (10–20 Gy with intraop electrons) and 13 treated without IORT. All pts rcv 45 Gy EBRT. LC improved with the addition of IORT (83% vs. 61%). (*Gieschen HL et al., IJROBP 2001*)

What did the ACOSOG Z9031 randomized trial try to address?

ACOSOG Z9031 randomized pts to **surgery alone vs. preop RT + surgery for primary retroperitoneal sarcoma.** The target accrual was 370 pts in 4.5 yrs. The primary endpoint was PFS. Unfortunately, this study closed due to poor accrual.

Summarize the outcomes of the Toronto Sarcoma Group and the MDACC prospective trials of preop EBRT for localized intermediate- or high-grade retroperitoneal sarcoma.

The Toronto Sarcoma Group and the MDACC prospective trials enrolled 72 pts with intermediate- or high-grade retroperitoneal sarcoma. 75% were primary, and 25% were recurrent. Pts were treated preoperatively to a median dose of 45 Gy with concurrent low-dose doxorubicin. 89% underwent laparotomy with curative intent 4–8 wks after RT. 60% had an intraop or postop boost. At median follow-up of 3.4 yrs, the recurrence rate was 52% after GTR. 5-yr LRFS was 60%, DFS was 46%, and OS was 61% (*Pawlik TM et al., Ann Surg Oncol 2006*). Results compared favorably to historical controls.

What EBRT dose is typically used for preop RT for retroperitoneal sarcoma? What phase I study tested tolerability of this preop RT dose with concurrent doxorubicin?

Retroperitoneal STS is typically treated to **50.4 Gy** preoperatively. Based on the **MDACC phase I trial** enrolling 35 pts with potentially resectable intermediate- or high-grade retroperitoneal sarcoma, preop RT can be safely administered to 50.4 Gy with concurrent weekly doxorubicin. At this dose, there was 18% grade 3–4 nausea. (*Pisters PW et al., JCO 2003*)

Summarize the outcomes of the retrospective study by the French Federation Cancer Sarcoma Group regarding adj RT for retroperitoneal sarcoma.

The French Federation Cancer Sarcoma Group retrospectively reviewed 145 pts with localized nonmetastatic retroperitoneal sarcoma. 65% underwent GTR, and 41% had adj RT. 5-yr OS was 46%. 5-yr LRC was 55% with adj RT vs. 23% with surgery alone (*Stoeckle E et al., Cancer 2001*). These results should be interpreted cautiously, as selection bias may have favored the RT arm in this study and adj RT is associated with significant RT-related morbidity.

In the preop radiotherapy management of retroperitoneal sarcoma, does the whole tumor volume need to be treated? What prospective study studied this question?

This is **uncertain.** *Bossi A et al.* was a prospective trial enrolling 18 pts with retroperitoneal sarcoma. Pts were treated with neoadj IMRT limited to the post abdominal wall, and planning was compared to standard RT fields. All pts successfully completed RT and surgery. There were 2 LRs, 1 within the high-dose region and 1 marginal recurrence that would not have been covered by the standard CTV. The authors concluded that limiting the CTV to the post abdominal wall is feasible. (*IJROBP 2007*)

What proportion of DM pts present with DM from an unknown melanoma primary?	**One third** of DM pts or 1%–2% of all pts present with mets from an unknown primary.
What are the 5 subtypes of melanoma?	Superficial spreading, nodular, lentigo maligna, acral lentiginous, and desmoplastic variant
Which of the 5 melanoma subtypes is the most common?	**Superficial spreading** (70%) is the most common subtype → nodular (25%).
What are typical features of desmoplastic melanoma?	Features of the desmoplastic subtype include older pts (60–70 yo), more infiltrative, higher rate of perineural invasion, **higher LF rates**, and **lower nodal met/DM rates.**
Which melanoma subtype has the best prognosis?	**Lentigo maligna** melanoma has the best prognosis.
What is the LN+ rate and 5-yr OS for lentigo maligna melanoma?	For lentigo maligna melanoma, the **LN+ rate is only 10%**, with **5-yr OS at 85%** after WLE alone.
What subtype commonly presents in dark-skinned populations, and what body locations does it commonly affect?	**Acral lentiginous**, which **commonly affects the palms/soles and subungual areas,** is the most common melanoma subtype in dark-skinned populations.
Which subtype of melanoma is most common and has the worst prognosis?	**Superficial spreading** is the most common subtype. This subtype also has the worst prognosis.
What is the name for lentigo maligna involving only the epidermis (Clark level I)?	**Hutchinson freckle** is lentigo maligna of the epidermis.
What are 3 commonly used immunohistochemical stains for melanoma?	**S100, HNB-45, and Melan-A** stains are commonly used for melanoma.

■ Workup/Staging

A pt presents with a pigmented lesion. What in the Hx can help to determine if this is a suspicious lesion?	Changes in **ABCDE: A**symmetry, **B**orders, **C**olor, **D**iameter (>6 mm), and **E**nlargement
What workup is necessary for tumors >1 mm thick?	For tumors >1 mm thick, provide a complete metastatic workup with CXR, LFTs, and CBC/CMP. CT C/A/P is needed for lesions >1 mm thick.

Per the latest NCCN guidelines, for what melanoma pts should imaging be performed?

Per the NCCN, imaging should be performed for **specific signs/Sx or stage ≥IIB** (not recommended for stages IA, IB, and IIA).

What is the typical workup for small (<1-mm) melanoma lesions?

The workup is the same as for other skin cancers: H&P, CN exam (if H&N), regional LN exam, CT/MRI for extent/bone involvement, and tissue Bx.

What are some common DM sites for melanoma?

The **skin, SQ tissues, distant LNs, lung, liver, viscera, and brain** are common melanoma DM sites.

What is the preferred method of tissue Dx for a suspected melanoma?

For suspected melanoma, **full-thickness or excisional Bx** (elliptical/punch) with a 1–3-mm margin is preferred for tissue Dx.

Why should wider margins on excisional Dx be avoided?

Avoid wide margins **to permit accurate subsequent lymphatic mapping.**

For what locations is full-thickness incisional or punch Bx adequate?

Full-thickness incisional and punch Bx are adequate for the **palms/soles, digits, face, and ears or for very large lesions.**

When is a shave Bx sufficient?

Shave Bx is sufficient **when the index of suspicion for melanoma is low.**

How do the Breslow thickness levels correspond to the latest AJCC T staging for melanoma?

The Breslow thickness levels are identical to and define the AJCC T staging of malignant melanoma:
T1: ≤1 mm
T1a: mitotic rate <$1/mm^2$
T1b: mitotic rate ≥$1/mm^2$
T2: 1.01–2 mm
T3: 2.01–4 mm
T4: >4 mm
T4a: no ulceration
T4b: ulceration

What is considered N1, N2, and N3 in melanoma staging?

All regional LN mets:
N1: 1+
N2: 2–3+
N3: ≥4+, or matted, or in-transit mets with mets to regional node(s)

For melanoma nodal groups, into what further categories are N1-N2 stages broken?

N1a: micromets
N1b: macromets
N2a: micromets
N2b: macromets
N2c: satellite or in-transit mets without nodal mets

How do M1a, M1b, and M1c differ in a pt with metastatic melanoma?

M1a: skin, SQ, distant LNs
M1b: lung only
M1c: viscera or other sites with ↑ LDH

Describe the overall stage groupings per the latest AJCC classification.

Stage 0: Tis
Stage IA: T1aN0
Stage IB: T2aN0 or T1bN0
Stage IIA: T3aN0 or T2bN0
Stage IIB: T4aN0 or T3bN0
Stage IIC: T4bN0
Stage III: any N+
Stage IV: any M1

With regard to the pathologic staging of melanoma, how does regional nodal involvement figure into stage IIIA, IIIB, and IIIC Dz?

Stage IIIA: nonulcerative primary with LN micromets
Stage IIIB: ulcerative primary + LN micromets or nonulcerative primary + LN macromets/in-transit mets
Stage IIIC: ulcerative primary + LN macromets/in-transit mets or N3 Dz

What are the Clark levels? Under what circumstance does the Clark level need to be known on the pathology report for a pt with melanoma?

Clark levels:
Level I: epidermis only
Level II: invasion of papillary dermis
Level III: filling papillary dermis, compressing reticular dermis
Level IV: invading reticular dermis
Level V: SQ tissue

The Clark level should be provided on the pathology report for lesions ≤1 mm.

What are the similarities and differences between clinical and pathologic staging for melanomatous lesions?

Both require microstaging of the primary after resection:
Clinical staging: clinical exam + radiology allowed (after complete resection)
Pathologic staging: pathology assessment of LN after dissection

What should the pathology report reveal about the primary tumor in a pt with a newly diagnosed melanoma after surgical resection?

The pathology report should list the **Breslow thickness, ulceration status, mitotic rate, deep/peripheral margins, evidence of satellitosis, and Clark level** (only for lesions ≤1 mm).

What are some adverse features on pathology after surgical resection for a melanoma?

Adverse pathology features after surgical resection include **+margins (+ deep margin), LVSI, and mitotic rate >1/mm^2.**

For clinical staging purposes, what stage designates regional nodal involvement?

Stage III designates nodal involvement in melanoma staging.

What is the most powerful prognostic factor for recurrence and survival for pts with melanoma?	**Sentinel LN status** is the most powerful prognostic factor.
What are 3 favorable clinical factors at presentation for pts with a newly diagnosed melanoma?	**Female gender, young age, and extremity location** are all favorable prognostic factors.
What are 5 poor prognostic factors on pathology in melanoma?	**Increasing thickness, # of nodes involved, ulceration, Clark level (if <1 mm), and satellitosis** are 5 poor prognostic factors in melanoma.
What are microsatellites as seen with melanoma?	With melanoma, microsatellites are **discrete nest of cells >0.05 mm that are separated from the body of the primary lesion by collagen or fat.**
In order of frequency, which melanoma sites have the highest LR rates after surgery?	Melanoma sites with highest LR rates after surgery (in descending order of frequency): **H&N (9.4%)** > distal extremities (5%) > trunk (3%) > proximal extremities (1%) (*Balch CM et al., Ann Surg Oncol 2001*)
What are the comparative OS rates of melanoma pts by stage at presentation?	OS rates of melanoma pts by stage: <u>Stage I</u>: 80%–90% <u>Stage II</u>: 40%–60% <u>Stage III</u>: 30% <u>Stage IV</u>: <10%

■ Treatment/Prognosis

What is the general paradigm for the management of melanoma lesions?	Melanoma lesion management paradigm: 1. WLE → sentinal LN Bx (if >0.6 mm thick or >0 mitotic rate). 2. If sentinal LN Bx is positive, then full LND is required.
When is WLE alone adequate as Tx of melanoma?	WLE alone is adequate for **in situ or stage IA lesions** without adverse features on Bx.
When should sentinel LN Bx be considered or recommended with WLE for melanoma?	Sentinel LN Bx with WLE for melanoma should be considered/recommended for **stage IA with adverse features, stage ≥IB, or Clark 4–5.**
What evidence demonstrates improved survival outcomes for prophylactic LND in the management of melanoma?	For lesions >1.6 mm thick, retrospective data by ***Milton et al.*** (*Br J Surg 1982*) and ***Urist et al.*** (*Ann Surg 1984*) have demonstrated improved survival. A randomized study by ***Balch et al.*** (*Ann Surg Oncol 2000*) has shown improved survival for pts with nonulcerated lesions, lesions 1–2 mm thick, and limb lesions.

What is the LN recurrence rate for pN+ melanoma pts after LND?

After LND, the LN recurrence rate for pN+ pts is **30% at 10 yrs** (*Lee RJ et al., IJROBP 2000*: no adj RT; 45% rcv chemo).

What min surgical margins are required by T stage for the optimal surgical management of melanoma?

Min surgical margins for optical surgical management:
Tis: 5 mm
T1: 1 cm
T2: 1–2 cm
T3-T4: 2 cm

Which randomized trials support the surgical margins currently used in the management of melanoma?

Balch et al. (*Ann Surg Oncol 2001*): 2 cm vs. 4 cm for >T2; no difference in outcome

Thomas et al. (*NEJM 2004*): 1 cm vs. 3 cm; 3 cm resulted in better LC for >T2 lesions, but no OS benefit

When is elective iliac or obturator LND necessary after resection of a lower extremity melanoma?

Elective iliac or obturator LND is necessary if there are **clinically positive superficial nodes, ≥3 superficial +LNs, or if pelvic CT shows LAD.**

When is primary RT ever indicated for Tx of melanoma?

Primary RT is indicated for **medically inoperable pts or lentigo maligna of the face** (cosmetic outcome better); this is given as 50 Gy/20 fx or 7–9 Gy × 6 biweekly (*Farshad A et al., Br J Dermatol 2002*), 1.5-cm margin, 100–250 kV photons.

If primary RT is used for medically inoperable pts, what modality can be added to improve the efficacy of RT?

Hyperthermia (*Overgaard J et al., Lancet 1995*) improves LC (46% vs. 28%) without added toxicity.

How were RT and hyperthermia administered to pts with melanoma in the Overgaard study?

In the Overgaard study, pts were given 24 or 27 Gy in 3 fx over 8 days +/− hyperthermia (43°C × 60 minutes), which improved LC.

When is adj RT indicated for resected melanoma?

Adj RT indications for resected melanoma:
Primary site: +/close margins, desmoplastic histology
Nodal site: >3 +LNs or matted LNs, >3 cm, +ECE, or incomplete nodal assessment

Note: Per the latest NCCN guidelines, consider RT for stage III pts.

Which studies suggest that RT can make up for lack of formal neck dissection in H&N pts?

MDACC data by *Ballo et al.* (*Head Neck 2005*): cN+ in neck s/p local excision only with adj RT; 5-yr LC 93%
Ang et al. (*IJROBP 1994*): high-risk pts +/− LND; 5-yr LC 88%

Note: The **ongoing Australia/TROG trial** is addressing this issue.

What is the only proven adj systemic therapy that improves DFS and OS in pts with resected high-risk stage III melanoma?

High-dose IFN-α, using the Kirkwood schedule (20 mU/m²/day intravenously, 5 to 7 days/wk for 4 wks → 10 mU/m²/day SQ, 3 × wk for 48 wks). However, **NCCTG 83-7052** did not demonstrate benefit of IFN (costly Tx at $50–$60K/pt).

When is high-dose IFN indicated for the management of melanoma? Which studies have demonstrated a benefit for these select pts?

High-dose IFN is indicated for **>4-mm or N+ lesions.** The **ECOG 1684, 1690, and 1694** studies have shown a 10% improvement in RFS, with an OS benefit in 2 of 3 trials.

Which study showed no benefit with moderate doses of IFN after surgical resection of melanoma?

EORTC 18952 (*Eggermont AM et al., Lancet 2005*): stage IIb–III, randomized to 13 mos or 25 mos of IFN or observation. There was no SS difference in OS; however, there was an SS difference in DMFS with 25 mos of INF.

What is the role of combining IFN with RT as adj Tx for high-risk resected stage III malignant melanomas?

Preclinical studies demonstrate **radiosensitization with IFN.** Retrospective reviews demonstrate feasibility but possible increased subacute/late toxicity (see Toxicity section below). Generally, 1 mo of high-dose induction INF → RT with an intermediate maintenance dose of INF is feasible.

What RT fractionation scheme is commonly used in the adj setting for melanoma of the H&N?

Biweekly 6 Gy/fx × 5 (30 Gy) based on the *Ang et al.* study (MDACC data): 5-yr LRC was 88%, OS was 47%, and there was min acute/late toxicity. (*IJROBP 1994*)

Is there a benefit to hypofractionating RT for melanoma in the adj setting?

No. RTOG 8305 (*Sause WT et al., IJROBP 1991*) showed no difference between 8 Gy × 4 and 2.5 Gy × 20.

What did the University of Florida experience/study (*Chang DT et al., IJROBP 2006*) demonstrate regarding adj nodal RT in pts with melanoma lesions of the H&N?

The University of Florida study showed excellent 5-yr LC (87%) and no difference between hypofractionation (6 Gy × 5 fx) and standard (60 Gy in 30 fx) dosing. The major cause of mortality was DM.

What is generally recommended for a pt with nodal recurrence after primary management for melanoma?

Recommendations for a pt with nodal recurrence after primary management include restaging, FNA or LN Bx → LND if no previous dissection → consideration for adj RT and/or INF, a clinical trial, or observation.

How is salvage RT delivered in melanoma pts with isolated axillary nodal recurrences?

After axillary LND, RT to the axilla alone is sufficient (the supraclavicular region may be omitted), using 6 Gy × 5 (30 Gy) per MDACC data (*Beadle BM et al., IJROBP 2009*). The 5-yr LC rate was 88%.

What are some active chemo agents currently in use for metastatic melanoma?

Temozolomide, dacarbazine, interleukin-2, Taxol, and platinum-doublet with Taxol (carboplatin or cisplatin) are currently used for metastatic melanoma.

■ Toxicity

What is the rate of lymphedema when treating different LN regions with hypofractionated RT?

The rates for lymphedema are **39% for the groin, 30% for the axilla, and 11% for H&N sites.** (MDACC data: *Ballo MT et al., Head Neck 2005*)

What is the α/β ratio of melanoma?

For melanoma, the α/β ratio is **2.5**. (*Overgaard J et al., Lancet 1995*)

When using a hypofractionated regimen (e.g., 6 Gy × 5 [30 Gy]), at what dose does the practitioner come off the spinal cord and small bowel?

2,400 cGy is the dose tolerance of the spinal cord/small bowel when hypofractionating with 6 Gy/fx.

What are the main toxicities of concurrent IFN and RT in the adj Tx of stage III melanoma?

In stage III melanoma, the use of concurrent IFN and RT in adj Tx can cause **acute skin toxicity as well as increased grade 3–4 subacute and late toxicities** (fibrosis, SQ necrosis, myelitis, mucositis, pneumonitis, lymphedema). Up to 50% of pts can develop grade 3 toxicities.

What are the latest NCCN follow-up recommendations for melanoma by stage?

NCCN melanoma follow-up recommendations:
1. Annual skin exam for life (all stages)
2. For stages IA–IIA: H&P q3–12mos for 5 yrs, then annually; routine labs/imaging not recommended
3. For stages IIB–IV: H&P q3–6mos for yrs 1–2, then q3–12mos for yrs 3–5, then annually; routine labs for 1st 5 yrs; consider imaging (CXR, PET/CT, annual MRI brain)

84
Squamous Cell and Basal Cell Carcinomas

Boris Hristov and Roland Engel

Background

Name the most common pathologic subtypes of squamous cell carcinoma (SCC).	Bowen Dz (SCC in situ), keratoacanthoma, adenosquamous, verrucous carcinoma (low grade in anogenital, oral, or plantar foot), spindle cell carcinoma
Name the most common pathologic subtypes of basal cell carcinoma (BCC).	Noduloulcerative, superficial, sclerosing morpheaform, infiltrative, pigmented, fibroepithelial tumor of Pinkus, and basosquamous
What area of the body is at highest risk for SCC and BCC?	The **H&N** region is at greatest risk for SCC and BCC.
What is the most common genetic mutation in both SCC and BCC?	In SCC and BCC, **p53** mutations are the most common.
What features of SCC confer a high risk of mets?	Large, deep lesions with PNI and those that appear on dorsum of hands, lips, ears, penis, or sites of chronic infection, ulceration, or RT have a high risk of mets.
What type of UV rays are most responsible for causing skin cancer?	**UVB** (medium wave) rays are most responsible for skin cancer.
What is more common: basal or squamous cell skin cancer?	**Basal cell** (80%) is more common than squamous cell (20%).
What is the sex predilection for skin cancers?	**Males** are more commonly affected than females (**4:1**).
What are the major risk factors for skin cancers?	Major risk factors include **sun exposure, chronic irritation, genetic disorders, and immunosuppression**.
What genetic/inherited disorders are associated with skin cancer?	**Phenylketonuria, Gorlin syndrome (PTCH), xeroderma pigmentosa, and albinism** have a genetic/inherited association with skin cancer.

What is the incidence of PNI and mets with BCC?

PNI: 1%
Mets: <0.1% (nodes > distant sites)

What is the incidence of PNI and mets with SCC?

PNI: 2%–15%
Mets: nodes: 1%–30% (1% grade 1, 10% grade 3, 30% from burns); distant: 2% (lung > liver > bones)

What are the major determinants of LN spread for SCC?

Poor differentiation, size/depth (>3 cm/>4 mm), PNI/LVI, location (lips, scars/burns, ear), and recurrent lesions

What LN regions are most commonly involved in SCC?

The **upper cervical and deep parotid regions** (with the H&N as the most frequent site) are most commonly involved in SCC.

Sun exposure at what stage of life correlates with BCC vs. SCC?

BCC: early in life/childhood
SCC: decade preceding Dx

What is Bowen Dz?

Bowen Dz is **SCC in situ.**

What is erythroplasia de Querat?

Erythroplasia de Querat is **Bowen Dz of the penis.**

What is a Marjolin ulcer?

Marjolin ulcer is **SCC arising in a burn scar.**

Which is more common when the ear is the primary site: BCC or SCC?

External ear: BCC more common
Internal/canal: SCC more common

■ Workup/Staging

On what is the latest AJCC T staging based for SCC/BCC?

T1: ≤2 cm (<2 high-risk features)
T2: >2 cm (≥2 high-risk features)
T3: invasion of maxilla, orbit, or temporal bone
T4: skeletal invasion, PNI of skull base

Per the latest AJCC classification, to what other site is N staging for skin cancer similar?

Skin cancer N staging is similar to that of the **H&N:**
N1: single, ipsi ≤3 cm
N2a: single, ipsi 3–6 cm
N2b: multiple, ipsi ≤ 6 cm
N2c: bilat or contralat LNs ≤6 cm
N3: LNs >6 cm

What defines stage groupings I, II, III, and IV?

Stage I: T1N0
Stage II: T2N0
Stage III: T3N0 or T1-3N1
Stage IV: N2-3, or T4, or M1

What defines a stage II(I) pt?

Stage II(I) represents a **pt with stage II Dz that is also immunosuppressed (I).** This is not part of formal staging but is allowed for studies/tumor registries.

What are considered high-risk features per the latest AJCC staging guidelines?

High-risk features include >2-mm DOI/thickness, Clark level ≥IV, +PNI, poor differentiation, an ear or hair-bearing lip site.

Where is the "H" zone anatomically, and why is it important?

The H zone is located in the **mid face where the embryologic fusion lines lie** (high risk for deep invasion and high risk for LR).

For what is a "pearly papule" lesion pathognomonic?

BCC lesions often appear as pearly papules.

How does SCC appear on the skin?

SCC is **flesh toned and variably keratotic.**

On H&P, what aspects should be the focus of the exam?

Palpate extent of tumor, CN exam for H&N lesions, regional LN evaluation, audiometry/otoscopy for cancers of the ear, and CT/MRI to verify extent

▌Treatment/Prognosis

Name 5 Tx options for SCC and BCC of the skin.

SCC/BCC of the skin Tx options:
1. Mohs surgery
2. Electrosurgery
3. Cryotherapy
4. Topical chemo
5. RT

Describe Mohs surgery.

In Mohs surgery, a superficial slice of skin is taken and then sectioned into quadrants. Additional layers are taken in the quadrants that show persistent Dz.

When are cryotherapy and curettage appropriate for skin cancer?

Cryotherapy and curettage are suitable for **small superficial BCC or superficial well-differentiated SCC.**

When is topical 5-FU used for SCC?

Topical 5-FU is used when the **lesion is confined to the epidermis.**

How can Bowen Dz be treated?

Bowen Dz Tx: surgery, cryotherapy, topical 5-FU, or RT (400 cGy × 10 [40 Gy])

What is the most commonly employed surgical technique for skin cancer?

Mohs micrographic surgery is the most common surgical technique for skin cancer.

When is Mohs surgery contraindicated for skin cancer?

Mohs surgery is not used for **central face lesions >5 mm or ear/scalp lesions >2 cm.**

What % of BCC recurs if margin+ at the time of resection?

BCC recurs in **30% for a + lat margin and >50% for a + deep margin.**

What % of SCC recurs if margin+ at the time of resection?

Nearly 100% of SCCs recur if margin+.

When is RT preferred as the primary Tx modality for skin cancer?

RT is preferred for lesions of the central face that are >5 mm at the nasal ala, lip, or eyelid and lesions >2 cm on the ears, forehead, or scalp. RT is also preferred for pts >55 yo.

What is the best predictor of LC after definitive RT?

T stage is the best predictor for LC (T1, 95%; T3, 50%).

What is the LC after definitive RT for BCC vs. SCC?

LC is similar for BCC and SCC with T1 lesions (95%) and lower for SCC than BCC if T2 (75%–85%) or T3 (50%).

What should be done if a BCC or SCC is resected to +margins?

Re-excise or use adj RT if margins are positive.

What are 4 indications for adj RT to the primary site with skin cancer?

Indications for adj RT to the primary in skin cancer:
1. +Margin
2. PNI of named nerve
3. >3-cm lesion and/or T4
4. Parotid SCC

What are relative contraindications to RT in the Tx of skin cancers?

Relative contraindications to RT for skin cancer include areas prone to trauma (hand dorsum or belt line) or with poor blood supply (below knees/elbows), age <50 yrs, post-RT recurrence, Gorlin syndrome, CD4 count <200, high occupational sun exposure, and exposed area of bone/cartilage.

When should adj nodal RT be considered after surgical resection for skin cancers?

Consider adj nodal RT after surgical resection for **multiple (>3) +LNs, large (>3 cm) LNs, ECE, a preauricular site (high rates of parotid LN involvement), and PNI.** (*Garcia-Serra A et al., Head Neck 2003*)

What fields and dose schemes are typically employed with photons/ orthovoltage in the Tx of skin cancers?

Treat the tumor/tumor bed + 1–2 cm to **60–66 Gy (2 Gy/fx),** especially for involvement of cartilage, or to **50–55 Gy (2.5–3 Gy/fx).** For the elderly/poor performance status, 3.5–4 Gy × 10 or 10 Gy × 2 can be used.

What is the margin/dose modification if electrons are used? Why?

If electrons are used, add an additional 0.5-cm margin on the skin surface and use 10%–15% higher daily/ total dose b/c of bowing out of isodose curves and a lower RBE (0.85–0.9) of electrons.

What is the Rx point if orthovoltage (100–200 kV) RT is employed?

Dmax (90% of the IDL has to encompass the tumor). Do not use this if the lesion is >1 cm deep.

When treating with electrons, how deep should the 90% IDL extend in relation to the lesion?

The IDL should extend at least **5–10 mm deeper than the deepest aspect of the lesion.**

When treating skin lesions with electrons, what rule is typically employed to choose the correct beam energy?

Electron energy (in MeV) should be **>3 times the lesion depth** (i.e., a 9-MeV beam is needed for a 2-cm lesion depth)

What is the RT volume if a named nerve is involved by SCC?

The RT volume should include nerve retrograde to the skull base. Consider IMRT/elective nodal RT.

Where do basosquamous skin cancers occur? What is the Tx paradigm?

Basosquamous skin cancers occur on the **face.** These are treated like SCC, as they have similar rates of nodal mets.

What kind of shields are used, and where should they be placed? Why?

Wax-covered lead shields are used b/c of backscattered electrons with low E beams. They are typically placed behind/downstream of tumor, as hotspots occur upstream of the shield.

How is SCC of the pinna approached?

For SCC of the pinna, use RT with **2.5–4 Gy/fx to 45–65 Gy in 2–3 fx/wk** to the lesion + a 1–2-cm margin (using bolus and shielding as necessary).

When should surgery be recommended for pinna lesions?

Recommend surgery **when cartilage is involved or with tumor extension to the canal.**

When is adj RT generally recommended for ear lesions?

Pinna: if +margin, ≥T3
Middle ear/mastoid: if ≥T2

Can definitive RT be done for canal/middle ear lesions?

Yes. Good outcomes have been reported with RT alone for T1 lesions. (*Ogawa K et al., IJROBP 2007*)

What RT fields/margins are used for middle ear/canal lesions?

For middle ear/canal lesions, include the **entire canal/temporal bone + a 2–3-cm margin and ipsi regional nodes** (preauricular, postauricular, level II).

How should fx size be tailored for skin cancer depending on the RT field size used?

The larger the field size, the smaller the fx size should be.

If simple excision is performed for BCC, what are the min margins required?

≤1-cm tumor: 4 mm
≥1-cm tumor: 5–10 mm

What is the 1st step to take when the pt has a +margin after excision?

Send the pt back to the surgeon to be evaluated for re-excision if the margin is positive.

What is the preferred RT modality for bone-invasive skin cancer? For cartilage invasion?	Megavoltage photons are the preferred Tx modality for bone invasion b/c of a more homogenous distribution compared to orthovoltage due to the f-factor; however, this is not so with cartilage invasion, as orthovoltage beams have little difference in distribution in cartilage regardless of energy.
If treating recurrent BCC or morpheaform BCC, what type of margins should be used?	Since these tumors infiltrate more extensively, an **extra 0.5–1-cm margin** should be added on the surface.
How long should be the wait for a skin graft to heal before starting RT?	**6–8 wks** of healing time is required after skin grafting before RT can be initiated.
How should an SCC of the mastoid be treated?	Treat SCC of the mastoid with **mastoidectomy or temporal bone resection → PORT.**
How should the RT doses be modified based on tumor size/extent for ear primaries?	Conventional fx of 1.8–2 Gy: Small thin lesions ≤1.5 cm: 50 Gy Larger tumors: 55 Gy Min cartilage/bone involvement: 60 Gy Cartilage/bone involvement: 65 Gy

▮ Toxicity

What are some toxicities expected after RT for skin cancer?	Telangiectasia, skin atrophy, hyperpigmentation, skin necrosis, fibrosis, osteonecrosis, chrondritis; xerostomia/hearing loss for the ear
If cartilage is in the RT field, what should the dose/fx be kept below?	The dose should be kept at **<3 Gy/fx** to reduce chondritis.
What is the incidence of skin necrosis after RT?	Skin necrosis occurs in **3%** of pts (in 13% if fx size is >4–6 Gy).
To what dose should middle ear/canal lesions be limited? Why?	Limit middle ear/canal lesions to **65–70 Gy** b/c of higher rates (>10%) of **osteoradionecrosis** with doses >70 Gy.
What must be done to reduce the toxicities to normal tissues from skin irradiation in the H&N region?	To reduce toxicities to normal tissues, use **lead shielding** to block the lens, cornea, nasal septum, teeth, and gums. Use **dental wax** on the side from which the beam enters to absorb backscatter.
Per the latest NCCN guidelines, what should be the follow-up intervals for pts with nonmelanoma skin cancers?	NCCN nonmelanoma skin cancer follow-up intervals: 1. Complete skin exam for life at least once/yr 2. For local Dz: H&P q3–6mos for yrs 1–2, q6–12 mos for yrs 3–5, then annually 3. For regional Dz: H&P q1–3mos for yr 1, q2–4mos for yr 2, q4–6mos for yrs 3–5, then q6–12mos for life

85
Merkel Cell Carcinoma
John P. Christodouleas and Benjamin D. Smith

Background

What is the annual incidence of Merkel cell carcinoma (MCC) in the U.S.?

~**500 cases/yr** of MCC in the U.S.

What is the median age of Dx for MCC?

The median age of Dx is ~**74 yrs** (90% >50 yrs).

What is the cell type of origin for MCC?

Neuroendocrine (dermal sensory cells)—aka trabecular or "small cell" cancer of the skin.

What is the prognosis of MCC as compared to other skin cancers?

Of skin cancers, MCC has the **worst prognosis** (even worse than melanoma).

What % of pts have LN involvement at Dx?

20% have LN involvement at Dx.

DMs develop in what % of pts with MCC?

50%–60% of MCC pts develop DMs.

Is MCC a radiosensitive or radioresistant tumor?

MCC is considered **radiosensitive.**

What demographic group does MCC affect predominantly?

Elderly whites are primarily affected by MCC.

Where do most MCCs arise anatomically?

H&N region (50%) > extremities (33%)

MCC tumors at which sites have a particularly poor prognosis?

Vulva and/or perineum MCC is associated with a particularly poor prognosis.

To what tumor type is the histologic appearance of MCC similar?

The histologic appearance of MCC is similar to **small cell carcinoma of the lung.**

What are the histologic subtypes of MCC?

Histologic subtypes of MCC:
1. Small cell
2. Intermediate cell
3. Trabecular

What histologic subtype of MCC has the best prognosis?

Trabecular MCC has the best prognosis.

What are 2 important prognostic factors in MCC?

Prognostic factors in MCC:
1. Thickness/DOI
2. LN status

■ Workup/Staging

What is the workup for MCC?

MCC workup: H&P, CBC, CMP, CT C/A/P, and MRI or **PET for H&N primaries** to assess nodal status

What imaging is required at a min for MCC staging?

CT chest/abdomen is required for staging.

Why is chest imaging paramount in the staging of MCC?

Chest imaging is important to **r/o mets and the possibility of small cell lung cancer with mets to the skin** as an etiology.

Outline the informal staging system commonly utilized by various institutions for MCC.

Informal staging system for MCC:
Stage I: localized
Stage II: LN+
Stage III: DMs

Outline the latest AJCC TNM staging for MCC.

T1: ≤2 cm
T2: >2 cm and ≤5 cm
T3: >5 cm
T4: invades bone, muscle, fascia, or cartilage
N1a: micromets
N1b: macromets
N2: in-transit mets (between primary and nodal basin or distal to primary)
M1a: mets to skin, SQ tissue, or distant LN
M1b: mets to lung
M1c: mets to all other visceral sites

What is the definition of in-transit mets or N2 Dz per the latest AJCC classification?

N2 Dz is defined as tumor distinct from the primary tumor and either between the primary and the nodal basin or distal to the primary.

Outline the latest AJCC stage groupings for MCC.

Stage IA: T1pN0
Stage IB: T1cN0
Stage IIA: T2-3pN0
Stage IIB: T2-3cN0
Stage IIC: T4N0
Stage IIIA: any TN1a
Stage IIIB: any TN1b-2
Stage IV: M1

▌Treatment/Prognosis

What is the Tx paradigm for MCC?

MCC Tx paradigm: surgery/WLE with sentinel LN Bx +/− LND +/− adj RT +/− adj chemo

What are some commonly used chemo agents for MCC?

Agents used in MCC: cisplatin or carboplatin with etoposide or irinotecan

What surgical margins are recommended?

Surgical margins of **3–4 cm** are recommended.

When is adj RT indicated for MCC?

Historically, adj RT has been included in the Tx course for the majority of MCC pts. A recent study by *Allen et al. (JCO 2005)* suggested that adj RT was of no benefit in margin− pts with surgically staged low-risk nodal Dz. Strong indications for RT include:
1. **Tumor >2 cm**
2. **+/Close margins**
3. **Angiolymphatic invasion**
4. **LN+ or no LN evaluation**
5. **Immunocompromised pts**

Per the NCCN, what RT doses are commonly used for MCC?

Commonly used total doses for MCC:
Negative margins: **50–56 Gy**
Positive margins: **56–60 Gy**
Gross residual or unresectable: **60–66 Gy**

What RT margins are typically used for MCC?

For MCC, the typical RT margin is **5 cm around the primary tumor** (i.e., not the scar).

When are regional LNs covered in the RT volume for MCC?

Regional LNs are typically covered for all MCC pts. Retrospective data suggests that the inclusion of regional LNs in the RT field is associated with superior outcomes (*Jabbour J et al., Ann Surg Oncol 2007; Eich HT et al., Am J Clin Oncol 2002*). However, the role of LN coverage in sentinel LN Bx–negative or LND-negative pts is controversial.

What is the evidence for concurrent CRT after surgery for MCC?

Data on concurrent CRT for MCC are **limited.** Phase II trials have shown that CRT is tolerable (*Poulsen MG et al., IJROBP 2006*), but no trials have established superior efficacy over RT alone.

What is the historical LF rate after surgery alone and with adj RT?

Historical rates are **45%–75%** with surgery alone and **15%–25%** with adj RT.

Estimate the 3-yr OS for MCC by informal staging.

3-yr OS by informal staging:
Stage I (localized): 70%–80%
Stage II (LN+): 50%–60%
Stage III (DM): 30%

▐ Toxicity

What specific follow-up studies do MCC pts require?	Frequent CXR imaging, consideration of serum neuron-specific enolase testing for recurrence, and total skin exam for life (high rates of 2nd skin cancers)
What follow-up intervals are recommended by the NCCN for MCC?	MCC recommended follow-up schedule: H&P and clinically indicated imaging q1–3mos for yr 1, q3–6mos for yr 2, and annually thereafter.
What are the major toxicities in pts receiving CRT for MCC?	**Skin** (grade 3–4) toxicity is ~60% and **neutropenia** is ~40%. (*Poulsen M et al., IJROBP 2001*)

86

Ear Cancer

Steven H. Lin and Vincent J. Lee

▐ Background

What structures constitute the outer and inner components of the ear?	Outer ear: pinna (auricle), external auditory canal, tympanic membrane, and middle ear Inner ear: temporal bone (mastoid bone of bony and membranous labyrinth)
What is the lymphatic drainage of the ear?	The ear drains to the **parotid, retroauricular, and cervical nodes.**
What are the most common cancer histologies of the outer vs. the inner ear?	Pinna: basal cell carcinoma Rest (canal, middle ear, mastoid): squamous cell carcinoma (SCC) (85%)
What % of pts with ear cancer present with nodal mets?	**<15%** of pts present with nodal mets.

▐ Workup/Staging

What is the general workup for tumors of the ear?	Tumor of the inner ear workup: H&P, otoscopy, LN exam, CT/MRI, tissue Bx, and audiometry
What staging system is used for cancer of the ear?	The **AJCC nonmelanoma skin cancer staging system** is used for ear cancer (refer to Chapter 84).

For cancer of the ear, what are considered high-risk features per the latest AJCC edition?	**DOI >2 mm, Clark level ≥IV, +PNI, and poor differentiation** are considered high-risk features for cancer of the ear.

Treatment/Prognosis

What is the general Tx paradigm for a pt with ear cancer?	Ear cancer Tx paradigm: surgery or definitive RT (surgery preferred for cartilage invasion)
What features of the primary tumor merit consideration of elective LN irradiation?	Elective LN irradiation is considered for **large tumors (>4 cm) and deep invasion of underlying structures (i.e., cartilage).**
How should SCC of the mastoid be treated?	SCC of the mastoid Tx: mastoidectomy or temporal bone resection → PORT
How are tumors of the pinna treated?	Tumor of the pinna Tx: electrons or orthovoltage RT (1-cm margin for <1-cm tumors; 2–3-cm margin for larger tumors)
How should tumors of the external auditory canal be treated?	External auditory canal Tx: Include in the Tx volume the entire external auditory canal and temporal bone with 2–3-cm margins, and include ipsi regional nodes (pre-/postauricular, level II); these tumors should be treated to **60–70 Gy.**
How should the RT doses be modified based on tumor size?	Conventional fx of 1.8–2 Gy: <u>Small thin lesions ≤1.5 cm</u>: 50 Gy <u>Larger tumors</u>: 55 Gy <u>Min cartilage/bone involvement</u>: 60 Gy <u>Cartilage/bone involvement</u>: 65 Gy
When should higher-energy electrons be used for ear lesions?	Higher-energy electrons should be used for **large, deep, unresectable tumors** (to cover the deepest extent).

Toxicity

What is the max dose allowed in order to minimize the likelihood of osteoradionecrosis?	Osteoradionecrosis can be minimized by keeping bone doses to **<70 Gy** (~10% rate for doses >65 Gy).
What are some complications in the Tx of the ear with RT?	RT complications include **osteo- or cartilage necrosis, hearing loss, chronic otitis, and xerostomia.**

PART XIV Palliative

87

Palliative Care: Brain Metastases

Bronwyn R. Stall and Kevin Camphausen

Background

What is the most common intracranial tumor?	**Brain mets** is the most common intracranial tumor.
What is the annual incidence of brain mets in the U.S.?	**170,000 cases/yr** of brain mets in the U.S.
What cancers are associated with hemorrhagic brain mets?	Hemorrhagic brain mets is associated with **melanoma, renal cell carcinoma, and choriocarcinoma.**
What does the term *solitary brain met* connote?	A solitary brain met is **only 1 brain lesion.**
What cancers are most likely to metastasize to the brain?	Cancers associated with brain mets: lung (40%–50%), breast (15%), melanoma (10%), and unknown primary (5%–10%)
What is more common type of brain met: single or multiple?	Most pts have **multiple** brain mets rather than a single lesion.
How do pts with brain mets present?	Presentation of pts with brain mets: Sx of ↑ ICP (HA, n/v), weakness, change in sensation, mental status changes, and seizure
Where do most brain mets occur?	Most brain mets arise in the **gray/white matter junction** due to narrowing of blood vessels. (*Delattre J et al., Arch Neurol 1988*)
Are most brain mets infra- or supratentorial?	The majority of brain mets are **supratentorial.**
What is the distribution of brain mets within the brain?	The distribution of brain mets correlates with relative weight and blood flow: <u>Cerebral hemispheres</u>: 80% <u>Cerebellum</u>: 15% <u>Brain stem</u>: 5% (*Delattre J et al., Arch Neurol 1988*)

If a pt presents with brain mets without a prior Dx of cancer, what is the most likely source?

Pts presenting with brain mets without a prior Dx of cancer most often have a **lung primary.**

What is the overall median time from initial cancer Dx to development of brain mets?

The median overall time from initial cancer Dx to development of brain mets is **1 yr.**

Do most pts with brain mets die from their CNS Dz?

No. ~30%–50% of pts with brain mets die from their CNS Dz.

■ Workup/Staging

Describe the workup of a brain met.

Brain met workup: H&P focus on characterization of any neurologic Sx, evaluation for infectious causes (fever, CBC), careful neurologic exam, MRI brain $+/-$ gadolinium, assessment for status of extracranial Dz, determination of Karnofsky performance status (KPS), and neurosurgery consult

What imaging test is 1st line in evaluating brain mets?

MRI is 1st line in the evaluation of brain mets.

What is the DDx for a new lesion in the brain?

Brain lesion DDx: mets, infection/abscess, hemorrhage, primary brain tumor, infarct, tumefactive demyelinating lesion, and RT necrosis

What imaging features are suggestive of brain mets?

Imaging features suggestive of brain mets include lesions at gray/white matter junction, multiple lesions, ring-enhancing lesions, and significant vasogenic edema

What is triple-dose gadolinium, and why is it used?

Triple-dose gadolinium: **0.3 mmol/kg.** It is used **to increase the sensitivity of MRI.**

■ Treatment/Prognosis

The RTOG recursive partitioning analysis (RPA) divides brain mets pts into how many prognostic classes?

The RTOG RPA divides brain mets pts into **3 prognostic classes.**

What prognostic factors are included in the RPA for brain mets?

Prognostic factors included in the RPA for brain mets include KPS, control of the primary, age <65 yrs, and the presence of mets outside the CNS. (*Gaspar L et al., IJROBP 1997*)

What pts are included in class I according to the RTOG for brain mets?

Brain met RPA class I: KPS ≥70, age <65 yrs, primary controlled, and no extracranial mets

What pts are included in class II according to the RTOG for brain mets?

Brain mets RPA class II: KPS ≥70 with 1 of the following—primary uncontrolled, age >65 yrs, or extracranial mets

What pts are included in class III according to the RTOG for brain mets?

Brain mets RPA class III: KPS <70

What is the MS time for RTOG RPA classes I, II, and III?

MS according to the RTOG brain met RPA:
    Class I: 7.2 mos
    Class II: 4.2 mos
    Class III: 2.3 mos

What is the Sperduto Index?

The Sperduto Index is a graded prognostic assessment based on age, KPS, # of brain mets, and the presence or absence of extracranial mets developed from an analysis of 1,960 pts in the RTOG database. Criteria is based on a point system:
    0 points: age >60 yrs, KPS <70, >3 brain mets, presence of extracranial mets
    0.5 points: age 50–59 yrs, KPS 70–80, 2 CNS mets
    1 point: age <50 yrs, KPS 90–100, 1 CNS met, no extracranial mets

The sum of points predicts MS in mos:
    0–1 point: 2.6 mos
    1.5–2.5 points: 3.8 mos
    3 points: 6.9 mos
    3.5–4 points: 11 mos

(*Sperduto P et al., IJROBP 2007*)

In pts with untreated brain mets, what is the MS?

MS of untreated brain mets is **1 mo.**

What Tx may be used for brain mets?

Brain met Tx: steroids, surgery, fractionated RT (WBRT), and SRS

In pts with brain mets treated with steroids alone, what is the MS?

MS in pts with brain mets treated with steroids alone is **2 mos.**

How are steroids for brain mets typically prescribed?

Steroid dose for newly diagnosed brain mets: **4 mg dexamethasone q6hrs;** may give initial loading dose of 10 mg.

Why are steroids used for symptomatic brain mets?

In pts with symptomatic brain mets, **steroids reduce leakage from tumor vessels,** therefore decreasing edema and mass effect.

What pharmacologic Tx should always accompany steroid Tx?

When prescribing steroids, also provide **GI prophylaxis with a proton-pump inhibitor or H2 blocker.**

Should anticonvulsants be used prophylactically?

No. In accordance with guidelines from the American Academy of Neurology, pts with newly diagnosed brain tumors should not be started on prophylactic anticonvulsants. (*Glantz M et al. Neurology 2000*)

Is there any randomized data on the dose for WBRT?

Yes. The RTOG conducted several RCTs from 1970–1995 of WBRT alone, assessing different fractionation schemes. The 1st 2 trials **(RTOG 6901 and 7361)** included >1,800 pts randomized to 40 Gy/20, 40 Gy/15, 30 Gy/15, 30 Gy/10, or 20 Gy/5. No significant difference was found in response rates, length of response, or OS. The MS in the 1st study was 4.1 mos and 3.4 mos in the 2nd. (*Borgelt B et al., IJROBP 1980*)

2 ultra-rapid fractionation schemes were also tested on these studies and reported separately; 10 Gy/1 **(RTOG 6901)** and 12 Gy/2 **(RTOG 7361)** in 26 and 33 pts, respectively. These schedules were associated with worse toxicity and time to neurologic progression than the standard fractionation. (*Borgelt B et al., IJROBP 1981*)

2 studies showed no MS advantage to giving a higher total dose. **RTOG 7606** randomized 255 pts to 30 Gy/10 vs. 50 Gy/20. MS was 4.1 and 3.9 mos, respectively (*Kurtz J et al., IJROBP 1981*). **RTOG 9104** randomized 429 pts to 30 Gy/10 vs. 54.4/1.6 Gy bid. MS was 4.5 mos in both arms (*Murray K et al., IJROBP 1997*).

What dose and fractionation schemes are considered standard for WBRT?

The most standard WBRT dose is **30 Gy/10.** Pts with a good KPS and longer life expectancy may be treated to 37.5 Gy/15, 40 Gy/20, or 50 Gy/20.

What % of brain met pts have Sx improvement with WBRT?

WBRT improves Sx from brain mets in ~**60%** of cases.

What is the rate of CR to WBRT for brain mets?

~**25%** of pts have a CR to WBRT for brain mets.

Should Bx be recommended if a new Dx of brain mets is suspected?

Yes. Bx should be considered if a new Dx of brain mets is suspected, as 11% of pts enrolled on the 1st Patchell trial were found not to have metastatic Dz on Bx despite MRI or CT findings consistent with metastatic Dz. (*Patchell R et al., NEJM 1990*)

What data supports surgery + RT rather than Bx + RT for brain mets?

The **1st Patchell study** for brain mets randomized 48 pts with 1 brain met and KPS ≥70 to surgery + WBRT vs. Bx + WBRT. WBRT in both arms was 36 Gy in 3 Gy/fx. Pts treated with surgery had a longer MS (40 wks vs. 15 wks, $p < 0.01$), longer functional independence (38 wks vs. 8 wks), and ↓LR (20% vs. 52%, $p < 0.02$). (*Patchell R et al., NEJM 1990*)

Did the Netherlands trial of WBRT +/− surgery support or refute the Patchell study?

The Noordijk study **supported** the findings of the 1st Patchell study. It randomized 63 pts to WBRT alone or surgery + WBRT. WBRT was 40 Gy in 2 Gy bid fx. Pts treated with surgery had improved MS (10 mos vs. 6 mos, $p = 0.04$) and longer functional independence (7.5 mos vs. 3.5 mos, $p = 0.06$). (*Noordijk E et at., IJROBP 1994*)

Does adj WBRT after surgical resection of a brain met improve OS?

No. Postop WBRT following resection of a brain met does not improve survival. In the 2nd Patchell study for brain mets, 95 pts following surgical resection of a single met were randomized to no further Tx or WBRT (50.4 Gy in 1.8 Gy/fx). WBRT decreased LR (10% vs. 46%), decreased the rate of any brain failure (18% vs. 70%), and decreased the rate of neurologic death (14% vs. 44%) but did significantly change MS (48 wks vs. 43 wks). (*Patchell R et al., JAMA 1998*)

Are there any current studies assessing the benefit of WBRT?

Yes. EORTC 22952 is an RCT of pts with 1–3 brain mets s/p surgery or SRS randomized to no further Tx vs. WBRT. This was closed to accrual in 2007 but has not yet been reported.

What was the 1st randomized study of WBRT +/− an SRS boost?

The 1st RCT of WBRT +/− an SRS boost was conducted at the **University of Pittsburgh.** 27 pts with KPS ≥70 and 2–4 mets ≤2.5 cm that were at least 5 mm from the chiasm were randomized to WBRT (30 Gy/12 fx) +/− a 16-Gy boost. The trial closed early b/c of significant difference in brain control. The SRS arm had a longer time to LF (36 mos vs. 6 mos, $p = 0.0005$) and longer time to any brain failure (34 mos vs. 5 mos, $p = 0.002$) but no difference in OS (11 mos vs. 7.5 mos, $p = 0.11$). (*Kondziolka D et al., IJROBP 1999*)

According to RTOG 9508, which pts had a survival advantage with the addition of an SRS boost to WBRT?

RTOG 9508 randomized 331 pts with 1–3 brain mets to WBRT + SRS boost vs. WBRT alone. WBRT on both arms was 37.5 Gy in 2.5 Gy/fx. The SRS boost dose was dependent on size in accordance with RTOG 9005. On univariate analysis, the addition of SRS improved the MS for pts with a single brain met (6.5 mos vs. 4.9 mos, $p = 0.39$). On subgroup multivariate analysis (MVA), RPA class I pts had improved survival with the SRS boost, as did pts with a lung cancer primary. (*Andrews D et al., Lancet 2004*)

What is the main determinant in selecting the Rx dose for SRS Tx of a brain met?

The SRS Rx dose for a brain met is determined by **size** in accordance with the results of **RTOG 9005,** a dose escalation study: 24 Gy if <2-cm diameter, 18 Gy if 2–3 cm, and 15 Gy if 3–4 cm. (*Shaw H et al., IJROBP 1996*)

What retrospective data supports the omission of upfront WBRT in pts treated with SRS for brain mets?

Sneed et al. compiled a database from 10 U.S. institutions to assess the effect of omitting upfront WBRT in pts treated with SRS for brain mets. 983 pts were analyzed and excluded pts treated with surgery (159 pts) and pts with a >1-mo interval between WBRT and SRS (179 pts). Of 569 evaluable pts, 268 had SRS alone and 301 had upfront WBRT + SRS. When adjusted for RPA class, there was no difference in survival. (*IJROBP 2002*)

According to randomized data, what is the effect of delaying WBRT after SRS for pts with 1–4 brain mets?

JROSG99-1 showed that the omission of WBRT after SRS for 1–4 brain mets does not affect survival but increases the risk of intracranial relapse (46% with SRS + WBRT vs. 76.4% with SRS alone) and thus increases the need for salvage Tx. (*Aoyama H et al., JAMA 2006*)

What was the 1st randomized trial to assess the effect of delaying WBRT after SRS?

The 1st trial to assess the effect of delaying WBRT after SRS was **JROSG99-1.** 132 pts with 1–4 mets were randomized to SRS or WBRT + SRS. The SRS dose was based on size (lesions ≤2 cm to 22–25 Gy; lesions >2 cm to 18–20 Gy) and randomization (30% SRS dose reduction for pts on the WBRT arm). The WBRT dose was 30 Gy in 10 fx. (*Aoyama H et al., JAMA 2006*)

In the RTOG SRS dose escalation study, did pts rcv WBRT?

No. In **RTOG 9005,** an SRS dose escalation study, pts did not rcv WBRT.

Is there any data on SRS dosing with planned WBRT?

Yes. Retrospective data from the **University of Kentucky** showed that optimal control of brain mets ≤2 cm was achieved with SRS of 20 Gy + WBRT. Pts treated with >20 Gy SRS + WBRT had higher rates of grade 3–4 neurotoxicity. (*Shehata M et al., IJROBP 2004*)

Is there any data comparing surgery + WBRT with SRS alone?

Yes. Retrospective data from **Germany** comparing RPA class I–II pts with 1–2 brain mets treated either with surgery + WBRT or SRS alone suggests that SRS is as effective. Of 206 pts treated from 1994–2006, 94 pts had SRS alone (18–25 Gy), and 112 pts had resection + WBRT (30 Gy/10 or 40 Gy/20). At 12 mos, there was no difference in OS (~50% in both groups), LC, or brain control. There was no difference according to the RPA group. (*Rades D et al., Cancer 2007*)

Can pts treated with WBRT for brain mets be reirradiated?

Yes. Reirradiation following WBRT may be considered in pts who initially responded well to WBRT and then develop worsening neurologic function at least 4 mos after initial WBRT. (*Cooper J et al., Radiology 1990*)

What dose should be used for reirradiation after WBRT for brain mets?

The optimal dose for reirradiation after WBRT is **unknown.** 20 Gy in 10 fx is often used.

How are the fields arranged for WBRT?

WBRT is delivered using opposed lat fields; a post gantry tilt of 3–5 degrees is used to avoid divergence into the eyes; and multileaf collimation or custom blocks are used to ensure adequate coverage of the cribriform plate, temporal lobe, and brain stem while protecting the eyes, nasal cavity, and oral cavity. The inf border is generally set at C1-2.

Should surgery be used for recurrent tumors?

Yes. Retrospective data from MDACC have suggested that reoperation for recurrent brain mets can prolong survival and improve QOL. MVA revealed several negative prognostic factors: presence of systemic Dz, KPS <70, short time to recurrence (<4 mos), age ≥40 yrs, and breast and melanoma primaries. (*Bindal R et al., J Neurosurg 1995*)

What is the advantage of tumor bed radiosurgery after brain met resection?

Retrospective data from the University of Sherbrooke in Canada have suggested that SRS to the tumor bed following resection for brain mets achieves LC rates that are comparable to WBRT but does not impact the development of remote brain mets. 40 pts underwent resection → SRS at a median of 4 wks post resection. 73% achieved LC, and 54% developed new brain mets. (*Mathieu D et al., Neurosurgery 2008*)

■ Toxicity

What are potential acute toxicities of WBRT?

Potential WBRT acute toxicities: alopecia, fatigue, HA, n/v, ototoxicity

What are potential long-term toxicities of WBRT?

Potential WBRT chronic toxicities: thinned hair, decline in short-term memory, altered executive function, leukoencephalopathy, brain atrophy, normal pressure hydrocephalus, RT necrosis

What is the relationship between WBRT-induced brain met shrinkage and neurocognitive function?

WBRT-induced brain met shrinkage correlates with improved neurocognitive function. This was demonstrated in an analysis of 208 pts with brain mets randomized to WBRT alone on a phase III trial of WBRT +/− motexafin gadolinium. Pts with a good response (>45% tumor volume reduction at 2 mos) to WBRT had a longer time to decline in neurocognitive function. (*Li J et al., JCO 2007*)

What daily fx size in WBRT is associated with RT necrosis?

WBRT administered in fx sizes **>300 cGy/day** are associated with RT necrosis. (*DeAngelis L et al., Neurology 1989*)

Name the potential acute toxicities of SRS for brain mets.

Potential acute toxicities of SRS for brain mets: HA, nausea, dizziness/vertigo, seizure

What is the risk of symptomatic RT necrosis after SRS for brain mets?

There is an ~**5%** risk of symptomatic RT necrosis secondary to SRS for brain mets. This is usually treated with steroids but may require surgery.

88

Palliative Care: Bone Metastases

Bronwyn R. Stall and William P. O'Meara

Background

What are the top 3 sites of metastatic Dz?	Top 3 sites of metastatic Dz: 1. Lung 2. Liver 3. Bone
What is the route of spread of cancer cells to the bone?	Most bone mets arise from **hematogenous** spread of cancer cells.
What part of the skeleton is more commonly affected by bone mets: axial or appendicular?	Bone mets more commonly affect the **axial** rather than the appendicular skeleton.
What part of the spine is most commonly affected by bone mets?	The **thoracic** spine is the most common site of bone mets. (*Bartels RH et al., CA Cancer J 2008*)
What 5 tumors are known to stimulate osteoclast activity?	Tumors known to stimulate osteoclast activity: 1. Breast 2. Prostate 3. Lung 4. Renal 5. Thyroid
In decreasing order, what 5 tumors carry the highest risk of bone mets?	Top 5 tumors with regard to the risk of bone mets (in decreasing order): 1. Prostate 2. Breast 3. Kidney 4. Thyroid 5. Lung
What is the most common presenting Sx of bone mets?	Most pts with bone mets present with **pain.**

▪ Workup/Staging

What is the workup for bone mets?

Bone met workup: H&P, characterization of pain, assessment of fracture risk, assessment for weight-bearing bone, orthopedic consult as necessary, plain films, and bone scan

What imaging test is 1st line in evaluating bone mets?

Initial imaging of asymptomatic bone mets usually involves a **bone scan** (skeletal scintigraphy). If symptomatic, directed plain films and bone scan as well as subsequent clinically directed CT and/or MRI may be beneficial.

When may plain films be useful when evaluating bone mets?

In the setting of **bone pain with a positive bone scan,** plain films may show an impending fracture or a pathologic fracture.

What cancer is associated with mixed lytic and sclerotic lesions?

Breast cancer is associated with mixed sclerotic and lytic lesions.

What cancers are associated with primarily blastic lesions?

Tumors with predominantly blastic lesions:
1. Prostate
2. Small cell lung cancer
3. Hodgkin lymphoma

What cancers are associated with primarily lytic lesions?

Tumors with predominantly lytic lesions:
1. Renal cell
2. Melanoma
3. Multiple myeloma
4. Thyroid
5. Non–small cell lung cancer
6. Non-Hodgkin lymphoma

What imaging test can help to differentiate degenerative Dz from mets?

CT and/or MRI can help to distinguish between degenerative Dz and bone mets.

When cord compression is suspected, what imaging is indicated?

MRI of the entire spine is indicated if cord compression is suspected.

What scoring system predicts for pathologic fracture?

The **Mirels scoring system** is a weighted system based on a retrospective review that predicts the risk of pathologic fracture through metastatic lesions in long bones. Score ranges from 4–12. A score <7 can be treated with RT alone, while a score ≥8 requires internal fixation prior to RT. (*Mirels H et al., Clin Ortho Res 1989*)

What are the components of the Mirels scoring system?

The Mirels scoring system consists of 4 variables:
1. Site (upper extremity, lower extremity, peritrochanteric)
2. Pain (mild, moderate, functional)
3. Lesion (blastic, mixed, lytic)
4. Size (less than one third, one third to two thirds, or more than two thirds cortex destruction)

Each variable receives 1–3 points for a total of 4–12 points. (*Mirels H et al., Clin Ortho Res 1989*)

What 2 risk factors predict for pathologic fracture of the femur?

Factors predicting for pathologic fracture of the femur:
1. Axial cortical involvement >30 mm
2. Circumferential cortical involvement >50%

(*Van der Linden Y et al., J Bone Joint Surg Br 2004*)

■ Treatment/Prognosis

What is the MS of pts with solitary or multiple bone mets?

RTOG 7402 reported that the MS with multiple bone mets is 24 wks, but 36 wks if there is only 1 met.

Name 6 Tx for bone mets.

Bone met Tx:
1. Chemo
2. Radionuclides
3. Local EBRT
4. Endocrine therapy
5. NSAIDs
6. Narcotics

What supportive measures can be used for pts with painful bone mets?

Supportive care for bone mets may include orthopedic braces such as **thoracolumbosacral orthosis (TLSO), canes, walkers, and wheelchairs.**

In what cancers may chemo eradicate bone mets?

Chemo can cure bone mets from **lymphomas and germ cell tumors.**

What is the chief action of bisphosphonates?

Bisphosphonates **inhibit osteoclast activity.**

What are the ASCO 2003 guidelines for bisphosphonates in the Tx of bone mets from breast cancer?

ASCO 2003 guidelines for bisphosphonate use state that bisphosphonates should be administered **q3–4wks** to breast cancer pts with destructive bone lesions seen on plain film.

Name 2 bisphosphonates	**Pamidronate and zoledronic acid** are 2 common bisphosphonates.
Name 3 radionuclides used to treat bone mets.	Radionuclides available in the U.S. for Tx of bone mets: 1. Strontium-89 2. Samarium-153 3. Phosphorus-32
Describe the decay of strontium-153.	Strontium-89 decays by **β emission to yttrium-89.**
What is the half-life of strontium-89?	The half-life of strontium-89 is **50.6 days.**
What is the max decay energy of strontium-89?	The max decay energy of strontium-89 is **β 1.4 MeV.**
What is the max particle range of strontium-89?	The max particle range of strontium-89 is **7 mm.**
Describe the decay of samarium-153.	Samarium-153 decays by **β and γ emission.**
What is the half-life of samarium-153?	The half-life of samarium-153 is **1.9 days.**
What is the max decay energy of samarium-153?	The max decay energy of samarium-153 is **β 0.81 MeV.**
What is the max particle range of samarium-153?	The max particle range of samarium-153 is **4 mm.**
Describe the decay of phosphorus-32.	Phosphorus-32 decays by **β emission.**
What is the half-life of phosphorus-32?	The half-life of phosphorus-32 is **14.3 days.**
What is the max decay energy of phosphorus-32?	The max decay energy of phosphorus-32 is **β 1.7 MeV.**
What is the max particle range of phosphorus-32?	The max particle range of phosphorus-32 is **8.5 mm.**
Describe some differences between strontium-89, samarium-153, and phosphorus-32.	1. Strontium is naturally occurring and is just below calcium on periodic table with the atomic number 38. It is metabolized like calcium and is incorporated into the bone matrix. 2. Samarium-153 is produced by neutron bombardment. Its mechanism of action is not fully understood, but it selectively accumulates in bone in association with hydroxyapatite. 3. Phosphorus-32 is a phosphate. 85% of total body phosphate is held within the skeleton, bound as inorganic phosphate to hydroxyapatite.

Describe the clinical implications of the differences in physical properties between strontium-89, samarium-153, and phosphorus-32.

1. Both strontium-89 and phosphorus-32 emit β particles with higher energy than those of samarium-153, causing deeper tissue penetration. Though these higher-energy β particles may have a therapeutic benefit, they can also cause greater marrow toxicity.
2. The half-life of samarium-153 is much shorter than that of strontium-89. Thus, the planned RT dose from samarium-153 is delivered more quickly, leading to faster time to pain relief in many published trials.
3. As the only gamma emitter, samarium-153 enables posttherapy scintigraphic imaging and dosimetry.

Why is phosphorus-32 seldom used for bone mets?

Phosphorus-32 was the 1st radionuclide to be used for bone mets, but it has **greater hematologic toxicity** compared to the other 2 agents (strontium-89 and samarium-153) available in the U.S.

When should radionuclides be considered?

Radionuclides should be considered in pts with **adequate blood counts and multifocal painful bone mets** imaged on bone scan.

What are some contraindications to radionuclides for bone pain?

Contraindications for using radionuclides for bone pain:
1. Myelosuppression
2. Impaired renal function
3. Pregnancy
4. Cord compression
5. Nerve root compression
6. Impending pathologic fracture
7. Extensive soft tissue component

What randomized data supports the use of samarium-153?

A **double-blind placebo controlled study** of samarium-153 supports its use. 118 pts with symptomatic bone mets were randomized to low-dose samarium-153 (0.5 mCi/kg), high-dose samarium-153 (1 mCi/kg), or placebo. Pts receiving high-dose samarium-153 had significant improvement in pain during the 1st 4 wks per pt and medical evaluation. Relief persisted until at least wk 16 in 43% of pts. There was a significant reduction in the pain score and analgesic use only in pts receiving the high dose. (*Serafini A et al., JCO 1998*)

What RTOG study originally reported no difference in bone pain relief between different fractionation schemes?

RTOG 7402 randomized 759 pts. Those with solitary bone mets were randomized to 40.5 Gy (270 cGy × 15) vs. 20 Gy (400 cGy × 5). Pts with multiple mets were randomized to 30 Gy (300 cGy × 10), 15 Gy (300 cGy × 5), 20 Gy (400 cGy × 5), or 25 Gy (500 cGy × 5). The initial report revealed that 90% of pts had some pain relief, and 54% had eventual CR of pain. There was no difference between regimens (*Tong D et al., Cancer 1982*). Reanalysis showed that a higher # of fx correlated with CR of pain, suggesting that a more protracted course was more effective. The analysis was based only on physician assessment of pain (*Blitzer P et al., Cancer 1985*).

What pts are generally excluded from RCTs of different fractionations for bone-met RT?

RCTs assessing different fractionation schemes for the Tx of bone mets have generally excluded **pts with cord compression and pathologic fracture.**

Did the study by the Bone Pain Trial Working Party support single- or multi-fx Tx of bone mets?

The Bone Pain Trial Working Party supported **single-fx** Tx. The study (UK/NZ) randomized 765 pts with painful bone mets to 8 Gy × 1 vs. a protracted regimen (200 cGy × 5 or 300 cGy × 10). Pain relief was evaluated for up to 1 yr post-Tx by the use of a validated pt questionnaire. There was no difference in pain control between the arms. Re-Tx was twice as common with single-fx Tx (23% vs. 10%), though this may have been due to a greater willingness to re-treat pts who rcv only 8 Gy × 1. (*No author, Radiother Oncol 1999*)

Did the Dutch Bone Metastasis Study support single- or multi-fx Tx of bone mets?

The Dutch Bone Metastasis Study supported **single-fx** Tx. 1,171 pts were randomized to 8 Gy × 1 vs. 4 Gy × 6. Pain relief was evaluated for up to 2 yrs post-Tx by the use of a validated pt questionnaire. No difference was seen with respect to pain relief. However, re-Tx was more common in the single-fx arm (25% vs. 7%) (*Steenland E et al, Radiother Oncol 1999*). Reanalysis suggested that the higher rate of re-Tx in the single-fx arm may be related to a greater willingness to re-Tx pts who rcv only 8 Gy × 1 (*Van der Linden YM et al., IJROBP 2004*).

Did RTOG 9714 support single- or multi-fx Tx of bone mets?

RTOG 9714 supported **single-fx Tx.** randomized 898 pts with breast or prostate cancer to 8 Gy × 1 vs. 3 Gy × 10. There was no difference in complete pain relief (15% vs. 18%) or partial pain relief (50% vs. 48%), but there was increased acute toxicity in the 3 Gy × 10 arm (10% vs. 17%). The re-Tx rate was significantly greater in the 8 Gy × 1 arm. (*Hartsell W et al., JNCI 2005*)

What were the results of the *Chow et al.* meta-analysis of trials comparing single- vs. multi-fx Tx of bone mets?

In a meta-analysis of trials comparing single- vs. multi-fx Tx of bone mets, *Chow et al.* showed no significant differences between fractionation schemes with respect to pain control. However, re-Tx was more common with single-fx Tx. (*JCO 2007*)

Is there data supporting 8-Gy single-fx Tx of bone mets rather than 4 Gy?

Yes. A **Royal Marsden** study randomized 270 pts with painful bone mets to 8 Gy × 1 vs. 4 Gy × 1. Pain was assessed by the pt prior to RT, then at 2, 4, 8, and 12 wks after Tx. The response rate wks was higher for 8 Gy (69% vs. 44%), but there was no difference in CR of pain at 4 wks or a duration of response. It was concluded that 8 Gy has higher probability of pain relief. (*Hoskin P et al., Radiother Oncol 1992*)

What study supported use of hemibody irradiation (HBI) after focal RT for bone mets?

RTOG 8206 randomized pts treated with focal RT to HBI (8 Gy) vs. no further Tx. HBI increased the time to progression as well as the time to re-Tx. (*Poulter C et al., IJROBP 1992*)

What are the published response rates of RT for palliation of symptomatic bone mets irrespective of the fractionation scheme?

The published response rates of RT for palliation of symptomatic bone mets are **60%–80%.**

What is the benefit of PORT after orthopedic stabilization?

PORT following orthopedic stabilization of impending or pathologic fracture decreases the need for 2nd surgery (2% vs. 15%) and increases the rate of regaining normal function (53% vs. 11.5%) for surgery alone. (*Townsend P et al., JCO 1994*)

How do NSAIDs alleviate pain from bone mets?

NSAIDS alleviate metastatic bone pain by **inhibiting prostaglandins,** which are released from osseous mets and can induce osteolysis.

What is the WHO analgesic ladder for cancer pain management?

3-Step WHO analgesic ladder for cancer pain:
1. Nonopioid (acetaminophen, aspirin, NSAIDs) +/− adj Tx
2. Opioid for mild to moderate pain (codeine, hydrocodone, oxycodone, propoxyphene) + nonopioid +/− adj Tx
3. Opioid for moderate to severe pain (morphine, oxycodone, hydromorphone, fentanyl) +/− nonopioid +/− adj Tx

(*Levy M et al., NEJM 1996*)

What is the relationship between oral, SQ, and intravenous opioid doses?

The oral dose is about one half the SQ dose and one third the intravenous dose.

▮ Toxicity

What are the expected acute and late RT toxicities associated with Tx of bone mets?

Potential toxicities from focal RT for bone mets:
    Acute: skin irritation
    Late: fibrosis, nerve damage, fracture, lymphedema

What is the main toxicity of radionuclide Tx?

Radionuclide Tx can cause **significant myelosuppression.**

89

Cord Compression

Bronwyn R. Stall and Kevin Camphausen

Background

What % of cancer pts develop cord compression?	**5%–10%** of cancer pts develop cord compression.
What are 3 routes of metastatic spread to the spine?	Routes of metastatic spread to the spine: hematogenous, direct extension, and CSF. (*Abeloff MD et al., Abeloff's clinical oncology. 4th ed. 2008*)
What malignancies commonly cause cord compression?	Cancers that commonly cause cord compression include lung, breast, prostate, renal cell, lymphoma, and multiple myeloma.
How do pts with cord compression present?	Presenting Sx of cord compression: back pain, radicular pain, weakness, altered sensation, bowel/bladder dysfunction, and paralysis
What is the most common presenting Sx of cord compression?	The most common Sx of cord compression is **back pain.**
What part of the vertebra is most commonly involved by metastatic Dz?	Metastatic Dz typically involves the **vertebral body** rather than the post elements.
What part of the spine is most often involved in cord compression?	The **thoracic** spine is most commonly affected by cord compression.

Workup/Staging

Describe the workup of cord compression.	Cord compression workup: H&P with careful attention to complete neurologic exam, evaluation of sensation to determine level of the lesion, assessment of pain, assessment of bowel/bladder function, and screening MRI spine
Why is a screening MRI of the spine ordered to evaluate cord compression?	Pts with suspected cord compression should be evaluated with a screening MRI of the spine b/c **multilevel involvement is not uncommon.**
Why is CT useful in evaluating cord compression?	CT evaluation of spinal cord compression **helps to delineate osseous structures**, including retropulsed fragments, and **aids in surgical planning.**

▌Treatment/Prognosis

What modalities are used to treat spinal cord compression?

Modalities used to treat spinal cord compression: steroids, surgery, and RT

What is the initial management of cord compression?

For initial management of cord compression, start steroids and consult neurosurgery or orthopedics, depending on the institution, to assess spine stability.

What initial bolus dose of steroids should be used in cord compression?

For newly diagnosed cord compression, a loading dose of 10 mg intravenously is generally given → 4 mg orally q6hrs. *Vecht et al.* randomized 37 pts to 10 mg intravenously vs. 100 mg intravenously, both → 16 mg daily in divided oral doses. There was no difference in pain control, rate of ambulation, or bladder function. (*Neurology 1989*)

Historically, what type of surgery was used to treat spinal cord compression?

Historically, **laminectomy** was used to treat spinal cord compression. However, this was abandoned b/c it can lead to instability, and improved surgical stabilization techniques have allowed for ant decompressive approaches.

What pts with cord compression are appropriate for decompressive surgery?

Pts with MRI evidence of cord compression in a single area and a life expectancy >3 mos who do not have radiosensitive tumors (lymphomas, leukemias, germ cell tumors, multiple myeloma) may be good candidates for decompressive surgery → RT. (*Patchell R et al., Lancet 2005*)

What was the trial design and outcome of the Patchell study of decompressive surgery for cord compression?

The Patchell cord compression trial was a multi-institutional RCT of 101 pts with MRI-confirmed spinal cord compression restricted to a single area with >3-mo life expectancy. Exclusion criteria included being paraplegic >48 hrs, radiosensitive tumors, Hx of prior cord compression, and other pre-existing neurologic conditions. Pts were randomized to decompressive surgery + RT vs. RT alone. RT was 30 Gy/10 delivered to the lesion + 1 vertebral body above and below. Surgery was tailored to the individual lesion to provide circumferential decompression and stabilization as needed. The study was stopped at interim analysis. Surgery significantly improved the ambulatory rate (84% vs. 57%), duration of ambulatory status (122 days vs. 13 days), and survival (122 days vs. 100 days). Pts nonambulatory prior to Tx were more likely to walk after surgery (62% vs. 19%). (*Patchell R et al., Lancet 2005*)

What data support the use of SRS for spinal mets?	Prospective nonrandomized data from the **University of Pittsburgh** support the use of SRS for spinal mets. 500 cases were treated with CyberKnife to a median dose of 20 Gy. SRS improved pain in 86% of cases (defined as a 3-point improvement on a 10-point pain scale). The majority of pts had prior Tx; however, in the 65 cases treated with SRS as the primary modality, the LC was 90%. (*Gerstzen P et al., Spine 2007*)
What pts with cord compression should be treated with RT alone?	Cord compression pts treated with RT alone: life expectancy <3 mos, no spinal instability or bony compression, and radiosensitive tumor
How are conventional RT fields arranged to treat the cervical, thoracic, and lumbar spine?	Field arrangement for cord compression: 　Cervical: opposed lats 　Thoracic: AP/PA or PA alone, respecting cord 　　tolerance 　Lumbar: AP/PA 　Encompass the lesion + 1–2 vertebral levels above 　　and below.
What fractionation schemes are used for cord compression?	Fractionation in cord compression: typically 300 × 10, but consider hypofractionation (400 × 5) in debilitated pts; protracted regimens such as 40/20 or 37.5/15 may be used in pts with a longer life expectancy.

▌Toxicity

What are potential acute toxicities of RT for cord compression?	Potential toxicities of RT for cord compression: odynophagia, globus, esophagitis, nausea, diarrhea, myelosuppression, rare spinal cord injury

90
Superior Vena Cava Syndrome
Bronwyn R. Stall and Brent A. Tinnel

▌Background

What vessels form the SVC?	The **right and left brachiocephalic veins** join to form the SVC.
What vessels form the brachiocephalic vein?	The **internal jugular and subclavian veins** join to form the brachiocephalic vein.

What is SVC syndrome?

SVC syndrome is extrinsic or intrinsic obstruction of blood flow through the SVC leading to proximal congestion.

At what bony landmark does the SVC begin?

The SVC begins at the level of the **sternal angle.**

Describe the course of the SVC.

The SVC begins at the sternal angle, extends inferiorly along the right lat side of the ascending aorta, and inserts into the right atrium.

What predisposes the SVC to compression?

The SVC is a thin-walled vessel with relatively low intravascular pressure and is therefore susceptible to compression by **surrounding rigid structures** including enlarged LNs and the trachea, sternum, pulmonary artery, and right mainstem bronchus.

What vessels form the collateral system of the SVC?

The collateral system of SVC is formed by the azygous, mammary, vertebral, lat thoracic, paraspinous, and esophageal vessels.

What vessels join to form the azygous vein?

The **right subcostal and right ascending lumbar veins** coalesce to form the azygous vein.

What is the most common cause of SVC syndrome?

Malignancy is the most common cause of SVC syndrome.

Name 4 benign causes of SVC syndrome.

Benign causes of SVC syndrome:
1. Catheter-induced thrombosis
2. Chronic mediastinitis
3. Retrosternal goiter
4. CHF

Name 6 cancers associated with SVC syndrome.

Cancers associated with SVC syndrome:
1. Non–small cell lung cancer (NSCLC)
2. Small cell lung cancer (SCLC)
3. Non-Hodgkin lymphoma (NHL)
4. Thymoma
5. Primary mediastinal germ cell tumors
6. Mesothelioma

What is the most common malignant cause of SVC syndrome?

The most common malignant cause of SVC syndrome is **NSCLC.**

Are NSCLC or SCLC pts more likely to develop SVC syndrome?

SCLC pts are more likely to develop SVC syndrome than NSCLC pts b/c of their propensity toward rapid growth in central airways.

What is the most common cause of SVC syndrome in pts <50 yo?

In pts <50 yo, the most common cause of SVC syndrome is **lymphoma.**

Which types of NHL are associated with SVC syndrome?	NHL types associated with SVC syndrome: 1. Diffuse large B-cell lymphoma 2. Lymphoblastic lymphoma 3. Primary mediastinal B-cell lymphoma with sclerosis
What is the typical duration of Sx prior to presentation with SVC syndrome?	Pts with SVC syndrome may have Sx over days to wks but usually present **within 1 mo of onset.**
Do most pts presenting with SVC syndrome have a prior cancer Dx?	**No.** Most pts presenting with SVC syndrome do not have a prior cancer Dx.
Why is SVC syndrome considered an emergency?	SVC syndrome **may cause airway obstruction and cerebral edema;** however, severe Sx are uncommon, and life-threatening Sx are rare.
How may pts with SVC syndrome present?	Presenting Sx of SVC syndrome: 1. Facial fullness 2. Facial and neck swelling, especially if bending forward 3. Stridor 4. Dyspnea
What is the most common Sx of SVC syndrome?	The most common Sx of SVC syndrome is **dyspnea.**
What physical exam findings are associated with SVC syndrome?	Signs of SVC syndrome: plethora, facial edema, jugular venous distension, and visible collateral venous drainage on the ant chest

■ Workup/Staging

Describe the workup of SVC syndrome.	SVC syndrome workup: H&P, assessment of respiratory status, CXR and/or CT chest with contrast (best to visualize the extent of blockage), determination of the best Bx route if Dx is unknown, labs (AFP, LDH, β-HCG), and BM aspirate and Bx
Name 5 ways to obtain tissue Dx for SVC syndrome.	Methods to obtain tissue Dx in SVC syndrome: 1. Sputum cytology 2. Bx of palpable LNs 3. Bronchoscopy 4. Mediastinoscopy 5. Video-assisted thorascopic surgery
What is usually seen on CXR in SVC syndrome?	CXR findings in SVC syndrome include a widened mediastinum and the presence of a mass near the SVC.
What CT finding is closely associated with SVC syndrome?	The **presence of collateral vessels** is a CT finding that closely relates to SVC syndrome.

Why should RT not be given prior to a histologic Dx in SVC syndrome?	RT **may obscure the histologic Dx** and should be deferred until diagnostic Bx is obtained in SVC syndrome.

■ Treatment/Prognosis

What is the 1st step in Tx of SVC syndrome?	The 1st step in treating SVC syndrome is to **establish a pathologic Dx,** which will determine further interventions.
What Tx may be used for SVC syndrome?	SVC syndrome Tx: RT, chemo, surgery, and stents
What is the role of steroids in SVC syndrome?	Steroids are **frequently used** in SVC syndrome, but there is limited data to support their use.
In which malignant causes of SVC syndrome is chemo 1st line?	Chemo is the Tx of choice in SVC syndrome caused by **lymphoma, germ cell tumors, and SCLC.**
Which pts with SVC syndrome may be appropriate for surgery?	Pts with SVC syndrome **who do not respond to chemo or RT** may be considered for surgical bypass with synthetic grafts or autologous tissue.
What is the most rapid way to manage SVC thrombosis?	The most rapid method to manage SVC thrombosis is by **intraluminal stenting.**
What Tx should be considered if a pt with SVC syndrome presents with thombosis?	Use **anticoagulation therapy** for pts with SVC syndrome presenting with thrombosis unless contraindications are present.
Which pts with SVC syndrome require emergent Tx?	SVC syndrome pts with central airway compromise, severe laryngeal edema, or coma secondary to cerebral edema require emergent Tx.
What fractionation is used to emergently treat SVC syndrome?	Fractionation for emergent SVC Tx is **250–400 cGy × 3**. There is conflicting retrospective data on the benefit of hypofractionation.
When treating SVC syndrome, what should the RT fields encompass?	RT fields for SVC syndrome include encompassing gross Dz and adjacent nodal tissue while respecting normal tissue toxicity, especially the lungs and heart.
What should guide the total RT dose used for SVC syndrome?	The total RT dose for SVC syndrome depends on the **underlying histology** (i.e., lung cancers are treated to ≥60 Gy, while lymphomas are treated to 35–45 Gy).
Does SVC syndrome portend a bad prognosis?	**No.** The prognosis in SVC syndrome depends on the underlying cause rather than the presence of the syndrome itself.
What is the overall symptomatic response to RT in SVC syndrome?	The overall response rate to RT for SVC syndrome is **~60%.**

Does RT for SVC syndrome restore normal flow in the SVC?

No. RT for SVC syndrome does not generally restore normal vascular flow despite improving Sx.

What non-Tx event likely contributes to symptomatic improvement in SVC syndrome?

The **development of collateral vessels** largely contributes to Sx improvement in SVC syndrome.

Toxicity

What are potential acute toxicities of emergent RT for SVC syndrome?

Potential acute toxicities of emergent RT for SVC syndrome: fatigue, skin irritation, cough, esophagitis

What are potential subacute and chronic toxicities of RT for SVC syndrome?

Potential subacute and chronic toxicities of RT for SVC syndrome: RT pneumonitis, pericarditis, pulmonary fibrosis, esophageal stenosis

PART XV Benign Disease

91
Heterotopic Ossification Prophylaxis

Jing Zeng and Michael J. Swartz

Background

What is heterotopic ossification (HO)?

HO refers to **abnl bone formation outside the skeleton.** It often appears after trauma or surgery in periarticular soft tissue and is commonly associated with injury to the hip.

What are common Sx of HO?

In HO, **functional impairment** such as joint stiffness is the most common Sx. **Pain** can also occur, beginning as early as a few days after surgery.

What is the etiology of HO?

The etiology of HO is not completely understood. It is assumed that pluripotent mesenchymal cells present in periarticular soft tissue and develop into osteoblastic stem cells, which then produce bone.

What are the highest risk factors for developing HO?

Pts who already have ipsi or contralat HO carry the greatest risk of developing further HO. Their risk is 80%–100%. Pts with osteophytes at the femoral head and socket, acetabular fractures, ankylosing spondylitis, and other hyperostosis conditions of the skeleton also carry a high risk for HO. This condition is more common in males than in females.

Workup/Staging

How soon after surgery can radiologic evidence of HO be detected?

Radiologic evidence of HO can be detected **2–6 wks** after surgery as calcified structures with blurred contours on x-ray. Bone scans typically show increased uptake in the soft tissues adjacent to the hip and can detect HO several days before it becomes apparent on plain film.

What is the most common staging system used for HO?	The most common staging system used for HO was developed by ***Brooker et al.***

Grade 1: bone islands in soft tissue around hip

Grade 2: exophytes in pelvis or proximal end of femur with at least 1 cm between opposing bone surfaces

Grade 3: exophytes in pelvis or proximal end of femur with <1 cm between opposing bone surfaces

Grade 4: bony ankylosis between proximal femur and pelvis

Grades 3–4 are considered clinically relevant even if there is no pain or impaired mobility.

▮ Treatment/Prognosis

What is the role of surgery in the Tx of HO?

Clinically relevant HO should be surgically removed. The risk of subsequent recurrence may be lower if the ectopic bone is removed after it has reached maturity. At the time of surgery, prophylaxis against future HO should be taken.

Other than RT, are there any other effective methods for prophylaxis against HO?

For prophylaxis against HO, **indomethacin and ibuprofen** (prostaglandin synthesis inhibitors) have been shown to decrease the incidence of HO compared to placebo. (*Fransen et al., Cochrane Database Syst Rev 2004*)

What should be the RT dose and fractionation for prophylaxis against HO?

There have been multiple randomized trials and retrospective series on the RT dose and fractionation for prophylaxis against HO:

Sylvester et al. (*IJROBP 1988*) compared 20 Gy in 10 fx vs. 10 Gy in 5 fx, and *Pellegrini et al.* (*J Bone Joint Surg Am 1992*) looked at 8 Gy in 1 fx vs. 10 Gy in 5 fx. There were no significant differences between those doses and fractionation schemes. More recent studies looked at using lower doses.

Healy et al. (*J Bone Joint Surg Am 1995*) compared 7 Gy × 1 against 5.5 Gy and concluded that 5.5 Gy is not a sufficient dose.

Padgett et al. (*J Arthroplasty 2003*) looked at 5 Gy in 2 fx or 10 Gy in 5 fx. There was a trend toward increased HO of any grade in the 5-Gy group.

What is the efficacy of preop RT for HO prophylaxis compared with PORT? What are the advantages and disadvantages of preop RT vs. PORT?

In 1 study, preop RT at 7–8 Gy in 1 fx gave the same rates of prophylaxis as the same dose given postop (*Gregoritch et al., IJROBP 1994*). Preop RT decreases pt discomfort associated with transport and positioning for RT but is often not feasible due to scheduling issues.

How soon should PORT be given after surgery for prophylaxis against HO?

PORT prophylaxis against HO should be given **no later than 4 days and ideally within 3 days** of surgery. (*Seegenschmiedt et al., IJROBP 2001*)

What is the time frame for giving preop RT for HO prophylaxis?

The randomized trial comparing preop RT vs. PORT for HO prophylaxis using 7–8 Gy in 1 fx (*Gregoritch et al., IJROBP 1994*) gave preop RT within 4 hrs of surgery. Other nonrandomized series have suggested that preop RT can be given as early as 8 hrs preop without a significant decrease in efficacy (*Seegenschmiedt et al., IJROBP 2001*).

Are there randomized trials comparing RT against indomethacin in HO prophylaxis?

**Yes. *Burd et al.* (*J Bone Joint Surg Am 2001*) randomized 166 pts to rcv either indomethacin or RT postoperatively for HO prophylaxis. Grade 3–4 HO occurred in 14% of the indomethacin group as compared with 7% of the RT group, but the results were not SS ($p = 0.22$).

A meta-analysis by ***Pakos et al.*** (*IJROBP 2004*) looked at 7 randomized trials comparing RT vs. NSAIDs. They concluded that RT postop >6 Gy tended to be more effective than NSAIDs in preventing Brooker 3 or 4 HO, but the absolute difference was only 1.2%.

What is the typical RT field for HO prophylaxis?

The RT fields for HO prophylaxis typically includes the usual area at risk for HO. When treating the hip for HO prophylaxis, the cranial border is usually 3 cm above the acetabulum and inferiorly includes two thirds of the shaft of the implant. Field size is usually around 14 × 14 cm. The prosthesis may be blocked from RT if a cementless fixation is used, but observational data suggest that this blocking strategy is associated with higher rates of subsequent HO.

■ Toxicity

What are the rates of increased wound-healing complications after RT for HO prophylaxis?

RT for HO prophylaxis has not been associated with an increased incidence of wound-healing complications.

Is there an increased risk of nonfixation of cementless implants after RT for HO prophylaxis?

No. There is not an increased risk of nonfixation of cementless implants after RT for HO prophylaxis based on multiple studies (*Seegenschmiedt et al., IJROBP 2001*). Animal studies have shown a transient decrease in force required to remove an implant after RT, but this difference resolved by wk 3 (*Konski et al., IJROBP 1990*).

What is the rate of RT-induced tumor after RT for HO prophylaxis?

There has yet to be a documented case of a RT-induced tumor after RT for HO prophylaxis. This is thought to be the effect of both low doses of RT as well as an older pt population. As RT is employed for younger pts, this concern is worth considering.

92
Keloids

Jing Zeng and Michael J. Swartz

Background

What is a keloid?

A keloid is a **benign fibroproliferative growth** resulting from a connective tissue response to a variety of proposed factors such as surgery, burns, trauma, inflammation, foreign body reactions, endocrine dysfunction, and occasional spontaneous occurrence.

Is there a racial predilection for keloid formation?

Yes. People of African descent are more likely to be predisposed to keloid formation than other ethnic groups. Any skin insult (piercings, lacerations, infected skin lesions, surgery) can cause keloid formation in predisposed individuals. Less commonly, lesions can occur de novo.

Name 3 common locations for keloids.

Keloids most commonly affect areas of increased skin tension, such as the ears, neck, jaw, presternal chest, shoulders, and upper back.

Name 3 Sx commonly associated with keloids.

Keloids can be asymptomatic but often are pruritic, tender to palpation, or occasionally cause pain.

Workup/Staging

What is the difference between a keloid and a hypertrophic scar?

Hypertrophic scars may initially appear similar to keloids but do not extend beyond the margins of the scar. Keloids are more infiltrative and can cause a local reaction such as pain and inflammation. Hypertrophic scars are much less likely to recur after resection.

Treatment/Prognosis

What are the indications for RT in keloid Tx?

The indications for RT in keloid Tx include demonstrated recurrence after resection, marginal or incomplete resection, an unfavorable location, or a larger lesion.

Within what time frame should RT be given postop after keloid resection?

PORT for keloids should be initiated **within 24 hrs** after resection.

What is the typical target RT volume for keloid Tx?

The typical target RT volume for keloid Tx is **scar + a 1-cm safety margin**.

What is the typical RT dose and fractionation for keloids?

The typical RT dose and fractionation for keloids is **3–4 Gy in 3–4 fx.** Single doses of 7.5–10 Gy are also effective (*Ragoowansi et al., Plast Reconstr Surg 2003*). Some series suggest that a dose of at least 9 Gy is required to maximize the benefit from RT (*Lo et al., Radiother Oncol 1990*; *Doornbos et al., IJROBP 1990*).

What RT modalities can be used in the Tx of keloids?

For RT Tx of keloids, the most common modalities are **lower megavoltage electrons, kilovoltage photons, or brachytherapy.**

Name 5 Tx options for keloids other than surgery and RT.

Tx options for keloids other than surgery and RT include steroid injections, pressure earrings, silicone gel sheeting, cryosurgery, laser therapy, imiquimod, and injections of fluorouracil or verapamil.

What is the recurrence rate for keloids after PORT?

The recurrence rate for keloids after PORT is typically **10%–35%.** This can vary depending on the size, location, extent of excision, etiology, and other factors.

Is there any randomized data comparing surgery + RT against surgery + steroid injection?

Yes. A prospective randomized trial conducted by Sclafani et al. looked at a series of 31 pts, comparing PORT vs. intralesional steroid injection. The recurrence rate after surgery + RT was 12.5%; the recurrence rate after surgery + steroid injection was 33%. (*Dermatol Surg 1996*)

For unresectable keloids, what is the efficacy of using RT alone?

Malaker et al. looked at 86 keloids in 64 pts treated with RT alone. 97% had significant regression 18 mos after completing radiotherapy. 63% of the pts surveyed were very happy with the outcome of their Tx. (*Clin Oncol 2004*)

■ Toxicity

What are the most common side effects after RT for keloids?

The most common side effects of RT for keloids are **hyperpigmentation, pruritis, and erythema.**

APPENDIX

Normal Tissue Constraint Guidelines

The radiation dose constraints below are meant to serve as a guide only and may not be applicable to all clinical scenarios. Most doses are derived from randomized studies or consensus guidelines and we have attempted to provide the sources for these recommendations. Please refer to the individual pediatric chapters for dose constraints in the pediatric population as these can vary greatly from protocol to protocol and tend to be particularly site- and age-dependent.

What are the recommended dose constraints for the following organs and clinical scenarios?	
ORGAN	*CONSTRAINTS*
CNS (1.8-2.0 Gy/fx)	
Spinal cord	**max 50 Gy** (full cord cross-section); tolerance increases by 25% 6 mos after 1st course (for re-irradiation) (QUANTEC)
Brain	**max 72 Gy** (partial brain); avoid >2 Gy/fx or hyperfractionation (QUANTEC)
Chiasm/optic nerves	**max 55 Gy** (QUANTEC)
Brainstem	**Entire brainstem <54 Gy, V59 Gy <1-10 cc** (QUANTEC)
Eyes (globe)	**Mean <35 Gy** (RTOG 0225), **max 54 Gy** (RTOG 0615)
Lens	**max 7 Gy** (RTOG 0539)
Retina	**max 50 Gy** (RTOG 0539)
Lacrimal Gland	**max 40 Gy** (Parsons)
Inner ear/cochlea	**mean ≤45 Gy** (consider constraining to ≤35 Gy with concurrent cisplatin) (QUANTEC)
Pituitary gland	**max 45 Gy** (for panhypopituitarism, lower for GH deficiency) (Emami)
Cauda equina	**Max 60 Gy** (Emami)
CNS (single fraction)	
Spinal cord	**max 13 Gy** (if 3 fxs, max 20 Gy) (QUANTEC)

What are the recommended dose constraints for the following organs and clinical scenarios? *(Continued)*	
ORGAN	*CONSTRAINTS*
CNS (single fraction)	
Brain	**V12 Gy** <5-10 cc (QUANTEC)
Chiasm/optic nerves	**max 10 Gy** (QUANTEC)
Brainstem	**max 12.5 Gy** (QUANTEC)
Sacral plexus	**V18** <0.035 cc, **V14.4** <5 cc (RTOG 0631)
Cauda equina	**V16** <0.035 cc, **V14** <5 cc (RTOG 0631)
H&N (1.8-2.0 Gy/fx)	
Parotid gland(s)	**mean** <25 Gy (both glands) or **mean** <20 Gy (1 gland) (QUANTEC)
Submandibular gland(s)	**mean** <35 Gy (QUANTEC)
Larynx	**mean** ≤44 Gy, **V50** ≤27%, **max 63-66 Gy** (when risk of tumor involvement is limited) (QUANTEC)
TMJ/mandible	**max 70 Gy** (if not possible, then V75 <1 cc) (RTOG 0615)
Oral cavity	Nonoral cavity cancer: **mean** <30 Gy, avoid hot spots >60 Gy (RTOG 0920)
	Oral cavity cancer: **mean** < 50 Gy, V55 <1 cc, max 65 Gy (RTOG 0920)
Esophagus (cervical)	**V45** <33% (RTOG 0920)
Pharyngeal constrictors	**Mean** <50 Gy (QUANTEC)
Thyroid	**V26** <20% (JHH)
Thoracic (1.8-2.0 Gy/fx)	
Brachial plexus	**max 66 Gy, V60** <5% (RTOG 0619)
Lung (combined lung for lung cancer treatment)	**mean** <20-23 Gy, **V20** <30%-35% (QUANTEC)
Lung (ipsilateral lung for breast cancer treatment)	**V25** <10% (JHH)
Single lung (after pneumonectomy)	**V5** <60%, **V20** <4-10%, **MLD** <8 Gy (QUANTEC)
Bronchial tree	**max 80 Gy** (QUANTEC)
Heart (lung cancer treatment)	**Heart V45** <67%; **V60** <33% (NCCN 2010)
Heart (breast cancer treatment)	**V25** <10% (QUANTEC)
Esophagus	**V50** <32% (Maguire), **V60** <33% (Emami)
Thoracic (hypofractionation)	Total recommended cumulative dose by the number of fractions per NCCN 2010. Note: the max dose limits refer to volumes >0.035 cc (~3 mm^3).
Spinal cord	1 fraction: 14 Gy 3 fractions: 18 Gy (6 Gy/fx) 4 fractions: 26 Gy (6.5 Gy/fx) 5 fractions: 30 Gy (6 Gy/fx)

What are the recommended dose constraints for the following organs and clinical scenarios? *(Continued)*	
ORGAN	*CONSTRAINTS*
Esophagus	1 fraction: 15.4 Gy 3 fractions: 30 Gy (10 Gy/fx) 4 fractions: 30 Gy (7.5 Gy/fx) 5 fractions: 32.5 Gy (6.5 Gy/fx)
Brachial plexus	1 fraction: 17.5 Gy 3 fractions: 21 Gy (7 Gy/fx) 4 fractions: 27.2 Gy (6.8 Gy/fx) 5 fractions: 30 Gy (6 Gy/fx)
Heart/Pericardium	1 fraction: 22 Gy 3 fractions: 30 Gy (10 Gy/fx) 4 fractions: 34 Gy (8.5 Gy/fx) 5 fractions: 35 Gy (7 Gy/fx)
Great vessels	1 fraction: 37 Gy 3 fractions: 39 Gy (13 Gy/fx) 4 fractions: 49 Gy (12.25 Gy/fx) 5 fractions: 55 Gy (11 Gy/fx)
Trachea/Large Bronchus	1 fraction: 20.2 Gy 3 fractions: 30 Gy (10 Gy/fx) 4 fractions: 34.8 Gy (8.7 Gy/fx) 5 fractions: 40 Gy (8 Gy/fx)
Rib	1 fraction: 30 Gy 3 fractions: 30 Gy (10 Gy/fx) 4 fractions: 32 Gy (7.8 Gy/fx) 5 fractions: 32.5 Gy (6.5 Gy/fx)
Skin	1 fraction: 26 Gy 3 fractions: 30 Gy (10 Gy/fx) 4 fractions: 36 Gy (9 Gy/fx) 5 fractions: 40 Gy (8 Gy/fx)
Stomach	1 fraction: 12.4 Gy 3 fractions: 27 Gy (9 Gy/fx) 4 fractions: 30 Gy (7.5 Gy/fx) 5 fractions: 35 Gy (7 Gy/fx)
GI (1.8-2.0 Gy/fx)	
Stomach	**TD 5/5 whole stomach: 45 Gy** (QUANTEC)
Small bowel	**V45 <195 cc** (QUANTEC)
Liver (metastatic disease)	**mean liver <32 Gy** (liver = normal liver minus gross disease)(QUANTEC)
Liver (primary liver cancer)	**mean liver <28 Gy** (liver = normal liver minus gross disease) (QUANTEC)
Colon	**45 Gy, max dose 55 Gy** (Emami)

What are the recommended dose constraints for the following organs and clinical scenarios? *(Continued)*	
ORGAN	**CONSTRAINTS**
Kidney (bilateral)	**mean <18 Gy, V28 <20%, V23 Gy <30%, V20 <32%, V12 <55%.** If mean kidney dose to 1 kidney > 18 Gy, then constrain remaining kidney to V6 <30%. (QUANTEC)
GI (single fraction)	Dose constraints per RTOG 0631
Duodenum	**V16 <0.035 cc, V11.2 <5 cc**
Kidney (Cortex)	**V8.4 <200 cc**
Kidney (Hilum)	**V10.6 <66%**
Colon	**V14.3 <20 cc, V18.4 <0.035 cc**
Jejunum/Ileum	**V15.4 <0.035 cc, V11.9 <5 cc**
Stomach	**V16 <0.035 cc, V11.2 <10 cc**
Rectum	**V18.4 <0.035 cc, V14.3 <20 cc**
GU (1.8-2.0 Gy/fx)	
Femoral heads	**V50 <5%** (RTOG GU Consensus)
Rectum	**V75 <15% , V70 <20%, V65 <25%, V60 <35%, V50 <50%** (QUANTEC)
Bladder	**V80 <15%, V75 <25%, V70 <35%, V65 <50%** (QUANTEC)
Testis	**V3 <50%** (RTOG 0630)
Penile bulb	**Mean dose to 95% of the volume <50 Gy. D70 ≤70 Gy, D50 ≤50 Gy** (QUANTEC 2010)
GU (LDR prostate brachytherapy)	
Urethra	Volume of urethra receiving 150% of prescribed dose **(Ur150) <30%** (JHH)
Rectum	Volume of rectum receiving 100% of prescribed dose **(RV100) <0.5 cc** (JHH)
GYN	
Bladder point (cervical brachytherapy)	**Max 80 Gy** (LDR equivalent dose) (ABS 2000)
Rectal point (cervical brachytherapy)	**Max 75 Gy** (LDR equivalent dose) (ABS 2000)
Proximal vagina (mucosa) (cervical brachytherapy)	**Max 120 Gy** (LDR equivalent dose) (Hintz)
Distal vagina (mucosa) (cervical brachytherapy)	**Max 98 Gy** (LDR equivalent dose) (Hintz)

Sources: **ABS 2000:** American Brachytherapy Society consensus statement for HDR brachytherapy for cervical cancer (Nag S, et al., *IJROBP*, 2000); **Emami:** Emami et al., *IJROBP* 31:5, 1995; **Hintz:** Hintz BL. et al., *IJROBP*, 1980; **JHH:** clinical practice at Johns Hopkins Hospital; **Maguire:** Maguire PD, Sibley GS, Zhou SM, et al: Clinical and dosimetric predictors of radiation-induced esophageal toxicity. *IJROBP* 45:97-103, 1999; **NCCN 2010:** www.nccn.org; Parsons: Parsons JT, et al., *Oncology*, 2006; **QUANTEC** (Quantitative Analyses of Normal Tissue Effects in the Clinic): *IJROBP*, 76 (2), Suppl, Mar 1, 2010; **RTOG** protocols: www.rtog.org; **RTOG GU** consensus: Lawton CAF et al., *IJROBP*, 2009.

INDEX

Page numbers followed by "t" indicate table, and "f" indicate figure.